Official "Do Not Use" List[1]

Do Not Use	Potential Problem	Use Instead
U (unit)	Mistaken for "0" (zero), the number "4" (four) or "cc"	Write "unit"
IU (International Unit)	Mistaken for IV (intravenous) or the number 10 (ten)	Write "International Unit"
Q.D., QD, q.d., qd (daily)	Mistaken for each other	Write "daily"
Q.O.D., QOD, q.o.d, qod (every other day)	Period after the Q mistaken for "I" and the "O" mistaken for "I"	Write "every other day"
Trailing zero (X.0 mg)* Lack of leading zero (.X mg)	Decimal point is missed	Write X mg Write 0.X mg
MS	Can mean morphine sulfate or magnesium sulfate	Write "morphine sulfate" Write "magnesium sulfate"
MSO_4 and $MgSO_4$	Confused for one another	

[1] Applies to all orders and all medication-related documentation that is handwritten (including free-text computer entry) or on pre-printed forms.

*Exception: A "trailing zero" may be used only where required to demonstrate the level of precision of the value being reported, such as for laboratory results, imaging studies that report size of lesions, or catheter/tube sizes. It may not be used in medication orders or other medication-related documentation.

Additional Abbreviations, Acronyms and Symbols
(For possible future inclusion in the Official "Do Not Use" List)

Do Not Use	Potential Problem	Use Instead
> (greater than) < (less than)	Misinterpreted as the number "7" (seven) or the letter "L" Confused for one another	Write "greater than" Write "less than"
Abbreviations for drug names	Misinterpreted due to similar abbreviations for multiple drugs	Write drug names in full
Apothecary units	Unfamiliar to many practitioners Confused with metric units	Use metric units
@	Mistaken for the number "2" (two)	Write "at"
cc	Mistaken for U (units) when poorly written	Write "mL" or "ml" or "milliliters" ("mL" is preferred)
µg	Mistaken for mg (milligrams) resulting in one thousand-fold overdose	Write "mcg" or "micrograms"

Institute for Safe Medication Practices (ISMP) Dangerous Abbreviations and Notations			
Abbreviation	Write	Abbreviation	Write
AD, AS, or AU	right ear, left ear, or both ears	X 3d	for 3 days
OD, OS, or OU	right eye, left eye, or both eyes	SC, SQ, or sub q	subcut or subcutaneous(ly)
BT	bedtime	ss	one half
cc	mL for milliliters	SSI	sliding scale (insulin)
HS	bedtime	µg	mcg
qhs	nightly	>	less than
		<	greater than
qid	4 times a day	+	plus or and
qn	nightly	@	at

Please note: This is a partial list. For a more complete list, refer to www.ISMP.org.

Drug Calculations

RATIO AND PROPORTION

PROBLEMS FOR CLINICAL PRACTICE

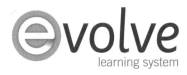
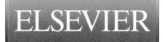

Drug Calculations

RATIO AND PROPORTION

PROBLEMS FOR CLINICAL PRACTICE

Ninth Edition

META BROWN SELTZER, M. ED, RN
Retired Colonel
U.S. Army Field Hospital
Former Director, Division of Nursing
Gateway Community College
Phoenix, Arizona

JOYCE M. MULHOLLAND, RNP
Nursing Education Consultant, Tucson, Arizona
M.S. California State University, Long Beach, California
M.A. Arizona State University, Tempe, Arizona
B.S. Fairleigh Dickinson College, Rutherford, New Jersey

3251 Riverport Lane
St. Louis, Missouri 63043

DRUG CALCULATIONS: RATIO AND PROPORTION
PROBLEMS FOR CLINICAL PRACTICE

ISBN: 978-0-323-07750-7

Notices

Knowledge and best practice in this field are constantly changing. As new research and experience broaden
our understanding, changes in research methods, professional practices, or medical treatment may become
necessary.

Practitioners and researchers must always rely on their own experience and knowledge in evaluating and
using any information, methods, compounds, or experiments described herein. In using such information
or methods they should be mindful of their own safety and the safety of others, including parties for whom
they have a professional responsibility.

With respect to any drug or pharmaceutical products identified, readers are advised to check the most
current information provided (i) on procedures featured or (ii) by the manufacturer of each product to be
administered, to verify the recommended dose or formula, the method and duration of administration, and
contraindications. It is the responsibility of practitioners, relying on their own experience and knowledge
of their patients, to make diagnoses, to determine dosages and the best treatment for each individual
patient, and to take all appropriate safety precautions.

To the fullest extent of the law, neither the Publisher nor the authors, contributors, or editors, assume
any liability for any injury and/or damage to persons or property as a matter of products liability, neg-
ligence or otherwise, or from any use or operation of any methods, products, instructions, or ideas
contained in the material herein.

Library of Congress Cataloging-in-Publication Data

Seltzer, Meta Brown.
  Drug calculations : ratio and proportion problems for clinical practice / Meta Brown Seltzer, Joyce M.
Mulholland. -- 9th ed.
    p. ; cm.
  Includes index.
  ISBN 978-0-323-07750-7 (pbk. : alk. paper)
  I. Mulholland, Joyce M. II. Title.
[DNLM: 1. Pharmaceutical Preparations--administration & dosage--Problems and Exercises. 2. Pharmaceuti-
cal Preparations--administration & dosage--Programmed Instruction. 3. Mathematics--Problems and Exercises.
4. Mathematics--Programmed Instruction. QV 18.2]

  615.1'401513--dc23

                                                                                                    2011035012

Sr. Editor: Yvonne Alexopoulos
Sr. Developmental Editor: Danielle M. Frazier
Publishing Services Manager: Deborah Vogel
Project Manager: Bridget Healy
Design Direction: Amy Buxton

Printed in the United States of America

Last digit is the print number: 9 8 7 6 5 4 3 2 1

Reviewers

Joy E. Ache-Reed, MSN, RN
Assistant Professor of Nursing
Indiana Wesleyan University
Marion, Indiana

Nancy Breed, MS, RN
Director of Nursing
Mountain View College
Dallas, Texas

Susan Carlson, MS, RN, NPP, APRN-BC
Assistant Professor of Nursing
Monroe Community College
Rochester, New York

Beth Carson EdD, RN, CNE
Dean for Undergraduate Affairs
Saint Anthony College of Nursing
Rockford, Illinois

Pamela J. Fowler, MS, RNC
Assistant Professor
Rogers State University
Caremore, Oklahoma

Kathleen K. Gudgel, RN, BSN, MSN
Retired Instructor of Nursing
School of Health Sciences
Pennsylvania College of Technology
Williamsport, Pennsylvania

Carolyn McCune, RN, MSN, CRNP
LPN Director
Columbia County Career and Technical Center
Staff Nurse in ED
Aultman Hospital
Louisville, Ohio

Kathleen Voeltzke, RN, MSN
Allied Health Coordinator
Tennessee Technology Center at Nashville
Nashville, Tennessee

Preface to Instructors

Drug Calculations was originally designed in the late 1970s as a basic practical resource for nursing students and faculty in classrooms and clinical areas. Since then, the content has been thoroughly reviewed and updated to be useful for refresher courses, practicing nurses in specialty areas, distance-learning students, nurses pursuing in-dependent learning, associate and baccalaureate nursing students, as well as practical nursing students.

This book primarily presents the ratio and proportion method, the easiest provable method of dose calculation for the majority of nursing students to master in a short time, and delivers all of the necessary material in a simple-to-complex sequence with brief rules, succinct examples, and logical steps to understanding and mastery of the underlying concepts.

A comprehensive, systematic arithmetic self-assessment quiz allows the student to focus on any basic mathematics areas that may need to review in preparation for dose calculations.

The first chapter offers a sufficient review of the basic arithmetic needed to solve all the calculations in the text. Students are referred to a general mathematics text if more practice is desired.

The text presents pharmacology principles and selected illustrations to enhance learning relevant to specific calculation areas. The reader is referred to current pharmacology texts, drug handbooks, and clinical skills manuals for complete coverage of those broad subjects.

As in prior editions, answers are completely worked out in the back of the book for all worksheets so that the learner can pinpoint areas of need. Concepts of the nursing process, logical thinking, and critical thinking are employed throughout the text, with highlighted Clinical Alerts to call the reader's attention to dose-related safety situations in actual practice that have resulted in medication errors. As with prior editions, the emphasis is on understanding rather than memorizing the medication math process.

Priorities are placed upon patient safety. Proofs and labels are requested for answers to all the basic problems to avoid errors and establish good habits. It is up to the faculty to make a decision about the use of calculators. Our recommendation is that the problems in the basic chapters be worked out in order to reinforce the students' understanding of the process and to enhance their ability to prove their answers. The goal is to be able to function independently, without a calculator, if that becomes necessary.

New Features for the 9th Edition

- Each chapter has been reviewed and updated for currency and accuracy. New labels and equipment for realistic practice have been included.
- New problems and labels, tables, equipment, and illustrations have been added to the chapters to give the students updated practice.
- Guidelines from The Joint Commission requirements (TJC) and Institute for Safe Medication Practices (ISMP) are included and emphasized in the text.
- ISMP High-Alert Medications have been assigned a special visual icon ▌ to reinforce recognition and safe practice.
- Quality and Safety Competencies (QSEN) patient safety goals are incorporated throughout the text.
- Additional Critical Thinking Exercises have been added for student analysis and guided discussion. A variety of responses can be elicited. Potential responses are not provided in the Answer Key.

- The Multiple-Choice Final and the Comprehensive Final contain updated labels and problems with an answer key to help students evaluate their progress.
- A Sample Verbal Communication Hand-Off Report is included in the appendix. It offers students a topical guideline and insight into reporting emphasis on patient needs and safety issues, communication of critical medication-related information during transfer of patient responsibilities is highlighted.

Ancillaries

Evolve resources for instructors and students can be found online at http://evolve.elsevier.com/BrownMulholland.

The Instructor Resources are designed to help instructors present the material in this text and include the following:
- Test Bank-Now with over 500 questions
- *NEW!* Power Point Slides—With over 350 slides
- *NEW!* Drug Label Glossary
- Suggested Class Schedules and Teaching Guidelines for First-Time Instructors
- *NEW VERSION!* **Romans & Daugherty's Dosages and Solutions Test Bank, Version 3.** This generic test-bank contains over 700 questions on general mathematics, converting within the same system of measurements, converting between different systems of measurement, oral dosages, parenteral dosages, flow rates, pediatric dosages, IV calculations, and more.

Student Resources provide students with additional tools for learning and include the following:
- *NEW VERSION!* **Drug Calculations Companion, version 4.** This is a completely updated, interactive student tutorial that includes an extensive menu of various topic areas within drug calculations, such as oral, parenteral, pediatric, and intravenous calculations. It contains over 600 practice problems covering ratio and proportion, formula, and dimensional analysis methods.

Acknowledgments

We extend our thanks to all the reviewers and users for their thoughts, time, and excellent suggestions. We followed them whenever practical, timely, and consistent with the style and space limitations of this text and the needs of a majority of practitioners. Full credit for the Power Point slides in this edition is attributed to Cynthia A. Dolata, MSN, RN, BC. Joyce Mulholland offers thanks to Penny Lutzi, computer software design consultant for her assistance with review and suggestions for improvement.

Meta Brown Seltzer
Joyce M. Mulholland

Preface to Students

Drug Calculations: Ratio and Proportion for Clinical Practice, provides all the information, explanation, and practice needed to competently and confidently calculate drug dosages. A review of basic arithmetic is provided to refresh math skills. The text also provides exclusive coverage of the ratio and proportion method of drug calculation in a full-color workbook format. Take a look at the features below so that you may familiarize yourself with this text and maximize its value.

A General Mathematics Self-Assessment and Math Review in Chapter 1 contain all necessary basic math for solving medication-related math problems. Be sure to complete this initial review.

Chapter 2 contains a general introduction to the ratio and proportion setup of problems to be applied to dose calculations. Be sure to master this brief chapter before continuing.

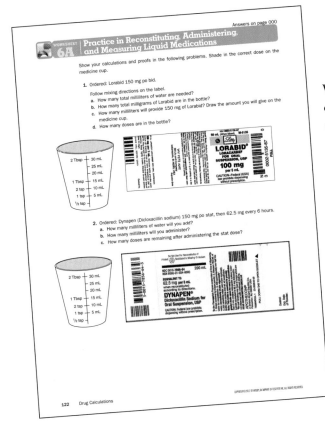

Worksheets with a series of practice problems follow each topical section, providing the practice you need to master math calculations.

The step-by-step format of problems includes a "proof" step to ensure that you understand the calculation and can double-check answers.

A high-alert medication icon ⌐ has been added as a visual reminder of high risk drugs identified by the Institute for Safe Medication Practices (ISMP).

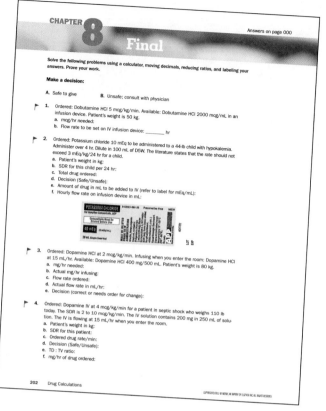

Critical Thinking Exercises at the end of most chapters include various patient medication-related scenarios, providing opportunity for discussion and analysis of commonly-encountered medication errors.

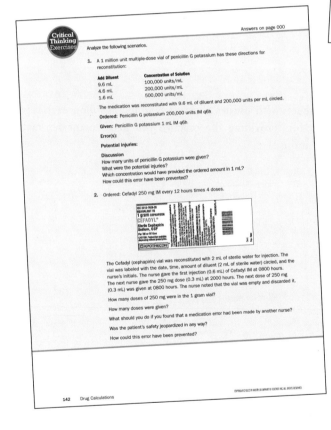

NEW VERSION! ***Drug Calculations Companion, version 4***. This is a completely updated, interactive student tutorial that includes an extensive menu of various topic areas within drug calculations, such as oral, parenteral, pediatric, and intravenous calculations. It contains over 600 practice problems covering ratio and proportion, formula, and dimensional analysis methods.

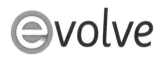

Look for this icon at the end of the chapters. It will refer you to ***Drug Calculations Companion, version 4*** for additional practice problems and content information.

Contents

General Mathematics Self-Assessment, 1

1 General Mathematics, 3
2 Ratio and Proportion, 31
3 Safe Medication Administration, 41
4 Drug Measurements and Oral Dose Calculations, 71
5 Injectable Medication Calculations, 99
6 Medications from Powders and Crystals: Oral and Intramuscular, 119
7 Basic Intravenous Therapy Calculations, 149
8 Advanced Intravenous Calculations, 181
9 Parenteral Nutrition, 205
10 Insulin Administration, 223
11 Anticoagulants, 257
12 Children's Dosages, 277

Multiple-Choice Final, 309
Comprehensive Final, 321
Appendix A, 333
Appendix B, 335
Answer Key, 337
Index, 441

General Mathematics Self-Assessment

In order to progress in the Drug Calculations text, students must know how to solve problems using fractions, addition, subtraction, multiplication, division, and percentage. Accurate medication dose calculations build on fundamental mathematics knowledge. Solve these basic problems and check your answers on page 337. Chapter 1, General Mathematics, provides a refresher for each type of problem.

FRACTIONS

Change to whole or mixed numbers.

1. $\frac{9}{2}$

2. $\frac{26}{5}$

Change to improper fractions.

3. $8\frac{1}{3}$

4. $5\frac{2}{5}$

Find the lowest common denominator in the following fractions.

5. $\frac{4}{11}$ and $\frac{1}{8}$

6. $\frac{2}{5}$ and $\frac{5}{9}$

Add the following.

7. $\frac{1}{5}, \frac{1}{6},$ and $\frac{2}{3}$

8. $1\frac{1}{2} + 3\frac{1}{8} + 2\frac{1}{6}$

Subtract the following.

9. $\frac{5}{7} - \frac{1}{3}$

10. $8\frac{1}{4} - 3\frac{3}{8}$

Multiply the following and reduce to lowest terms.

11. $\frac{1}{6} \times \frac{1}{3}$

12. $\frac{2}{8} \times 1\frac{1}{3}$

Divide the following and reduce to lowest terms.

13. $\frac{1}{3} \div \frac{2}{5}$

14. $1\frac{1}{8} \div 2\frac{1}{2}$

Express the following fractions reduced to lowest terms (numbers).

15. $\frac{4}{120}$

16. $\frac{3}{7}$

DECIMALS

Write the following as decimals.

17. Twelve hundredths

18. Three and sixteen thousandths

Add the following.

19. 3.04 + 1.864

20. 25.7 + 3.008

Subtract the following.

21. $3 - 0.04$

22. $0.96 - 0.1359$

Multiply the following.

23. 0.05×2

24. 3×0.4

Divide the following and carry to the third decimal place.

25. $500 \div 15$

26. $20.6 \div 0.21$

Change the following to decimals and carry to the third decimal place.

27. $\frac{24}{44}$

28. $9\frac{1}{8}$

PERCENTAGES

Find the following percentages.

29. 25% of 300

30. 1% of 50

Change the following decimals to fractions and reduce to lowest terms.

31. 0.005

32. 0.05

Change the following fractions to a decimal and a percentage.

33. $\frac{3}{4}$

34. $\frac{1}{8}$

Rounding

Round the following decimals.

	Decimal	Nearest Whole Number	Nearest Hundredth	Nearest Tenth
35.	0.8734			
36.	0.842			
37.	0.553			
38.	0.689			
39.	2.75			

Answer the following questions.

40. What is 25% of 2?   Ans: fraction _____   Ans: decimal _____

41. What is $\frac{1}{4}$ of 2?   Ans: fraction _____   Ans: decimal _____

42. What is 75% of 2?   Ans: fraction _____   Ans: decimal _____

43. Divide 0.5 by 0.25:

44. Divide 0.2 by 0.1:

45. Divide $\frac{1}{100}$ by $\frac{1}{200}$:

General Mathematics

Objectives

- Add, subtract, multiply, and divide fractions and mixed numbers.
- Convert improper fractions and mixed numbers.
- Reduce fractions to lowest terms.
- Create equivalent fractions and compare values.
- Add, subtract, multiply, and divide decimals.
- Compare decimal values.
- Round decimals.
- Convert decimals, fractions, and percentages.

Introduction

This chapter provides a thorough and easy-to-follow review of the arithmetic needed for accurate medication dose calculations. Many examples, practice problems, and answers related to fractions, decimals, rounding, and percentages are offered. Your ability to avoid medication errors and solve medication dose-related problems starts with competence in basic arithmetic. If you need further review, refer to a general basic mathematics text. Mastery of these concepts is essential before you proceed to the following chapters and medication-related calculations.

Fractions

A fraction is part of a whole number. The fraction $\frac{6}{8}$ means that there are 8 parts to the whole number (bottom number, or denominator), but you want to measure only 6 of those parts (top number, or numerator).

The fraction $\frac{6}{8}$ can be reduced by dividing both the numbers by 2.

$$\frac{6 \div 2}{8 \div 2} = \frac{3}{4} \quad \begin{array}{l} \text{numerator} \\ \text{denominator} \end{array}$$

Changing Improper Fractions to Whole or Mixed Numbers

An improper fraction has a numerator that is larger than the denominator, as in $\frac{8}{4}$.

Steps for Changing Improper Fractions to Whole or Mixed Numbers

1. When the top number (numerator) is larger than the bottom number (denominator), divide the bottom number (denominator) into the top number (numerator).
2. Write the remainder as a fraction and reduce to lowest terms.

Examples $\frac{8}{4} = 8 \div 4 = 2$ *This is a whole number.*

$\frac{16}{6} = 16 \div 6 = 2\frac{4}{6} = 2\frac{2}{3}$ This is a *mixed number* because it has a whole number plus a fraction.

Answers on page 338

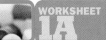 **WORKSHEET 1A** | ## Changing Improper Fractions to Whole or Mixed Numbers

Change the following to whole numbers or mixed fractions and reduce to lowest terms.

1. $\frac{6}{6} =$ 2. $\frac{10}{2} =$ 3. $\frac{13}{4} =$

4. $\frac{14}{9} =$ 5. $\frac{34}{6} =$ 6. $\frac{100}{20} =$

7. $\frac{9}{4} =$ 8. $\frac{120}{64} =$ 9. $\frac{18}{3} =$

10. $\frac{41}{6} =$

Changing Mixed Numbers to Improper Fractions

Steps for Changing Mixed Numbers to Improper Fractions

1. Multiply the whole number by the denominator of the fraction.
2. Add this to the numerator of the fraction.
3. Write the sum as the numerator of the fraction; the denominator of the fraction remains the same.

Examples $2\frac{3}{8} = \frac{8 \times 2 + 3}{8} = \frac{19}{8}$ numerator denominator

$4\frac{2}{5} = \frac{5 \times 4 + 2}{5} = \frac{22}{5}$ numerator denominator

| **Changing Mixed Numbers to Improper Fractions**

Change the following to improper fractions.

1. $3\frac{1}{2} =$ **2.** $1\frac{1}{6} =$ **3.** $4\frac{1}{8} =$

4. $3\frac{7}{12} =$ **5.** $13\frac{3}{5} =$ **6.** $16\frac{1}{3} =$

7. $3\frac{5}{6} =$ **8.** $2\frac{5}{8} =$ **9.** $10\frac{3}{6} =$

10. $125\frac{2}{3} =$

Finding a Common Denominator for Two or More Fractions

To add and subtract fractions, the denominators must be the *same*.

Example   Fractions with same denominators

$\frac{5}{16} - \frac{2}{16}$ or $\frac{3}{8} + \frac{1}{8}$ or $\frac{3}{4} + \frac{1}{4}$

These fractions can be added and subtracted. Each set's value is also easier to compare because of the common denominators.

Example   Different denominators in fractions with the same value as the fractions in example A:

$\frac{5}{16} - \frac{1}{8}$ or $\frac{3}{8} + \frac{2}{16}$ or $\frac{3}{4} + \frac{2}{8}$

These fractions cannot be added or subtracted until they are converted to *equivalent* fractions with a *common* denominator. The relative value of each set is harder to compare until they are converted to equivalent fractions. A *common* denominator is a number that can be divided evenly by *all* the denominators in the problem. It is easier to add or subtract fractions if the lowest common denominator is used.

Steps for Finding a Common Denominator for Two or More Fractions

1. Examine the largest denominator in the group to determine whether the other denominators will divide *evenly* into it.
2. If any of the denominators will not divide evenly into the largest denominator, begin multiplying the largest denominator by 2. If the other denominators cannot be divided by 2 evenly, then proceed to multiply the denominator by 3, 4, 5, 6, and so on until all denominators can be divided into the number equally. This becomes the common denominator.

Example $\frac{5}{16}$ and $\frac{1}{8}$: the largest denominator, 16, can be divided by 8 without a remainder. 16 is the common denominator.

Example $\frac{2}{8}$ and $\frac{3}{4}$ and $\frac{1}{2}$: the largest denominator, 8, can be divided by 4 and by 2 without a remainder. 8 is the common denominator.

Example $\frac{3}{8}$ and $\frac{2}{3}$ and $\frac{1}{4}$: 3 will *not* divide evenly into 8.

The largest denominator in the group is **8**.
$8 \times 2 = 16$ 3 will *not* divide evenly into 16.
$8 \times 3 = 24$ Both 3 and 4 will divide evenly into **24**.
$8 \times 4 = 32$ 3 will *not* divide evenly into 32.
$8 \times 5 = 40$ 3 will *not* divide evenly into 40.
$8 \times 6 = 48$ Both 3 and 4 will divide evenly into **48**.

Therefore 24 and 48 are common denominators for $\frac{3}{8}$ and $\frac{2}{3}$ and $\frac{1}{4}$, but 24 is the *lowest* common denominator for the three numbers.

Example $\frac{1}{7}$, $\frac{1}{6}$, and $\frac{1}{3}$
3 and 6 will *not* divide evenly into 7.

Multiples of 7: 14, 21, 28, 35, and 42.
42 is the lowest number that can be divided evenly by 6 and 3. Therefore **42** is a common denominator, the lowest common denominator.

Changing Fractions to Equivalent Fractions

RULE   Whatever you do to the denominator (multiply or divide by a number), you must do the *same* to the numerator so that the value does not change.

To maintain equivalence, the numerator and the denominator must be divided (or multiplied) by the *same* number.

Example $\frac{3}{8}$, $\frac{2}{3}$, and $\frac{1}{4}$

Steps for Changing Fractions to Equivalent Fractions

1. Find the common denominator—in this case 24.
2. Multiply each *numerator* by the *same* number used to obtain the common denominator for that fraction.

$\frac{3}{8} \underset{(\times 3)}{=} \frac{?}{24}$ $3 \times 3 = 9$ Therefore $\frac{3}{8} = \frac{9}{24}$

$\frac{2}{3} \underset{(\times 8)}{=} \frac{?}{24}$ $2 \times 8 = 16$ $\frac{2}{3} = \frac{16}{24}$

$\frac{1}{4} \underset{(\times 6)}{=} \frac{?}{24}$ $1 \times 6 = 6$ $\frac{1}{4} = \frac{6}{24}$

Reducing Fractions to Lowest Terms

A fraction is in lowest terms when the numerator and denominator cannot be divided by any other number except one.

RULE   To reduce a fraction to *lowest* terms, **divide** the numerator and denominator by the *largest* same whole number that will divide evenly into both. When there are no whole numbers that can be used except one, the fraction is in lowest terms.

The fraction $\frac{6}{8}$ is not in lowest terms because it can be reduced by dividing both the numerator and the denominator by 2, a common denominator. $\frac{3}{4}$ is expressed in lowest terms.

Example $\frac{6 \div 2 = 3}{8 \div 2 = 4}$ Note that both 6 and 8 are divided by 2.

Example $\frac{10 \div 5 = 2}{15 \div 5 = 3}$ Note that both 10 and 15 are divided by 5.

Example $\frac{4 \div 4 = 1}{24 \div 4 = 6}$ Note that both 4 and 24 are divided by 4.

$\frac{3}{4}$ and $\frac{2}{3}$ and $\frac{1}{6}$ cannot be further reduced. No other number than one will divide evenly into both the numerator and denominator. They are now in their simplest or *lowest* terms.

Changing to Equivalent Fractions Using Higher Terms

RULE To change a fraction to **higher** terms and maintain equivalence, **multiply** both the numerator and the denominator by the **same** number.

Example $\frac{6 \times 2 = 12}{8 \times 2 = 16}$ $\frac{6}{8} = \frac{12}{16}$

The value has not changed because the multiplier 2 is used for both the numerator and the denominator, and $\frac{2}{2} = 1$.
  Multiplying or dividing numbers by one does *not* change the value. Equivalence is maintained.

Addition of Fractions and Mixed Numbers

RULE If fractions have the same denominator, add the numerators, write over the denominator, and reduce.

Example

$$\begin{array}{r} \frac{1}{5} \\ + \frac{2}{5} \\ \hline \frac{3}{5} \end{array}$$

$$\begin{array}{r} \frac{2}{6} \\ + \frac{1}{6} \\ \hline \frac{3}{6} = \frac{1}{2} \end{array}$$

RULE If fractions have different denominators, convert each fraction to an equivalent fraction using the lowest common denominator and then add the numerators.

Example

$$\begin{array}{r} \frac{3}{5} = \frac{9}{15} \\ + \frac{2}{3} = + \frac{10}{15} \\ \hline \frac{19}{15} = 19 \div 15 = 1\frac{4}{15} \end{array}$$

$$\frac{3\,(\times 3)}{5\,(\times 3)} = \frac{9}{15}$$
$$\frac{2\,(\times 5)}{3\,(\times 5)} = \frac{10}{15}$$

RULE To add mixed numbers, first add the fractions by converting to a common denominator and then add this to the sum of the whole numbers.

Example

$$\begin{array}{r} 9\frac{5}{8} = 9\frac{15}{24} \\ + 6\frac{1}{6} = + 6\frac{4}{24} \\ \hline 15\frac{19}{24} \end{array}$$

$$\frac{5\,(\times 3)}{8\,(\times 3)} = \frac{15}{24}$$
$$\frac{1\,(\times 4)}{6\,(\times 4)} = \frac{4}{24}$$

WORKSHEET 1C | Addition of Fractions and Mixed Numbers

Add the following fractions and mixed numbers, using the common denominator, and reduce to lowest terms.

1.
$$\dfrac{2}{5}$$
$$+\dfrac{2}{5}$$

2.
$$\dfrac{4}{5}$$
$$+\dfrac{2}{3}$$

3.
$$6\dfrac{1}{6}$$
$$+9\dfrac{5}{8}$$

4.
$$2\dfrac{1}{4}$$
$$+3\dfrac{1}{8}$$

5.
$$1\dfrac{3}{4}$$
$$+9\dfrac{9}{10}$$

6.
$$\dfrac{1}{8}$$
$$\dfrac{1}{4}$$
$$+\dfrac{3}{9}$$

7.
$$\dfrac{7}{9}$$
$$\dfrac{4}{5}$$
$$+\dfrac{9}{10}$$

8.
$$3\dfrac{1}{4}$$
$$+9\dfrac{3}{4}$$

9.
$$8\dfrac{2}{5}$$
$$14\dfrac{7}{10}$$
$$+9\dfrac{9}{10}$$

10.
$$2\dfrac{1}{3}$$
$$+4\dfrac{1}{6}$$

Subtraction of Fractions and Mixed Numbers

RULE If fractions have the same denominator, find the difference between the numerators and write it over the common denominator. Reduce the fraction if necessary.

Example
$$\dfrac{27}{32}$$
$$-\dfrac{18}{32}$$
$$\dfrac{9}{32}$$

The difference between the numerators (27 minus 18) equals 9. The denominator is 32.

RULE If fractions have different denominators, find the lowest common denominator and proceed as above.

Example
$$\dfrac{7}{8}=\dfrac{21}{24}$$
$$-\dfrac{2}{3}=\dfrac{16}{24}$$
$$\dfrac{5}{24}$$

The difference between the numerators (21 minus 16) equals 5. The lowest common denominator is 24.

RULE To subtract mixed numbers, first subtract the fractions and then find the difference in the whole numbers. If the lower fraction is larger than the upper fraction, you cannot subtract it. *You must borrow from the whole number before subtracting the fraction.*

Example

$21\frac{7}{16}$
$-7\frac{12}{16}$

You cannot subtract 12 from 7 because 12 is larger than 7. Therefore you must borrow a whole number (1) from the 21, make a fraction out of 1 ($\frac{16}{16}$), and add the 7.

$$\frac{16}{16} + \frac{7}{16} = \frac{23}{16}$$

Because you added a whole number to the fraction, you must take a whole number away from 21 and make it 20. The problem is now set up as follows:

$$21\frac{7}{16} = 20\frac{16}{16} + \frac{7}{16} = \ 20\frac{23}{16}$$
$$-7\frac{12}{16}$$
$$13\frac{11}{16}$$

RULE Reduce your answer to lowest terms.

Answers on page 338

WORKSHEET 1D | Subtraction of Fractions and Mixed Numbers

Subtract fractions and mixed numbers, and reduce the answers to lowest terms.

1.
$\frac{2}{3}$
$-\frac{1}{2}$

2.
$\frac{27}{32}$
$-\frac{18}{32}$

3.
$10\frac{2}{5}$
$-6\frac{1}{4}$

4.
$7\frac{16}{24}$
$-3\frac{1}{8}$

5.
$6\frac{3}{10}$
$-2\frac{1}{5}$

6.
$\frac{7}{8}$
$-\frac{1}{3}$

7.
$3\frac{5}{8}$
$-1\frac{3}{8}$

8.
$5\frac{3}{7}$
$-1\frac{6}{7}$

9.
7
$-1\frac{3}{4}$

10.
$2\frac{7}{8}$
$-\frac{3}{4}$

Multiplication of Fractions and Mixed Numbers

Steps for Multiplication of Fractions and Mixed Numbers

1. Change the mixed number to an improper fraction if necessary.
2. Cancel, if possible, by dividing the numerators and denominators by the largest common divisor contained in each.
3. Multiply the remaining numerators to find a result, or product.
4. Multiply the denominators to find a result, or product.
5. Reduce the answer to lowest terms.

Example $\qquad \dfrac{4}{5} \times \dfrac{15}{16} = \dfrac{\overset{1}{\cancel{4}}}{\underset{1}{\cancel{5}}} \times \dfrac{\overset{3}{\cancel{15}}}{\underset{4}{\cancel{16}}} = \dfrac{3}{4}$

$\qquad 4\dfrac{1}{2} \times 2\dfrac{1}{4} = \dfrac{9}{2} \times \dfrac{9}{4} = \dfrac{81}{8} = 10\dfrac{1}{8}$

$\qquad 6 \times \dfrac{3}{8} = \dfrac{6}{1} \times \dfrac{3}{8} = \dfrac{\overset{3}{\cancel{6}}}{1} \times \dfrac{3}{\underset{4}{\cancel{8}}} = \dfrac{9}{4} = 2\dfrac{1}{4}$

Answers on page 339

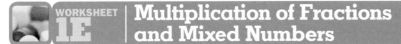

WORKSHEET 1E | Multiplication of Fractions and Mixed Numbers

Multiply the following fractions and mixed numbers, and reduce the answers to lowest terms.

1. $\dfrac{1}{5} \times \dfrac{2}{4} =$ **2.** $\dfrac{1}{5} \times \dfrac{1}{6} =$ **3.** $1\dfrac{3}{4} \times 3\dfrac{1}{7} =$

4. $4 \times 3\dfrac{1}{3} =$ **5.** $\dfrac{2}{4} \times 2\dfrac{1}{6} =$ **6.** $5\dfrac{1}{2} \times 3\dfrac{1}{8} =$

7. $\dfrac{3}{5} \times \dfrac{5}{8} =$ **8.** $\dfrac{5}{6} \times 1\dfrac{9}{16} =$ **9.** $\dfrac{5}{100} \times 900 =$

10. $2\dfrac{1}{10} \times 4\dfrac{1}{3} =$

Division of Fractions and Mixed Numbers

Steps for Division of Fractions and Mixed Numbers

1. Change mixed numbers to improper fractions if necessary.
2. Invert the number after the ÷ (division) sign.
3. Follow the steps for multiplication, and reduce any fractions.

Examples $\qquad \dfrac{1}{2} \div \dfrac{1}{3} = \dfrac{1}{2} \times \dfrac{3}{1} = \dfrac{3}{2} = 1\dfrac{1}{2}$

$\qquad 8\dfrac{3}{4} \div 15 = \dfrac{\overset{7}{\cancel{35}}}{4} \times \dfrac{1}{\underset{3}{\cancel{15}}} = \dfrac{7}{12} *$

---

*Reducing fractions $\left(\dfrac{7}{4} \times \dfrac{1}{3} \right)$ makes the math easier and reduces errors.

WORKSHEET 1F | Division of Fractions and Mixed Numbers

Divide the following fractions and mixed numbers, and reduce the answers to lowest terms.

1. $\frac{1}{5} \div \frac{1}{8} =$

2. $\frac{1}{3} \div \frac{1}{2} =$

3. $\frac{3}{4} \div \frac{1}{8} =$

4. $\frac{1}{16} \div \frac{1}{4} =$

5. $8\frac{3}{4} \div 15 =$

6. $\frac{3}{4} \div 6 =$

7. $2 \div \frac{1}{5} =$

8. $3\frac{3}{8} \div 4\frac{1}{2} =$

9. $\frac{3}{5} \div \frac{3}{8} =$

10. $4 \div 2\frac{1}{8} =$

Value of Fractions

RULE The denominator determines the number of parts into which the whole numbers divided. The smaller the denominator of a fraction, the greater the fraction's value if the numerators are the same.

Example Which would you rather have, $\frac{1}{6}$ or $\frac{1}{9}$ of your favorite candy bar? $\frac{1}{6}$ is greater than $\frac{1}{9}$. It represents a larger part of the whole unit.

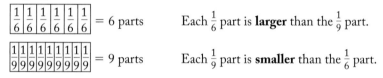

$\boxed{\frac{1}{6}\frac{1}{6}\frac{1}{6}\frac{1}{6}\frac{1}{6}\frac{1}{6}}$ = 6 parts   Each $\frac{1}{6}$ part is **larger** than the $\frac{1}{9}$ part.

$\boxed{\frac{1}{9}\frac{1}{9}\frac{1}{9}\frac{1}{9}\frac{1}{9}\frac{1}{9}\frac{1}{9}\frac{1}{9}\frac{1}{9}}$ = 9 parts   Each $\frac{1}{9}$ part is **smaller** than the $\frac{1}{6}$ part.

WORKSHEET 1G | Value of Fractions

Answer the following questions by circling the correct answer.

1. Would you rather own $\frac{1}{10}$ or $\frac{1}{20}$ of a lottery ticket?

2. Would you rather have 2 out of 7 or 2 out of 14 days off?

3. If you had a choice of a bonus of $\frac{1}{20}$ or $\frac{1}{30}$ of your annual salary, which would you prefer?

4. Which would be the *greater* incidence of a disease, 1 out of approximately every 100,000 people $(\frac{1}{100,000})$ or 1 out of approximately 250,000 people $(\frac{1}{250,000})$?

5. If a tablet was ordered for a patient at grain $\frac{1}{4}$ and you had tablets labeled grain $\frac{1}{8}$, would you need to give *more* or *less* than what is on hand?

6. Which is **greater?** $\frac{1}{5}$ or $\frac{1}{8}$

7. Which is **smaller?** $\frac{1}{100}$ or $\frac{1}{150}$

8. Which is **greater?** $\frac{1}{250}$ or $\frac{1}{300}$

9. Which is **smaller?** $\frac{1}{7}$ or $\frac{1}{9}$

10. Which is **smaller?** $\frac{1}{50}$ or $\frac{1}{200}$

Value of Decimals

A decimal fraction is a fraction whose denominator (bottom number) is 10, 100, 1000, 10,000, and so on. It differs from a common fraction in that the denominator is *not* written but is expressed by the proper placement of the decimal point.

Observe the scale below. All whole numbers are to the left of the decimal point; all decimal fractions are to the right.

RULE All whole numbers are to the left of the decimal; all decimal fractions are to the right of the decimal point.

To read a decimal fraction, read the number to the right of the decimal and use the name that applies to "place value" of the *last* figure other than zero. Decimal fractions read with a *ths* on the end.

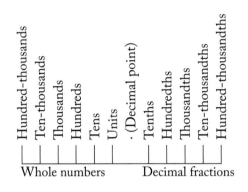

Examples	0.2	= Two Ten*ths*
	0.25	= Twentyfive hundre*ths*
	0.257	= Two hundred fifty-seven thousand*ths*
	0.2057	= Two thousand fifty-seven ten-thousand*ths*
	0.20057	= Twenty thousand fifty-seven hundred thousand*ths*

RULE For a whole number and a fraction, read the decimal point as an **and**.

Example 327.006 = Three hundred twenty-seven *and* six thousand*ths*

Comparison of Decimals

To determine which decimal is larger or smaller, compare the decimals from left to right, starting with the tenths place value, then the hundredths if needed, and so on.

Examples	0.4 and 0.5	5 is larger than 4. 0.5 is greater than 0.4.
	0.123 and 0.234	2 is larger than 1 in the tenths place so 0.234 is greater than 0.123.
	0.189 and 0.194	Both have 1 in the tenths column, but comparing the hundredths column reveals that the 9 is greater than 8. Therefore 0.194 is greater than 0.189.
	0.34 and 0.269	Avoid distraction because of the difference in lengths. Compare the tenths place value first. 3 is greater than 2. Therefore 0.34 is greater than 0.269.

Rounding Decimals

Steps for Rounding Decimals

1. Calculate *one* decimal place beyond the desired place.
2. If the final digit is **4** or less, make no adjustment. If the final digit is **5** or more, *increase* the prior digit by one number.
3. Drop the final digit.

Examples

- Round 2.7 to the nearest whole number. Examine the tenths column.
- Because 7 is greater than 5, the answer is 3 and 0.7 is dropped.

- Round 2.55 to the nearest tenth.
  Examine the second decimal place (hundredths column).
  Because the hundredths column is 5, the 2.5 is rounded up to 2.6 and the final 0.05 (hundredths) is dropped.
- Round 3.762 to the nearest hundredth.
  Examine the third decimal place (thousandths column).
  Because 2 is less than 5, no adjustment will be made in the hundredths column and the 2 is dropped. 3.76 is the answer.

	Nearest Whole Number	Nearest Tenth	Nearest Hundredth
1.689	2	1.7	1.69
204.534	205	204.5	204.53
7.87	8	7.9	7.87
3.366	3	3.4	3.37
0.845*	1	0.8	0.85

*To reduce reading errors, maintain the habit of placing a zero (0) in front of the decimal when a whole number is absent.

⊖ CLINICAL ALERT

Do **not** round medication dosages to the nearest whole number. This could result in an overdose. Syringes are calibrated in tenths and hundredths of a milliliter; therefore rounding to a whole number could result in an overdose. For instructions on how to round medication doses, refer to Chapter 4 (page 74).

WORKSHEET 1HA | Rounding Decimals

Round the decimal to the nearest whole number, the nearest tenth, and the nearest hundredth.

	Nearest Whole Number	Nearest Tenth	Nearest Hundredth
1. 93.489	_____	_____	_____
2. 25.43	_____	_____	_____
3. 38.1	_____	_____	_____
4. 57.8888	_____	_____	_____
5. 0.0092	_____	_____	_____
6. 3.144	_____	_____	_____
7. 8.999	_____	_____	_____
8. 77.788	_____	_____	_____
9. 12.959	_____	_____	_____
10. 5.7703	_____	_____	_____

WORKSHEET 1HB | Value of Decimals

Read the following decimals and write out in words.

1. 0.06 _____

_____

2. 0.092 _____

_____

3. 0.005 _____

_____

4. 100.01 _____

_____

5. 0.9 _____

_____

Write the following as decimals.

6. Thirty-four hundredths   _____

7. Three thousandths   _____

8. Two and seventeen thousandths _____

9. Nine and two ten-thousandths _____

10. Thirty-four and one tenth _____

⊜ CLINICAL ALERT

Make it your habit to always insert a zero (0) in front of decimal fractions when a whole number is absent. This draws attention to the decimal and avoids two potentially critical errors: missing the decimal or mistaking it for a number "1."

Answers on page 340

WORKSHEET 11A | Rounding Decimals

Round to tenths 0.0

1. 0.297 _____

2. 4.435 _____

3. 2.754 _____

4. 0.845 _____

5. 6.766 _____

Round to thousandths 0.000

11. 8.9374 _____

12. 5.6256 _____

13. 10.8976 _____

14. 4.6255 _____

15. 3.7386 _____

Round to hundredths 0.00

6. 0.297 _____

7. 4.435 _____

8. 2.754 _____

9. 0.835 _____

10. 6.766 _____

Round to ten-thousandths 0.0000

16. 8.93749 _____

17. 5.62568 _____

18. 10.89763 _____

19. 4.62557 _____

20. 3.73869 _____

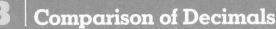

Comparison of Decimals

One of the keys to avoiding decimal errors when calculating medication doses is to know at a glance whether the amount you will give is *more* or *less* than the amount provided. Refer to page 12 for a review.

Which is *smaller*? Circle the correct answer.

1. 0.4 or 0.3

2. 0.5 or 0.25

3. 0.125 or 0.25

4. 2.309 or 2.07

5. 1.465 or 1.29

Which is *larger*? Circle the correct answer.

6. 0.9 or 0.1

7. 0.07 or 0.7

8. 0.58 or 0.09

9. 0.25 or 0.05

10. 0.001 or 0.1

Addition of Decimals

Steps for Adding Decimals

1. Write decimals in a column, keeping the decimal points under each other (A).
2. Add as in whole numbers, from right to left.
3. Place the decimal point in the answer directly under the decimal points in the numbers to be added.
4. Insert zeros as placeholders if desired within the problem after the last number (B).

	A	B	C
Examples	0.8	1.64	2.42
	+ 0.5	+ 2.10	+ 1.08
	1.3	3.74	3.5̸0

remember   Line up the decimal points.
Remove trailing zeros from the answer (C).

WORKSHEET 1J | Addition of Decimals

Add the following decimals.

1. 0.4 + 0.7 =

2. 5.03 + 2.999 =

3. 1.27 + 0.06 + 4 =

4. 15.6 + 0.19 + 500 =

5. 210.79 + 2 + 68.41 =

Subtraction of Decimals

Steps for Subtracting Decimals

1. Write decimals in a column, keeping the decimal points under each other.
2. Subtract as in whole numbers, from right to left.
3. Place the decimal point in the answer directly under the decimal points in the numbers to be subtracted (zeros can be added *after* the decimal point without changing the value).

Examples

$$\begin{array}{r} 0.604 \\ -\ 0.524 \\ \hline 0.080 \end{array}$$

$$\begin{array}{r} 0.500 \\ -\ 0.123 \\ \hline 0.377 \end{array}$$

remember Line up the decimal points.

WORKSHEET 1K | Subtraction of Decimals

Subtract the following decimals.

1. 2.5 − 1.25 =

2. 0.5 − 0.25 =

3. 0.45 − 0.367 =

4. 108.56 − 5.4 =

5. 1.25 − 0.75 =

Multiplication of Decimals

Steps for Multiplying Decimals

1. Multiply as with whole numbers.
2. Count the total number of decimal places in the multiplier and in the number to be multiplied.
3. Start from the right and count off the same number of places in the answer.
4. If the answer does not have enough places, supply as many zeros as needed, counting from right to left as illustrated on the following page. Eliminate trailing zeros in the answer.

Example $2.6 \times 0.0002 =$ 2.5   (1 decimal place)
                                          $\times\, 0.0002$ (4 decimal places)
                                ───────────
                                   0.00050̸   (5 decimal places from right to left in the answer
                                                before the trailing zero is deleted)

Answers on page 340

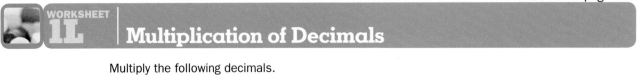

WORKSHEET **1L** | ## Multiplication of Decimals

Multiply the following decimals.

1. $100 \times 0.5 =$

2. $0.25 \times 2 =$

3. $3.14 \times 0.002 =$

4. $2.14 \times 0.03 =$

5. $36.8 \times 70.1 =$

Division of Decimals

Examine the divisor—the number you are dividing by. Is it a *whole* number or a *decimal?*

RULE   If the divisor is a *whole* number, the dividend decimal place is unchanged. Immediately place the decimal point prominently on the answer line directly *above* the decimal point in the dividend. Use zeros in the answer to hold places until you can divide. Prove your answer.

Examples $\cdot\ 1.20 \div 15$

$$
\begin{array}{r}
0.08 \leftarrow \text{Answer} \\
\text{Divisor} \rightarrow 15\overline{)1.20} \leftarrow \text{Dividend} \\
1\ 20
\end{array}
$$

PROOF	(Divisor × answer = dividend)
	0.08
	× 15
	────
	1.20̸

$\cdot\ 3.15 \div 7$

$$
\begin{array}{r}
0.45 \\
7\overline{)3.15} \\
2\ 8 \\
\hline
35 \\
35 \\
\hline
\end{array}
$$

PROOF	0.45
	× 7
	────
	3.15

RULE   If the divisor has a *decimal*, you must make it a whole number by moving the decimal point to the right. Move the decimal point in the dividend the same number of places to the right and immediately place the decimal point directly above on the answer line. Then divide as with whole numbers. Prove your answer.

Example   10 ÷ 4.4

$$
\begin{array}{r}
2.27 \\
4.4\overline{)10.0\,00} \\
8\,8 \\
\hline
1\,2\,0 \\
8\,8 \\
\hline
3\,2\,0 \\
3\,08 \\
\hline
1\,2 \quad \text{Remainder}
\end{array}
$$

Example   30 ÷ 5.2

$$
\begin{array}{r}
5.7 \\
5.2\overline{)30.0\,0} \\
26\,0 \\
\hline
4\,0\,0 \\
3\,6\,4 \\
\hline
3\,6 \quad \text{Remainder}
\end{array}
$$

Note that, as with whole division, a remainder is not just added to the answer in decimal division. Additional division will allow the remainder to be converted to a decimal fraction.

Example   2.6 ÷ 4

$$
\begin{array}{r}
0.6 \\
4\overline{)2.6} \\
2\,4 \\
\hline
2 \quad \text{Remainder}
\end{array}
\qquad
\begin{array}{r}
0.65 \\
4\overline{)2.60} \\
2\,4 \\
\hline
20 \\
20 \\
\hline
\end{array}
$$

remember   Keep all your decimals dark.

Answers on page 341

 WORKSHEET 1M | **Division of Decimals**

In the following problems, the divisor is a whole number. Place the decimal point on the answer line as illustrated in red in #1. Do NOT do the math in these problems.

1. $60\overline{)1.35}$

2. $20\overline{)15.6}$

3. $19\overline{)10.14}$

4. $7\overline{)60.5}$

5. $25\overline{)35.9}$

In the following problems, the divisor has a decimal. Make the divisor a whole number, move the decimal place in the dividend, and place the decimal point on the answer line as illustrated in red in #6. Calculate the answer to the *nearest tenth*. Add zeros to the dividend as necessary.

6. $0.25\overline{)0.50}$

7. $0.1\overline{)0.5}$

8. $4.8\overline{)2.04}$

9. $0.5\overline{)0.25}$

10. $0.12\overline{)0.44}$

Answers on page 341

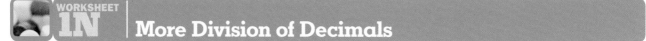

More Division of Decimals

Divide the following and carry to the *third* decimal place if necessary, and prove your answers.

1. $200 \div 6 =$ **2.** $15.06 \div 6 =$

3. $79.4 \div 0.87 =$ **4.** $158.4 \div 48 =$

5. $670.8 \div 0.78 =$

Changing Decimals to Fractions

RULE   The numbers to the *right* of the decimal can be written as a fraction because they are only part of the whole number.

remember   The first number past the decimal to the **right** is ten*ths*, the second is hundred*ths*, the third is thousand*ths*, the fourth is ten-thousand*ths*, and so on.

So if your problem has 3 numbers to the *right* of the decimal, just remove the decimal and put the number over 1000.

Examples   • 0.376 has 3 numbers to the *right* of the decimal. To make a fraction out of 0.376 and also get rid of the decimal, place it over 1000.

0.376 written as a fraction is $\frac{376}{1000}$.

• It's easy to remember: 3 numbers on top and 3 zeros on the bottom.

0.95 written as a fraction is $\frac{95}{100}$.

The idea is the same as above: 2 numbers on top and 2 zeros on the bottom. The fraction $\frac{90}{100}$ can be reduced to $\frac{9}{10}$ by dividing the numerator and the denominator by 10.

WORKSHEET 10 | Changing Decimals to Fractions

Change the following decimals to fractions, and reduce to lowest terms.

1. 0.8 =

2. 0.4 =

3. 0.25 =

4. 1.32 =

5. 4.08 =

6. 0.5 =

7. 0.75 =

8. 0.2 =

9. 0.65 =

10. 0.7 =

Changing Common Fractions to Decimals

RULE To change a common fraction to a decimal, divide the numerator by the denominator and place the decimal point in the proper position on the answer line.

Examples

WORKSHEET 1P | Changing Common Fractions to Decimals

Carry out the following division problems to the *third* decimal place as needed.

1. $\frac{1}{5}$ =

2. $\frac{2}{3}$ =

3. $\frac{1}{2}$ =

4. $\frac{1}{12}$ =

5. $\frac{6}{8}$ =

Percentages, Decimals, and Fractions

The term "percent" and its symbol (%) means parts per hundred. A percent number is a fraction whose numerator is already known and whose denominator is always understood to be 100. 25% means 25 parts per hundred.

Changing a Percentage to a Decimal

RULE To change a percentage to a decimal, divide the percentage by 100, moving the decimal point two places to the *left*. Remove the percent sign. (Remember that an implied decimal point immediately follows a whole number.)

Examples
$5\% \div 100 = 0.05$ (5% has an implied decimal point after the 5)
$0.5\% = 0.005$
$10\% = 0.1$ (10% has an implied decimal point after the 10)

Changing a Percentage to a Fraction

RULE To change the percentage to a fraction, *first* change the percentage to a decimal by dividing the percentage by 100, moving the decimal point two places to the *left*. Write the decimal as a fraction.

Examples
$5\% (\div 100) = 0.05 = \frac{5}{100}$
The fraction can then be further reduced to $\frac{1}{20}$
$0.1\% = 0.001 = \frac{1}{1000}$
$10\% = 0.1 = \frac{1}{10}$

Converting a Decimal to a Percentage

RULE To change a decimal to a percentage, multiply the decimal by 100 by moving the decimal point 2 places to the *right* and add the percent sign.

Examples
$0.1 (\times 100) = 10\%$
$0.01 = 1\%$
$0.5 = 50\%$

Answers on page 342

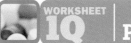

Percentages, Decimals, and Fractions

Fill in the following blanks with the appropriate equivalents.

	Fraction	Decimal	Percentage
1.	$\frac{1}{2}$		
2.			50%
3.		0.05	
4.	$\frac{1}{12}$		
5.	$\frac{3}{1000}$		
6.		0.10	
7.			250%

8. _____ 0.35 _____

9. _____ $\frac{4}{5}$ _____ _____

10. _____ _____ 75%

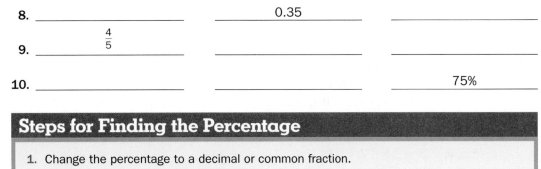

Steps for Finding the Percentage

1. Change the percentage to a decimal or common fraction.
2. _Multiply_ the number by this decimal.

Examples 50% of 120 = 0.5 × 120 = 60 or $\frac{1}{2}$ × 120 = 60

10% of 120 = 0.1 × 120 = 12 or $\frac{1}{10}$ × 120 = 12

Answers on page 343

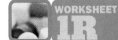 WORKSHEET **1R** | **Finding the Percentage**

Solve the following problems.

1. 2% of 1500 =   **2.** 114% of 240 =

3. 28% of 50 =   **4.** 9% of 200 =

5. $\frac{1}{2}$% of 9328 =   **6.** $\frac{1}{3}$% of 930 =

7. 120% of 400 =   **8.** 5% of 105.80 =

9. 10% of 520 =   **10.** 3% of 40.80 =

Answers on page 343

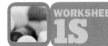 WORKSHEET **1S** | **Using Fractions to Percentages to Make Solutions**

In the hospital you might be asked to prepare a baby formula diluted to 50% ($\frac{1}{2}$) strength from a full-strength formula. If the baby was to receive 120 mL (4 oz) at each feeding, the nurse would multiply 0.5 (or $\frac{1}{2}$) × 120 for a result of 60 mL. 60 mL of full-strength formula would be measured and 60 mL of water added (120 mL − 60) for the total 120 mL to make a 50%-strength formula.

For 10% strength, the nurse would multiply 0.1 × 120 for a result of 12 mL full-strength formula. The nurse would measure 12 mL of full-strength formula and add 108 mL of water (120 mL total − 12 mL formula = 108 mL) for the total of 120 mL of 10%-strength formula.

Another way to do the math would be by ratio and proportion. This method will be introduced in Chapter 2. It is simpler to convert percentages, decimals, and fractions using basic arithmetic.

10 mL : 100 mL ∷ x mL : 120 mL

100 x = 10 × 120

x = 12 mL of full-strength formula

120 − 12 = 108 mL of water to be added

Make 150 mL of a 50% Betadine solution using normal saline (NS). 50% can be written as 50 : 100 or 1 : 2. The Betadine solution is the active solution and the NS is the solvent.

1 mL : 2 mL :: X mL : 150 mL multiply the two inside numbers and then the 2 outside numbers. Always divide the X number into the number on the right to get the answer. The resulting answer is the amount of solvent (Betadine) needed to make a 50% solution. The formula is called a ratio and proportion 1 mL : 2 mL :: X mL : 150 mL.

Example $2x = 1 \times 150 = 150$
$2x = 150$
$x = 75$ ml Betadine $+ 75$ mL of NS $= 150$ mL of a 50% solution.

Make the following solutions using Betadine solution as the active ingredient and NS as the diluent.

1. Make 450 mL yielding a $\frac{2}{3}$ strength solution.
2. Make 6 oz of a $\frac{1}{3}$ strength solution.
3. Make a $\frac{1}{4}$ strength solution for a total of 500 mL.
4. Make 800 mL yielding a $\frac{3}{4}$ strength solution.
5. Make a $\frac{2}{3}$ ratio solution for a total of 120 mL.

Answers on page 343

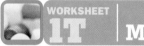

WORKSHEET 1T | Multiple-Choice Practice

Solve the following problems and select the correct answer. Estimate the correct answer before working the problem.

1. $\frac{30}{9}$ can be converted to which whole and mixed number?

   a. $3\frac{3}{9} = 3\frac{1}{3}$ **c.** $2\frac{1}{8}$

   b. $2\frac{1}{30}$ **d.** $4\frac{2}{9}$

2. Select the *fraction* equivalent for $3\frac{5}{6}$.

   a. $\frac{15}{6}$ **c.** $4\frac{1}{6}$

   b. $\frac{23}{6}$ **d.** $\frac{8}{6}$

3. $\frac{7}{8}$ and $\frac{3}{5}$ have which lowest common denominator?

   a. 8   **c.** 13

   b. 10   **d.** 40

4. $5\frac{1}{8} + 1\frac{1}{4} + 4\frac{1}{2} =$

   a. $10\frac{7}{8}$ **c.** $12\frac{1}{2}$

   b. $9\frac{1}{6}$ **d.** $10\frac{3}{4}$

5. $6\frac{3}{4} - 5\frac{1}{3} =$

   a. $\frac{1}{2}$ **c.** $1\frac{5}{12}$

   b. $1\frac{1}{2}$ **d.** $1\frac{5}{8}$

6. $\frac{5}{6} \times \frac{2}{8} =$

    a. $\frac{1}{12}$ c. $\frac{7}{14}$

    b. $\frac{5}{24}$ d. $\frac{10}{44}$

7. Divide the following fraction and reduce the lowest term: $\frac{1}{6} \div \frac{1}{3}$

    a. $\frac{2}{12}$ c. $\frac{1}{6}$

    b. $\frac{1}{2}$ d. $\frac{1}{3}$

8. Divide the following fraction and reduce the lowest term: $\frac{5}{6} \div \frac{1}{3}$

    a. $\frac{1}{6}$ c. $1\frac{1}{6}$

    b. $\frac{5}{18}$ d. $2\frac{1}{2}$

9. Two and eighteen thousandths can be written in decimal form as:

    a. 2.0018   c. 2.18

    b. 2.018   d. 2.118

10. $0.41 - 0.2538 =$

    a. 0.1562   c. 0.4138

    b. 0.2503   d. 0.6638

11. $5 \times 0.9 =$

    a. 0.45   c. 5.09

    b. 4.5   d. 45

12. $79.4 \div 0.87 =$

    a. 12.024   c. 80.276

    b. 21.084   d. 91.264

13. Change $\frac{1}{6}$ to a decimal and round the answer to the nearest *hundredth*.

    a. 0.02   c. 0.166

    b. 0.0625   d. 0.17

14. 20% of 450 =

    a. 90   c. 150

    b. 135   d. 185

15. $6\frac{1}{4}$% of 9328 =

    a. 0.56   c. 583

    b. 540   d. 5596

16. Change 0.285 to a fraction.

    a. $\frac{285}{1000}$ c. $\frac{285}{100}$

    b. $\frac{28}{100}$ d. $\frac{29}{1000}$

17. Change $\frac{2}{5}$ to a decimal to the nearest *tenth*.

    a. 0.4   c. 0.04

    b. 0.25   d. 0.025

18. Change $\frac{1}{8}$ to a decimal to the nearest *hundredth.*
   a. 0.13
   b. 0.12
   c. 0.17
   d. 0.125

19. Round 58.09 to the nearest *tenth.*
   a. 58
   b. 58.07
   c. 58.1
   d. 58.7

20. Change 4% to a decimal.
   a. 0.4
   b. 0.04
   c. 0.25
   d. 0.2

CHAPTER 1

Answers on page 344

Final

Change to whole or mixed numbers.

1. $\frac{25}{4}$

2. $\frac{32}{8}$

Change to an improper fraction.

3. $10\frac{1}{5}$

4. $3\frac{5}{6}$

Find the lowest common denominator in the following pairs of fractions.

5. $\frac{17}{20}$ and $\frac{4}{5}$

6. $\frac{7}{8}$ and $\frac{3}{5}$

Add the following.

7. $\frac{1}{18} + \frac{1}{4} + \frac{2}{9}$

8. $5\frac{1}{8} + 1\frac{1}{4} + 4\frac{1}{2}$

Subtract the following.

9. $\frac{7}{8} - \frac{2}{3}$

10. $6\frac{2}{4} - 5\frac{1}{2}$

Multiply the following.

11. $\frac{1}{5} \times \frac{1}{6}$

12. $\frac{5}{6} \times \frac{2}{8}$

Divide the following.

13. $\frac{3}{4} \div \frac{1}{8}$

14. $3\frac{3}{8} \div 4\frac{1}{2}$

Reduce the following fractions to lowest terms (numbers).

15. $\frac{2}{500}$

16. $\frac{9}{27}$

Write the following as decimals.

17. Five one hundredths

18. Two and seventeen thousandths

Add the following.

19. 5.01 + 2.999

20. 36.87 + 8.26 + 15.84

Subtract the following.

21. $4 - 0.176$ **22.** $0.41 - 0.2538$

Multiply the following.

23. 0.0005×0.02 **24.** 5×0.7

Divide the following and carry to the third decimal place.

25. $158.4 \div 48$ **26.** $79.4 \div 0.87$

Change the following to decimals.

27. $\frac{57}{48}$ **28.** $8\frac{1}{16}$

Find the following percentages.

29. 24% of 52   **30.** $6\frac{1}{4}$% of 9328

Change the following decimals to fractions.

31. 0.4   **32.** 0.285

Fill in the following blanks with the appropriate equivalents.

	Fraction	Decimal to Nearest Tenth	Decimal to Nearest Hundreths	Percentage
33.	$\frac{1}{3}$			
34.				5%
35.	$\frac{2}{5}$			
36.				22%
37.	$\frac{1}{8}$			
38.				10%
39.	$\frac{1}{12}$			
40.				$\frac{1}{2}$%
41.	$\frac{5}{16}$			
42.				15%
43.	$\frac{1}{4}$			
44.				12%
45.	$\frac{1}{100}$			
46.				80%
47.	$\frac{1}{200}$			
48.				33%
49.	$\frac{1}{250}$			
50.				75%

evolve Refer to the Mathematics Review section of Drug Calculations Companion, version 4 on Evolve for additional practice problems.

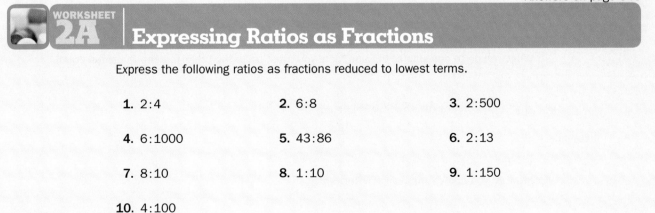

Ratio and Proportion

Objectives
- Express ratios as fractions.
- Reduce fractions to lowest numerical terms.
- Solve verbal and numerical ratio/proportion problems for x.
- Solve one-step ratio/proportion problems.
- Estimate answers.
- Prove answers.

Introduction
Ratio and proportion is an easy, provable method of drug dose calculation. The setup of problems is logical and systematic. Answers can be proven if the setup is correct.

Ratio

A ratio indicates the relationship of one quantity to another. It indicates *division* and may be expressed in fraction form.

Example $\frac{1}{3}$ may be expressed as the ratio $1:3$.

Answers on page 345

WORKSHEET 2A | Expressing Ratios as Fractions

Express the following ratios as fractions reduced to lowest terms.

1. 2:4	**2.** 6:8	**3.** 2:500
4. 6:1000	**5.** 43:86	**6.** 2:13
7. 8:10	**8.** 1:10	**9.** 1:150
10. 4:100		

Proportion

A proportion shows the relationship between two equal ratios. A proportion may be expressed as $3 : 5 :: 6 : 10$ or $3 : 5 = 6 : 10$.

To solve the ratio and proportion problems, do the following:

Steps for Solving Ratio and Proportion Problems

1. Multiply the two inside numbers.
2. Multiply the two outside numbers.
3. Check to see that the answers are the same.

Example $3 : 5 :: 6 : 10$

multiply

Multiply the two *inside* numbers: $5 \times 6 = 30$.
Multiply the two *outside* numbers: $3 \times 10 = 30$.

Solving Proportion Problems When One of the Numbers Is *Unknown,* or *x*

Example $2 : 8 :: x : 24$

multiply

Multiply the two *inside* numbers (means).

$8 \times x = 8x$

Multiply the two *outside* numbers (extremes).

$2 \times 24 = 48$

Move the x product to the **left** side of the equation. It will now look like this:

$8x = 48$

Now you must get x to stand alone.

RULE   To solve for the value of x, *divide* both sides of the equation by the number *next* to x. Those numbers will cancel each other. The result will be that x will stand alone.

What you do to one side of the equation, you must do to the other to keep the sides equal.

Example $\dfrac{\cancel{8}}{\cancel{8}}x = \dfrac{48}{8}$ This means $48 \div 8$ or $8\overline{)48}$ = 6 ; $\dfrac{48}{0}$

$x = 6$

How do you know your answer is correct?

To check your answer, substitute the answer for the x in the problem, multiply the inside numbers together, and then multiply the outside numbers together. The products should be equal.

PROOF	$8 \times 6 = 48$	(product of inside numbers, or means)
	$2 \times 24 = 48$	(product of outside numbers, or extremes)

Another way to view this example is:

$$\frac{2}{8} \underset{\times}{\overset{\times}{=}} \frac{x}{24}$$

Cross-multiplication solves this equation: $8x = 48$

$$x = 6$$

Example $2 : 3 :: 6 : x$ $\frac{2}{3} \underset{\times}{\overset{\times}{=}} \frac{6}{x}$ $2 : 3 :: 6 : 9$

multiply

PROOF	$2 \times 9 = 18$	(product of outside numbers)
	$3 \times 6 = 18$	(product of inside numbers)

$$2x = 18$$
$$\frac{\cancel{2}}{\cancel{2}}x = \frac{18}{2} \quad 18 \div 2 \quad \text{or} \quad 2\overline{)18} = 9$$

remember Divide both sides by the number next to x.

Answers on page 346

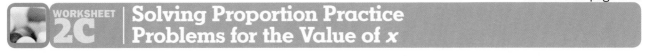

WORKSHEET 2B | Solving Proportion Practice Problems for the Value of x

Multiply the two inside numbers, multiply the two outside numbers, then move the x product to the left side of the equation. Solve for x.

1. $5 : 300 :: 9 : x$

2. $9 : 27 :: 300 : x$

3. $1 : 8 :: \frac{1}{2} : x$

4. $\frac{1}{4} : 500 :: x : 1000$

5. $6 : 24 :: 0.75 : x$

6. $36 : 12 :: \frac{1}{100} : x$

7. $4 : 120 :: x : 600$

8. $0.7 : 70 :: x : 1000$

9. $\frac{1}{1000} : \frac{1}{100} :: x : 60$

10. $6 : 12 :: \frac{1}{4} : x$

Answers on page 346

WORKSHEET 2C | Solving Proportion Practice Problems for the Value of x

Solve the following proportions for x, and prove your answers.

1. $\frac{1}{2} : \frac{1}{6} :: \frac{1}{4} : x$

2. $15 : 30 :: x : 12$

3. $1.5 : 10 :: 15 : x$

4. $6 : 12 :: 0.25 : x$

5. $300 : 5 :: x : \frac{1}{60}$

6. $\frac{1}{150} : \frac{1}{200} :: 2 : x$

7. $1 : 800 :: \frac{1}{200} : x$

8. $7.5 : 12 :: x : 28$

9. $\frac{1}{1000} : \frac{1}{100} :: x : 30$

10. $0.4 : 12 :: 10 : x$

Setting Up Ratios and Proportions

HINTS To set up a ratio and proportion problem, you must always put on the *left*-hand side what you already *have*, or what you already *know*.
On the *right*-hand side, you will put your *x*, or what you *want* to know.
Each side of the equation is set up the *same way*.

Examples Apples : *Pears* :: Apples : *x Pears*

Steps for Solving Ratio and Proportion Problems

1. Multiply the two inside numbers. Multiply the two outside numbers.
2. Place x product to the left side of the equal sign.
3. Divide both sides by the number next to x.
4. Prove all answers and label them.

Examples You wish to make a floral bouquet of 6 daffodils for every 4 roses. How many daffodils will you use for 30 roses?

KNOW WANT TO KNOW
6 daffodils : 4 roses :: *x* daffodils : 30 roses
(inside: ×; outside: multiply)

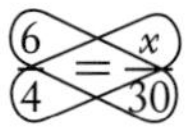

PROOF $4 \times 45 = 180$
$6 \times 30 = 180$

$$\frac{\not{4}}{\not{4}}x = \frac{180}{4} = 180 \div 4 = 45 \text{ daffodils}$$

remember **Place the x product on the left side of the equation to solve:**

$4x = 180$
$x = 45$ daffodils

- Make a necklace that has 19 blue beads for every yellow bead. How many blue beads are needed if you have 8 yellow beads?
(Prove your answer.)

KNOW   WANT TO KNOW
19 blue beads : 1 yellow bead ∷ x blue beads : 8 yellow beads

— multiply —

x = 152 blue beads needed

PROOF 19 × 8 = 152
          1 × 152 = 152

Answers on page 348

Setting Up Ratios and Proportions

Set up a proportion for each of the following problems. Label and prove your answers.

1. You have to make a fruit basket with 6 bananas for every 9 apples. How many bananas will there be for 72 apples?

2. You are making coffee, and 7 scoops make 8 cups. How many scoops make 40 cups?

3. You have a recipe for cocoa: 4 scoops make 6 cups of cocoa. You want to make 18 cups for a party. How many scoops of cocoa are needed? Set up a proportion.

4. Ordered: 4 pills each day. The patient will be taking the medication for 21 days. How many pills will you give the patient?

5. You wish to plant 8 bushes for every 2 trees in your yard. How many bushes will there be if there are 36 trees? (Estimate and prove.)

6. Ordered: 4 cups of bran every day. How many days would it take to consume 84 cups of bran? (Estimate and prove.)

7. It takes 4 cups of flour to make 3 loaves of bread. How many loaves of bread can be made from 24 cups of flour?

8. Your recipe for punch calls for 3 cups of soda for every $\frac{1}{2}$ cup of fruit juice. How many cups of soda will be needed for 2 cups of fruit juice?

9. You need 4 tablespoons of sugar for every glass of lemonade you prepare. How many tablespoons of sugar will be needed for 6 glasses of lemonade?

10. Ordered: 4 capsules every day. How many capsules would be needed for 14 days?

Answers on page 349

Ratio and Proportion Practice

Use ratio and proportion to solve the following problems, and label and prove your answers.

1. The office needs 4000 envelopes. The boxes on hand contain 200 envelopes per box. How many boxes will you send to the office?

2. The order is for 300 computer disks. The packages on hand contain 10 disks per package. How many packages will you send?

3. If one computer is allocated for every 18 students, how many computers will be needed for an enrollment of 1260 students?

4. Your doctor tells you to drink 3 glasses of water and eat 2 apples every day. How many apples will you have eaten when you have drunk 24 glasses of water?

5. If all the teachers were to receive 6 pens for every 8 pencils, how many pens would you give them if the teachers have 72 pencils?

6. The nurse is assigned 6 patients per shift. How many nurses will be needed for 36 patients?

7. If each baby formula calls for 4 tablespoons of powdered formula for every 8 ounces of water, how many tablespoons of powdered formula would be needed for 56 ounces of water?

8. The hospital requires 2 nurses for every unit for each 12-hour shift. How many nurses are needed for each unit for 72 hours?

9. If a patient takes 8 aspirin tablets per day, how many aspirin tablets will the patient need for a 2-week vacation?

10. If a multidose liquid medication contains 100 mL, and the patient takes 5 mL (1 teaspoon) per day, how many days will the medication last?

Answers on page 350

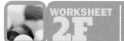

WORKSHEET
2F | **Multiple-Choice Practice**

Use ratio and proportion to solve the following problems. Label and prove your answers.

1. If you need 10 diapers a day, how many days will a package of 50 diapers last?
   a. 5 days
   b. 10 days
   c. 15 days
   d. 20 days

2. Ordered: 120 insulin syringes. They are delivered in units of 10 per package. How many packages will you receive?
   a. 10 packages
   b. 12 packages
   c. 15 packages
   d. 20 packages

3. You have to take 4 teaspoons of medicine every day. The bottle contains 80 teaspoons. How many days will the bottle last?
   a. 2 days
   b. 5 days
   c. 10 days
   d. 20 days

4. Ordered: 3 capsules per day. How many capsules will the patient need for 21 days?
   a. 12 capsules
   b. 20 capsules
   c. 31 capsules
   d. 63 capsules

5. You have a vial holding 30 mL of liquid. If the average dose given is 5 mL, how many doses are available?
   a. 5 doses
   b. 6 doses
   c. 8 doses
   d. 10 doses

6. The hospital has allotted 120 days of inservice for 15 departments. How many days of inservice can each department use?
   a. 4 days
   b. 8 days
   c. 12 days
   d. 15 days

7. The hospital staffs every 8 patients with one RN. How many RNs will be needed when the census is 240?
   a. 30 RNs
   b. 60 RNs
   c. 90 RNs
   d. 120 RNs

8. The directions state that for every $\frac{1}{2}$ cup portion of baby cereal you will need 4 ounces of milk. How many ounces of milk will you need to prepare 20 portions?
   a. 20 ounces
   b. 40 ounces
   c. 80 ounces
   d. 100 ounces

9. If you receive $15 an hour overtime, how many hours would you need to work overtime to receive $450 in overtime earnings?
   a. 3 hours
   b. 15 hours
   c. 30 hours
   d. 45 hours

10. One nurse assistant is employed for every 20 beds. How many nurse assistants are employed for a 360-bed hospital?
    a. 18 assistants
    b. 20 assistants
    c. 25 assistants
    d. 30 assistants

CHAPTER 2

Answers on page 351

Final

Solve each problem using ratio and proportion. Label and prove your answers.

1. The hospital assigns 5 nursing supervisors per shift. How many supervisors are needed for 3 shifts?

2. Each nurse is assigned 6 patients. How many nurses are needed for 150 patients in a hospital?

3. The hospital laundry provides 4 sheets per bed per day. How many sheets are needed per day for a 200-bed hospital?

4. The average number of discharges is 32 patients per day. How many patients are discharged each week?

5. A nurse earns $20 an hour extra pay for overtime hours. How much will the nurse earn for 24 hours of overtime in a pay period?

6. A CNA is hired for every 12 beds in the hospital. How many CNAs would be hired for a 360-bed hospital?

7. There is 1 nursing supervisor or administrator for every 30 nurses. How many supervisors or administrators would be needed for 150 nurses?

8. The hospital rents 25 portable oxygen canisters a week for $750. How much will a 4-week supply of canisters cost?

9. Approximately 1 resident and 2 interns are assigned for every 20 patients. How many interns are needed for 210 patients?

10. Some studies show that approximately 1 of every 6 medications given involves an error. Approximately how many medication errors would occur for every 240 medications given?

11. If a patient has to take 1 antiinflammatory tablet every 6 hours, how many tablets will he or she need for 3 days?

12. If a patient is discharged with a 1-week supply of antibiotic capsules and is to take 4 capsules per day, how many capsules will the patient need?

13. Ordered: 2 tablets, 3 times daily. How many days will a bottle of 60 tablets last?

14. The patient is to drink 4 ounces of water every $\frac{1}{2}$ hour. How much water will the patient have consumed in 8 hours?

15. The budget permits 48 inservice days per year. There are 12 units. How many inservice days could each unit receive for a year?

16. A multidose vial contains 20 mL. If each dose is 2.5 mL, how many doses are in the vial?

17. If the average adult weight is 150 pounds and the elevator can hold 1800 pounds, how many people, on average, can ride the elevator?

18. If each orientation for an RN costs approximately $3000, how many RNs can the hospital plan to hire with an annual orientation budget of $96,000?

19. If a guest speaker is paid a $50 honorarium, how many guest speakers can be invited if the budget is $600?

20. If a patient needs a 30-day supply of tablets and takes 2 tablets four times a day, how many tablets will the patient need at discharge?

ⓔvolve **Refer to the Mathematics Review section of Drug Calculations Companion, version 4 on Evolve for additional practice problems.**

Safe Medication Administration

Objectives
- Identify the knowledge and skills needed for safe administration of medications.
- Describe safe nursing practices that reduce medication errors.
- Interpret medication-related abbreviations and medication labels.
- Identify equipment for oral medication administration.
- Identify solid and liquid forms of medications.
- Identify key characteristics of medication administration records (MARs).
- Convert time to military hours.
- Explain the need for incident reports.
- Analyze medication errors using critical thinking.

Introduction **Safe medication administration involves more than accurate dose measurement and calculations. Prior to calculation, the nurse must be able to interpret the medication-related documents that will be encountered. This interpretation includes knowledge of medical terminology, hospital forms and abbreviations used in medication orders, drug forms, drug label contents, medication-related patient records, and current drug references. Attention to detail and patient rights are necessary elements for the protection of each patient.**

Patient Rights

There are many patient rights related to safe medication administration. As you read through these seven rights, think about the implications should one of these rights be violated.

Right Patient

The patient for whom the medication is ordered must be the patient who receives the medication. Similar names and lack of attention to patient identification when the medication is in hand can result in a medication being administered to the wrong patient. There are strict agency and The Joint Commission procedures for safe patient identification. They include using two separate written identifiers, such as the *patient name* and medical record number or *birth date*.

Right Drug

The nurse must be able to interpret orders for the drug, identify and clarify incomplete or unclear orders by conferring with the prescriber, and compare supplied drugs by matching them exactly to the order. Drugs may have a trade name in addition to a generic and chemical name. The nurse needs to become familiar with these alternative names. There are many similar-sounding drugs on the market, and they must be distinguished from each other.

Right Dose

Knowledge of abbreviations and measurement systems commonly used in the preparation and administration of medications is essential. The nurse must ascertain that it is a safe dose for the intended patient and must calculate and measure the precise dose ordered. Attention to decimals and zeros is vital for the prevention of errors.

Right Time

If a medication is omitted, delayed, or given too early, there can be serious consequences. A nurse must be able to interpret the 24-hour clock as well as read traditional time. Prioritizing emergency and stat drugs and identifying drugs that have to be given before, with, or after a meal are abilities that must be acquired through clinical practice and supervision. Knowledge of each drug's purpose and action is required. It is important to ask for help if the workload is too heavy to allow for perfect attention to detail.

⊕ CLINICAL ALERT

Always document the medication promptly *after* it is administered. Never document *before* a medication is administered. Doing so may lead to double dosing a medication.

Right Route

The nurse must prepare the medication so it can be administered via the route ordered. Abbreviations are usually used for medication routes. Many medications are available in solid and liquid forms for oral, intramuscular, or intravenous routes of administration. If the patient refuses or is unable to tolerate the route ordered, the nurse must obtain an order for change from the prescriber.

Right Documentation

Accurate and timely reporting and documentation in the patient medical records is an essential protection for the patient and the nurse.

Right to Refuse a Medication

Patients are entitled to refuse medications (and treatments). The reason should be ascertained, reported, and documented in a timely fashion so that corrective action can be taken if necessary. Include a comment on mental status when reporting and recording refusals.

Medication Errors

Several studies have shown that many medications are given in error; the rate ranges from 2% to well over 10% when underreporting and wrong time of administration are considered.

Errors may occur in the prescriber's order, in the interpretation of the order by the pharmacy or the nurse, in the copying of the order into a computer or onto a record, on the label or with the medication supplied by the pharmacy, or during the preparation and administration of the medication. Check agency policies pertaining to reporting medication errors.

There are many Internet references well worth reading that pertain to medication errors. The following is a sampling of on-line sources:

www.nlm.nih.gov/medlineplus/drugsafety.html
www.fda.gov/cder/drug/MedErrors
www.ismp.org
www.jointcommission.org/PatientSafety/DoNotUseList
www.medscape.com
www.nccmerp.org/aboutMedErrors.html

Note: It is recommended that you subscribe to the ISMP free medication safety newsletter: www.ismp.org/newsletters/nursing/default.asp

⊙ CLINICAL ALERT

The nurse who prepares and administers the medication offers the last protection to the patient.

Abbreviations

In order to interpret prescriber orders, drug literature, and drug labels, the nurse must learn treatment-related and medication-related abbreviations; they are listed on the inside front cover. The nurse must also avoid writing the abbreviations that are on The Joint Commission's Do Not Use list (Table 3-1). These abbreviations have been misinterpreted and have led to medication errors. Only approved abbreviations may be used, and they must be written precisely. You will have to review them several times in order to memorize them. Use these worksheets to help yourself remember them. Abbreviations for drugs have led to errors and are best avoided. The trend is to reduce the number of approved abbreviations.

Answers on page 351

WORKSHEET 3A | Abbreviations for Time and Route

Study the approved and recommended abbreviations and their patterns of similarities and differences as well as The Joint Commission's Do Not Use list in Table 3-1 and the Institute for Safe Medication Practices (Table 3-2). Then enter the approved or recommended abbreviation in the space provided.

Worksheet 3A: Abbreviations for Time and Route Table

Time	Abbreviation (if Applicable)	Time	Abbreviation (if Applicable)
before		after	
before meals		after meals	
daily	Write out daily	three times a day	
twice a day		every other day	Write out every other day
every day	Write out every day	every 6 hours	
every 4 hours		every 12 hours	
whenever necessary		as desired, freely	
immediately, at once		bedtime	Write out bedtime
with		without	

Continued on page 46

Table 3-1 The Joint Commission's Official "Do Not Use" List

Official "Do Not Use" List[1]

Do Not Use	Potential Problem	Use Instead
U (unit)	Mistaken for "0" (zero), the number "4" (four) or "cc"	Write "unit"
IU (International Unit)	Mistaken for IV (intravenous) or the number 10 (ten)	Write "International Unit"
Q.D., QD, q.d., qd (daily)	Mistaken for each other	Write "daily"
Q.O.D., QOD, q.o.d, qod (every other day)	Period after the Q mistaken for "I" and the "O" mistaken for "I"	Write "every other day"
Trailing zero (X.0 mg)* Lack of leading zero (.X mg)	Decimal point is missed	Write X mg Write 0.X mg
MS	Can mean morphine sulfate or magnesium sulfate	Write "morphine sulfate" Write "magnesium sulfate"
MSO_4 and $MgSO_4$	Confused for one another	

[1] Applies to all orders and all medication-related documentation that is handwritten (including free-text computer entry) or on pre-printed forms.

*Exception: A "trailing zero" may be used only where required to demonstrate the level of precision of the value being reported, such as for laboratory results, imaging studies that report size of lesions, or catheter/tube sizes. It may not be used in medication orders or other medication-related documentation.

Additional Abbreviations, Acronyms and Symbols
(For <u>possible</u> future inclusion in the Official "Do Not Use" List)

Do Not Use	Potential Problem	Use Instead
> (greater than) < (less than)	Misinterpreted as the number "7" (seven) or the letter "L" Confused for one another	Write "greater than" Write "less than"
Abbreviations for drug names	Misinterpreted due to similar abbreviations for multiple drugs	Write drug names in full
Apothecary units	Unfamiliar to many practitioners Confused with metric units	Use metric units
@	Mistaken for the number "2" (two)	Write "at"
cc	Mistaken for U (units) when poorly written	Write "mL" or "ml" or "milliliters" ("mL" is preferred)
μg	Mistaken for mg (milligrams) resulting in one thousand-fold overdose	Write "mcg" or "micrograms"

© The Joint Commission, 2010 Reprinted with permission.

Institute for Safe Medication Practices

ISMP's List of *Error-Prone Abbreviations, Symbols,* and *Dose Designations*

The abbreviations, symbols, and dose designations found in this table have been reported to ISMP through the ISMP Medication Error Reporting Program (MERP) as being frequently misinterpreted and involved in harmful medication errors. They should NEVER be used when communicating medical information. This includes internal communications, telephone/verbal prescriptions, computer-generated labels, labels for drug storage bins, medication administration records, as well as pharmacy and prescriber computer order entry screens.

The Joint Commission has established a National Patient Safety Goal that specifies that certain abbreviations must appear on an accredited organization's "do-not-use" list; we have highlighted these items with a double asterisk (**). However, we hope that you will consider others beyond the minimum Joint Commission requirements. By using and promoting safe practices and by educating one another about hazards, we can better protect our patients.

Abbreviations	Intended Meaning	Misinterpretation	Correction
μg	Microgram	Mistaken as "mg"	Use "mcg"
AD, AS, AU	Right ear, left ear, each ear	Mistaken as OD, OS, OU (right eye, left eye, each eye)	Use "right ear," "left ear," or "each ear"
OD, OS, OU	Right eye, left eye, each eye	Mistaken as AD, AS, AU (right ear, left ear, each ear)	Use "right eye," "left eye," or "each eye"
BT	Bedtime	Mistaken as "BID" (twice daily)	Use "bedtime"
cc	Cubic centimeters	Mistaken as "u" (units)	Use "mL"
D/C	Discharge or discontinue	Premature discontinuation of medications if D/C (intended to mean "discharge") has been misinterpreted as "discontinued" when followed by a list of discharge medications	Use "discharge" and "discontinue"
IJ	Injection	Mistaken as "IV" or "intrajugular"	Use "injection"
IN	Intranasal	Mistaken as "IM" or "IV"	Use "intranasal" or "NAS"
HS	Half-strength	Mistaken as bedtime	Use "half-strength" or "bedtime"
hs	At bedtime, hours of sleep	Mistaken as half-strength	
IU**	International unit	Mistaken as IV (intravenous) or 10 (ten)	Use "units"
o.d. or OD	Once daily	Mistaken as "right eye" (OD-oculus dexter), leading to oral liquid medications administered in the eye	Use "daily"
OJ	Orange juice	Mistaken as OD or OS (right or left eye); drugs meant to be diluted in orange juice may be given in the eye	Use "orange juice"
Per os	By mouth, orally	The "os" can be mistaken as "left eye" (OS-oculus sinister)	Use "PO," "by mouth," or "orally"
q.d. or QD**	Every day	Mistaken as q.i.d., especially if the period after the "q" or the tail of the "q" is misunderstood as an "i"	Use "daily"
qhs	Nightly at bedtime	Mistaken as "qhr" or every hour	Use "nightly"
qn	Nightly or at bedtime	Mistaken as "qh" (every hour)	Use "nightly" or "at bedtime"
q.o.d. or QOD**	Every other day	Mistaken as "q.d." (daily) or "q.i.d. (four times daily) if the "o" is poorly written	Use "every other day"
q1d	Daily	Mistaken as q.i.d. (four times daily)	Use "daily"
q6PM, etc.	Every evening at 6 PM	Mistaken as every 6 hours	Use "daily at 6 PM" or "6 PM daily"
SC, SQ, sub q	Subcutaneous	SC mistaken as SL (sublingual); SQ mistaken as "5 every;" the "q" in "sub q" has been mistaken as "every" (e.g., a heparin dose ordered "sub q 2 hours before surgery" misunderstood as every 2 hours before surgery)	Use "subcut" or "subcutaneously"
ss	Sliding scale (insulin) or ½ (apothecary)	Mistaken as "55"	Spell out "sliding scale;" use "one-half" or "½"
SSRI	Sliding scale regular insulin	Mistaken as selective-serotonin reuptake inhibitor	Spell out "sliding scale (insulin)"
SSI	Sliding scale insulin	Mistaken as Strong Solution of Iodine (Lugol's)	
i/d	One daily	Mistaken as "tid"	Use "1 daily"
TIW or tiw (also BIW or biw)	TIW: 3 times a week BIW: 2 times a week	TIW mistaken as "3 times a day" or "twice in a week" BIW mistaken ad "2 times a day"	Use "3 times weekly" Use "2 times weekly"
U or u**	Unit	Mistaken as the number 0 or 4, causing a 10-fold overdose or greater (e.g., 4U seen as "40" or 4u seen as "44"); mistaken as "cc" so dose given in volume instead of units (e.g., 4u seen as 4cc)	Use "unit"
UD	As directed ("ut dictum")	Mistaken as unit dose (e.g., diltiazem 125 mg IV infusion "UD" misinterpreted as meaning to give the entire infusion as a unit [bolus] dose)	Use "as directed"
Dose Designations and Other Information	**Intended Meaning**	**Misinterpretation**	**Correction**
Trailing zero after decimal point (e.g., 1.0 mg)**	1 mg	Mistaken as 10 mg if the decimal point is not seen	Do not use trailing zeros for doses expressed in whole numbers
No leading zero before a decimal point (e.g., .5 mg)**	0.5 mg	Mistaken as 5 mg if the decimal point is not seen	Use zero before a decimal point when the dose is less than a whole unit

© ISMP 2010

Used with permission, Institute for Safe Medication practice (ISMP) http://www.ismp.org.

Time	Abbreviation (if Applicable)	Time	Abbreviation (if Applicable)
by mouth		nothing by mouth	
intravenous		intramuscular	
sublingual		subcutaneous	
intradermal		suppository*	
left eye	Write out left eye	right ear	Write out right ear
nasogastric		per gastrostomy tube	

*Orders for suppositories require further route identification per vagina, per rectum, or per urethra.

Measurement Abbreviations

Metric abbreviations are commonly used for medication orders.

Metric measurement abbreviations are *not* pluralized. Two kilograms would be written as 2 kg, not 2 kgs; 2 grams would be written as 2 g, not 2 gs. Insert a space between the number and the metric unit: 10 g (not 10g).

Answers on page 351

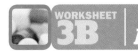

WORKSHEET 3B | Abbreviations for Drug Measurements

Study the abbreviations on the inside front cover. Pay attention to upper and lower case letters when learning the abbreviations. There are only a few instances when upper case is employed. Then provide the approved abbreviations for the measurements.

Metric Measurement Term*	Abbreviation (if Applicable)
microgram(s)	
milligram(s)	
gram(s)	
kilogram(s)	
milliliter(s)	
milliequivalent(s)	
unit	Write out unit
international unit	Write out international unit
liter	
square meter	
Other Measurement Term	**Abbreviation (if Applicable)**
one half	Write out one half
teaspoon	
tablespoon	
pound	

*The metric abbreviations are the same for singular and plural measurements.

CLINICAL ALERT

mcg, micrograms, may also be encountered written as μg. Write mcg for micrograms because μg has been misread as mg (milligrams) when poorly written; that is a thousandfold error.

cc is sometimes written interchangeably with mL (milliliters). It means cubic centimeters and has been mistaken for aa (of each) and u (units). Write mL instead. Do *not* write cc. Do *not* make up your own abbreviations for metric terms.

Answers on page 352

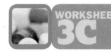

WORKSHEET 3C | **Abbreviations for Drug Forms**

Study the abbreviations on the inside front cover. Then provide the abbreviations in the spaces provided.

Term	Recommended Abbreviation
capsule*	
tablet	
fluid	
solution	
suspension	
elixir	
teaspoon	
tablespoon	
liquid	
ounce	
double-strength	
extended release*	
long acting*	
sustained release*	
controlled release*	

*Do not crush these medications.

CLINICAL ALERT

Study examples of abbreviations that have caused errors and are best written out. Refer to Tables 3-1 and 3-2.

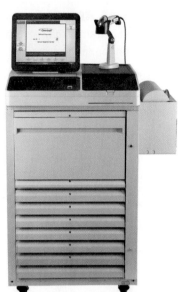

FIGURE 3-1 The OmniRx with OmniDispenser unit is an example of a computerized unit dose medication cabinet. Each dose is released individually, recorded automatically, and requires no counting when issued or at the end of a shift. The OmniRx is used for managing controlled substances, first doses, as-needed doses, floor stock, supplies, and other charge items. (From Omnicell, Inc., Mountain View, CA.)

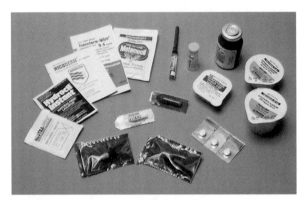

FIGURE 3-2 Unit does packages. (From Clayton BD, Stock YN, Cooper S: Basic pharmacology for nurses, ed 15, St Louis, 2010, Mosby. Courtesy of Chuck Dresner.)

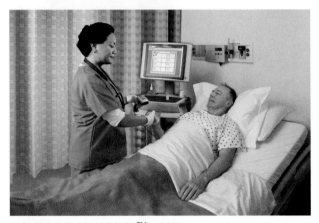

FIGURE 3-3 The Savvy ™ mobile medication system streamlines the medication administration process and provides safe and secure transportation of medications from the automated dispensing cabinet (ADC) to the patient's bedside. (From Omnicell, Inc, Mountain View, CA.)

Medication Delivery

Many hospital pharmacies stock supply and resupply computerized medication carts as shown in Figure 3-1. Computerized carts with bar scanners are thought to provide greater security and reduce the chances of medication errors by providing unit dose (single-serving) medications for one to three shifts at a time and one bottle of multidose liquid medications (Figure 3-2). The bar scanner is used to compare the bar code on the medication with the patient ID at the bedside (Figure 3-3).

Drug Forms: Solids and Liquids

As can be seen in the list and figures that follow, drugs can be provided in a variety of forms for both oral and other routes—tablets, capsules, suspensions, suppositories, and so forth. It is very important to distinguish among the forms and to ascertain the precise form intended by the prescriber. The form affects the rate of absorption of the drug and the route of administration.

Solids

- Plain tablets (Figure 3-4, *A*): compressed powdered drugs.
- Scored tablets (Figure 3-4, *B*): tablets with indentation; the only kind of tablet that may be broken. Use a pill cutting device for an accurate cut. (Figure 4-2)

- Enteric-coated tablets (Figure 3-4, *C*): tablets with coating for delayed dissolution.
- Capsules (caps) (Figure 3-4, *D*): soluble case, usually gelatin, that holds liquid or dry particles of drug.
- Extended-release capsules (S-R, slow-release) (Figure 3-4, *E*): capsules that contain beaded particles of drug for delayed absorption.
- Powders/granules (Figure 3-4, *F*): loose or molded drug substance; usually to be dissolved in liquid or food.

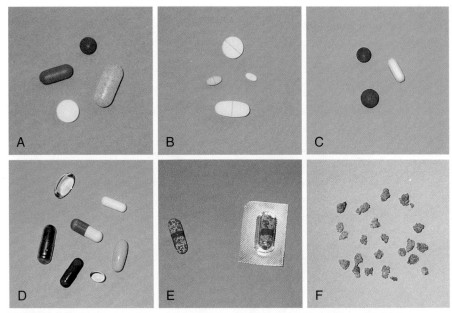

FIGURE 3-4   Various solid oral drug forms. **A,** Plain tablets. **B,** Scored tablets. **C,** Enteric-coated tablets. **D,** Capsules. **E,** Extended-release capsules. **F,** Granules. (Courtesy Amanda Politte, St Louis, MO.)

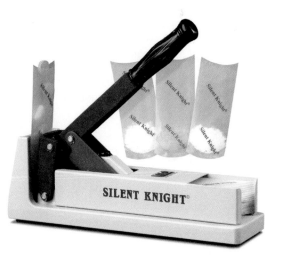

FIGURE 3-5   Silent Knight® Tablet Crushing System. A pill crusher that contains disposable pouches for each tablet to prevent cross contamination with prior crushed medications. (Used with permission by Links Medical Products, Inc., Irvine, CA.)

Liquids

- Aqueous suspensions: solid particles suspended in liquid that must be mixed well before administration
- Elixirs: sweetened alcohol and water solutions
- Emulsions: fats or oils suspended in liquid by an emulsifier
- Extracts: syrups or derived forms of active drugs
- Fluid extracts: concentrated alcoholic liquid extracts of plants or vegetables

⟳ CLINICAL ALERT Some tablets may be crushed if needed, and mixed with a liquid. Check current drug reference (Fig 3-5).

Reminder: Never cut unscored tablets. Never crush enteric-coated, E-R, S-R, XR, or gel-coated medications. Do not crush capsules. Check with prescriber if it is deemed necessary to alter the ordered form of medication, for example, when the patient develops difficulty swallowing.

Oral liquids are supplied in individual prepacked unit dose cups, bottles, calibrated plastic spoons, oral syringes, and so forth. Medicine cups with metric measurements are commonly used.

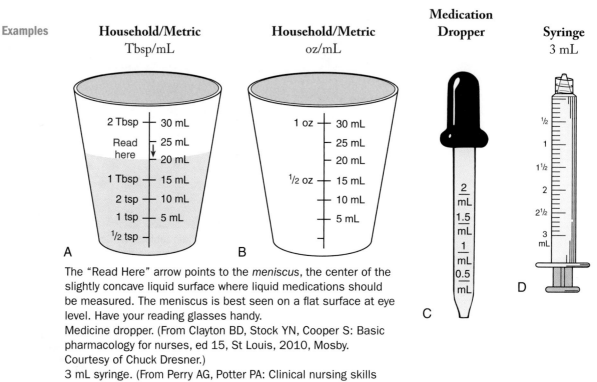

The "Read Here" arrow points to the *meniscus*, the center of the slightly concave liquid surface where liquid medications should be measured. The meniscus is best seen on a flat surface at eye level. Have your reading glasses handy.
Medicine dropper. (From Clayton BD, Stock YN, Cooper S: Basic pharmacology for nurses, ed 15, St Louis, 2010, Mosby. Courtesy of Chuck Dresner.)
3 mL syringe. (From Perry AG, Potter PA: Clinical nursing skills and techniques, ed 7, St Louis, 2010, Mosby.)

⟳ CLINICAL ALERT

Do not substitute the ordered form of a drug for another form. Do not substitute household utensils, such as spoons, cups, and droppers, when measuring medications. Medication utensils are calibrated for exact doses according to the metric system of measurement.

Liquid Injectables

Liquids may also be supplied in injectable (also known as *parenteral*) forms in ampules, vials, and prefilled syringes these are covered in Chapter 5.

Medication Labels

It is helpful to study the information provided on medication labels so as to facilitate your interpretation of prescriber orders and of medication administration records. Some of the label information is already familiar because of personal experience with medication prescriptions and over-the-counter (OTC) products. The label must be read carefully to ensure that the medication is precisely what the prescriber ordered.

Interpreting Medication Labels

Medication labels can be confusing because of the vast amount of information they contain and the small print. Some labels are prepared in-house by pharmacists or pharmacy technicians. The most important information is as follows:

- Name, both generic (the first letter is usually lowercase) and proprietary, brand, or trade (the first letter is usually capitalized)
- Route
- Form
- Unit dose (drug concentration) per milliliter(s), per tablet, or per capsule
- *Total* amount in the container
- Instructions for preparation (if applicable)
- Instructions for storage
- Expiration date (stamped by firm or pharmacist after manufacture)

Example

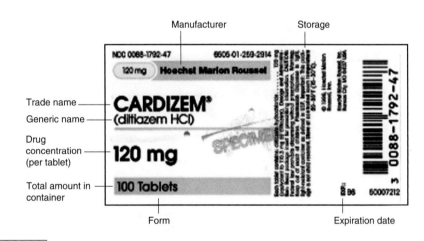

Note: The metric measurement mg is the abbreviation of milligrams.

Cardizem is the proprietary, or trade, name for this Hoechst Marion Roussel product. Diltiazem is the generic name used by all companies that produce this drug. There are 100 tablets total in the multidose container; each tablet contains 120 mg (unit dose). Tablets are usually given by mouth. The route is not specified, but the storage directions are given and space is provided for an expiration date. When calculating a dose, place the 120 mg : 1 tab on the left side of your ratio and proportion.

Example

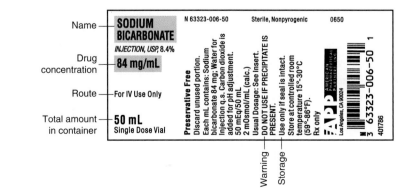

This vial of sodium bicarbonate contains 50 mL of 84 mg per mL intravenous injection fluid for emergencies. Note that it can permit much more than 1 to 2 times the concentration of 84 mg per mL, yet it is labeled a "single" dose vial. This is a type of drug that will call for a wide range of doses depending on patient condition and response to the drug, but it also is a drug that deteriorates upon standing so must be discarded after use. When calculating a dose, enter the *drug concentration* on the label, 84 mg : 1 mL, on the (left) side of the equation.

⊝ CLINICAL ALERT

Single dose vials must be discarded according to hospital policy after use no matter how much of the medication is unused.

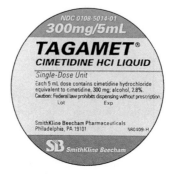

This is an example of packaging of a liquid with the "usual adult dose." Oral liquid medications often need more than 1 mL to be dissolved and palatable. This anti-ulcer drug label has a concentration of 300 mg per 5 mL (or 1 medication teaspoon), which is the usual dose for an adult. When calculating a dose, place the *drug concentration* seen on the label, *300 mg : 5 mL*, on the left side of the equation for what you *have* on hand. This can be reduced (simplified) to 50 mg : 1 mL by dividing both of the numbers by 5 before completing the calculation.

Example

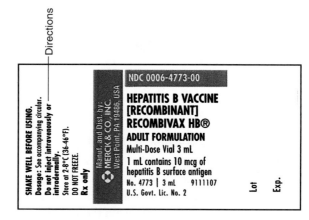

This hepatitis B vaccine label emphasizes that it is for adult use. The routes to be avoided are also emphasized. You would have to read the accompanying literature to determine whether it is to be given po or IM. (It is to be administered IM.) Also note the dose concentration: 10 mcg : 1 mL. The nurse must be very aware of the difference between micrograms and milligrams (mg). This vaccine, like many medications, is also issued in other strengths. It is important to note that this is a small *multidose* 3 mL vial, *not* a single-use vial.

⊝ CLINICAL ALERT

A lethal error can be made if the *total* dose in a multidose container is mistaken for the single dose or if an intramuscular preparation is given intravenously because the administrator failed to check the route.

HIGH-ALERT MEDICATIONS

This flag icon ⚑ is placed in front of medications and medication classes used in the text which appear on the Institute for Safe Medication Practices List of High-Alert Medications in the appendix. The icon is a visual reminder that will help the reader to become familiar with some of the specific types of medications which can cause significant harm to patients when used in error.

Please refer to the ISMP's List of High Alert Medications in the appendix for a complete list of these drugs as you work through this text, study pharmacology, and prepare care plans for your patients. Most are parenteral drugs, but there are also oral medications. Some agencies will require a manual independent second-nurse check for the preparation of some of these medications. Check your agency's policies.

Answers on page 352

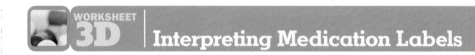

WORKSHEET 3D | Interpreting Medication Labels

Examine the label and fill in the requested information. Check your answers in the Answer Key before moving on to the next problem.

What you have or know (unit dose), 100 mg : 1 tab or 50 mg : 1 mL, is determined from the label and is inserted on the left side of your ratio and proportion.

1.

```
NDC 0028-0051-10          FSC 3602
6505-01-071-6557

Lopressor® 50 mg
metoprolol tartrate USP

EXP
LOT

1000 tablets
Keep this and all drugs out
of the reach of children.

Dispense in tight, light-resistant
container (USP).

Caution: Federal law prohibits
dispensing without prescription.

Geigy

PHARMACIST: Container closure is not child-resistant.
Dosage: See package insert.
Store between 59°- 86°F (15°- 30°C).
Protect from moisture.

Ciba-Geigy Corporation
Pharmaceuticals Division
Summit, NJ 07901

645120
```

    a. Trade name (registered patent or brand name, capital first letter)

    b. Generic name (common name, *usually* lowercase and in parentheses)

    c. Drug concentration and form (tab/cap/mL)

    d. Total amount in container

    e. Ratio for "what you have or know" (left side of your proportion)

2.

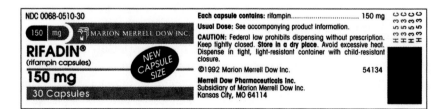

    a. Trade (brand) name

    b. Generic (common) name

    c. Drug concentration and form

    d. Total amount in container

    e. Ratio for "what you have or know"

3.

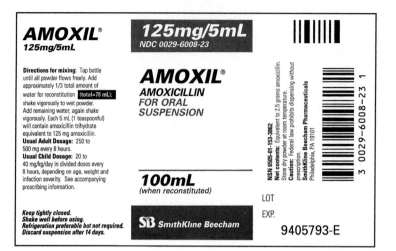

a. Trade name

b. Total amount (mL) of sterile water to add for reconstitution

c. Drug concentration and form

d. Total amount (mL) in container after reconstitution

e. Ratio for "what you have"

f. Length of time permitted for storage

Note: This is a multidose container commonly used by pharmacies and patients at home so that the patient does not have to go to a pharmacy for each dose of the medication. Most *oral* antibiotic suspensions and many other liquid oral medicines require more than 1 mL to be dissolved, palatable, and fully administered while accounting for some loss. One mL is only ⅕ of a medication teaspoon, and allowing for some loss or remainder in the equipment could involve a large amount of the medication.

4.

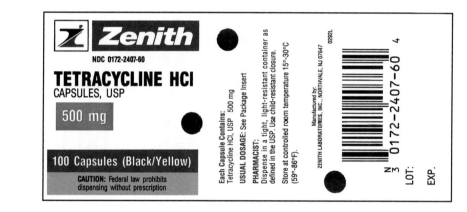

a. Generic name

b. Drug concentration and form

c. Total amount in container

d. Ratio for "what you have"

⊘ CLINICAL ALERT

The drug concentration (500 mg per capsule or tablet) (or 125 mg per 5 mL), also known as the unit dose, is usually the average dose ordered for the target population. If your calculations call for more than one or two times the drug concentration provided, double check the order and your math and research the reason. This commonsense approach can save lives. If the dose is appropriate, give the medication. If there is a question, contact your instructor, the prescriber, and/or the pharmacy.

5.

2.5 mL	2.5 mL
Streptomycin Sulfate Injection, USP	**Streptomycin Sulfate Injection, USP**
1 g/2.5 mL	**1 g/2.5 mL**
(400 mg/mL) (of streptomycin) *For IM use only* Store under refrigeration at 36° to 46°F (2° to 8°C) **CAUTION: Federal law prohibits dispensing without prescription.**	(400 mg/mL) (of streptomycin) *For IM use only* Store under refrigeration at 36° to 46°F (2° to 8°C) **CAUTION: Federal law prohibits dispensing without prescription.**
LOT **EXP**	**LOT** **EXP**
Pfizer **Roerig** Division of Pfizer Inc, NY, NY 10017	*Pfizer* **Roerig** Division of Pfizer Inc, NY, NY 10017

a. Generic name
b. Route
c. Drug concentration (mg per mL)
d. Total amount in container
e. Storage directions

Note that two concentrations are on the label: 1g per 2.5 mL and 400 mg per mL. If the order is for a gram, calculate the dose using the 1 g per 2.5 mL, and if the order is for milligrams (less than a gram), use the 400 mg per mL concentration for the "have" on the left side of the equation.

⊘ CLINICAL ALERT

Note the 400 mg/mL drug concentration on the label. If no number appears in front of mL, it is assumed to be the number one (1).

24-Hour Clock

Most health care agencies use the 24-hour clock, also known as "international time" and "military time."

The 24-hour clock runs sequentially from 0001, which is one minute after midnight, to 2400, which is midnight. Each hour is written in increments of 100. It is written with four digits, the first two for hours and the second two for minutes. No number is repeated.

Comparison of the 12-hr Clock and the 24-hr Clock*

12-hr Clock	24-hr Clock	12-hr Clock	24-hr Clock
Midnight 12:00 a.m.	2400	Noon 12:00 p.m.	1200
1:00 a.m.	0100	1:00 p.m.	1300
2:00 a.m.	0200	2:00 p.m.	1400
3:00 a.m.	0300	3:00 p.m.	1500
4:00 a.m.	0400	4:00 p.m.	1600
5:00 a.m.	0500	5:00 p.m.	1700
6:00 a.m.	0600	6:00 p.m.	1800
7:00 a.m.	0700	7:00 p.m.	1900
8:00 a.m.	0800	8:00 p.m.	2000
9:00 a.m.	0900	9:00 p.m.	2100
10:00 a.m.	1000	10:00 p.m.	2200
11:00 a.m.	1100	11:00 p.m.	2300

*The 24-Hour clock does not use colons or a.m., p.m.
**Adding or subtracting 1200 is the constant that converts PM hours between the two systems.

The system is computer-compatible and helps avoid the confusion of duplication of numbers (1 AM, 1 PM; 12 AM, 12 PM, etc.) in the traditional AM/PM 12-hr clock time.

At 2400 hours, midnight, the clock is reset to 0000 for counting purposes only so that 0001 will be one minute after midnight.

The AM clock begins at midnight, 2400 hours (12:00 AM), and it ends at 1159 hours (11:59 AM).

The PM clock begins at noon, 1200 hours (12:00 PM), and it ends at 2359 hours (11:59 PM).

Observe the chart on the prior page: The major difference from traditional time begins at 1300 hours or 1:00 PM. This is when duplication is avoided. Focus on the PM hours.

Seconds may be designated as follows: 1830:20 (6:30 PM and 20 seconds).

Observe the chart once more and memorize the 24-hour time for noon and midnight: 1200 hours (noon) and 2400 hours (midnight).

_____

Note: 24-hour time is always stated in hundreds (twelve hundred). Do not say, "one thousand two hundred.")

Examples

1159 = 1 minute before noon	2359 = 1 minute before midnight
1201 = 1 minute after noon	0001 = 1 minute after midnight

It is very helpful to study some key times in your daily schedule. Fill in the space provided in 24-hour clock time.

Your usual breakfast hour: _____

The time your shift begins: _____

The time your shift ends: _____

Your usual dinner hour: _____

Your usual bedtime hour: _____

Noon (12 PM):   _____

Midnight (12 AM):   _____

Physician's Orders

Medication orders may be entered into a computer by the prescriber or pharmacy and printed by the pharmacy or handwritten by the prescriber.

All medication orders must contain the complete date and time, the name of the patient and the medication, the total dose and form (if supplied in more than one form) of each administration of the medication, the route, the frequency schedule, and the prescriber's signature.

Examples   Patient: Mary Lopez

12/01/12   1800   Aspirin tablets 650 mg PO at bedtime daily with a snack. John Doe, MD.

OR

12/01/12   0900   Aspirin suppository 325 mg per rectum q6h for fever over 38° C. John Doe, MD.

Orders must be legible to avoid errors or misinterpretation. Questions pertaining to orders should be clarified with the prescriber and documented. Students should contact their instructor.

In most agencies, the pharmacy provides a printed daily medication administration record (MAR) to the unit for the patient record. It is based on the prescriber's order and includes additional information for the nurse who will administer the medication.

⊕ CLINICAL ALERT

Consult The Joint Commission's and clinical agency's policies and limitations pertaining to verbal and telephone orders.

Understanding Medication Administration Records (MAR)

Every nursing institution has its own medication administration record (MAR) forms, and the trend is to record the medications on computer. Similar in content, most of these forms are self-explanatory. All contain places to record identifying patient data; allergies; medication orders, including the dose, route, and frequency and hour desired for administration; and full signature (with date) of the person administering the medication. Most MAR forms list suggested codes for data entry.

During orientation, a new employee must identify hospital policies that are not stated on the form. These include how to add a new order, how to indicate discontinuance of a medication, procedures for data entry and reporting of medication errors, and additional documentation required to support the MAR. Examples of MARs are shown in Figures 3-9 and 3-10.

Entering the time on the wrong MAR or entering the wrong date or wrong shift may result in time-consuming frustration. To avoid entry errors on MARs, it is recommended that you use the following order when checking or entering data concerning a patient:

1. Patient ID
2. Correct date on MAR
3. Correct medication and allergies
4. Time when the medication was last given
5. Correct shift column

If the last dose of a scheduled medication was given late, it may be necessary to delay the next dose that you are preparing. This is done to protect the patient from a drug-overload injury.

Many hospitals have policies for charting by "exception," meaning entering a narrative explanation of data that requires more explanation than is allowed for on a flow sheet.

If a medication is withheld, follow agency policy for notation. In Figure 3-10, the first medication, Digoxin, was withheld, circled and initialed, and the code, R, was entered.

Any time a nonscheduled medication is given, such as a stat or prn medication, it is necessary to document prompt follow-up assessments and the time. This can be recorded on the nurse's notes or flow sheet, according to hospital policy—for example, "1630 states nausea is relieved."

If an entry error is made, follow hospital policy for corrections; an example of a medication incident report is shown in Figure 3-11. Handwritten data must be legible. It is *illegal* to discard a record or to erase, back date or obscure any entry on medical records.

As with all medical records, the MAR is considered confidential information, and permission to make photocopies must be specifically obtained.

Some institutions preprint the *exact* times for administration on the MAR. Refer to the MAR if the medication is administered at a *different* time; the time printed should be *circled,* and the actual time written in next to it, with the nurse's initials. Computer-generated MARs (CMAR) data entry varies and must be learned during orientation to each facility.

Realistically, it is impossible to give five different patients their medications at, for instance, 0900. Some institutions' MARs allow the nurse to initial the printed time if the actual time is within one half hour. An experienced nurse knows which medications do not permit flexible administration times and *prioritizes* the medication administration order.

Brown, John
ID# 45764304
DOB: 01-10-50   Sex: M   Rm: 406A
Dr. Marin, Cruz

ALLERGIES: DRUGS: *IV iodine, Aspirin*
FOODS: ___Denies___

RN Verification: ___*FD*___

MAR Date: 05-07-12 0700 - 05-08-12 0659

MEDICATION: Dose Route Freq   Time of Administration, Site, and Initials

	START	**STOP**	**0700 TO 1459**	**1500 TO 2259**	**2300 TO 0659**
SCH	05-05-12 Digoxin 0.125 mg po Q AM	05-12-12	(0900) *JM* R		
SCH	05-05-12 Tylenol (acetaminophen) 500 mg po BID	05-12-12	0800 *JM*	2000	
SCH	05-05-12 Clotrimazole 1% CR TOP bid to affected area	05-12-12	0900 *JM* L	2100	

This is a pharmacy-generated MAR for a 24-hr period stated in military time beginning with the day shift, 5-7-12. The RN who signs the verification is verifying that the medication orders accurately match the provider orders and that the allergies have been noted. SCH means a regularly scheduled medication versus a PRN order. You must use the agency *code* for administration sites. A circled time denotes med NOT given. Additional documentation may need to be added elsewhere in the nurse's record. PRN meds and one time only meds have *separate* placeholders. You may add new orders by writing them in (refer to promethazine). This pharmacy prints instructions for diluting intravenous medications. The narcotic (morphine sulfate) has an automatic 48-hr limit and then must have a written renewal order. This hospital policy calls for a yellow highlight to denote discontinued/expired orders. All discontinued orders, automatic or other, must be renewed if it is necessary to continue them. On the SITE CODES note that if a medication is withheld other than for NPO or surgery, the reason must be documented on the patient record, e.g.: "refused acetaminophen and states it 'doesn't do anything for him.' Dr. Marin notified."

ONE TIME ONLY AND PRN MEDS

	Start	**Stop**	**Time**	**Initials**	**Full Name/Title**
PRN	05-07-12 Morphine sulfate 25 mg IV q6h PRN Dilute in 5 mL NS and give over 5 min	05-09-12 0700	*2300* C	*FD*	*Florence Dane, RN*
	05-07-12 promethazine 25 mg IM STAT	*5/7/12*	*1900 J*	*TR*	*T Robbins, RN*

Sign: *Joe Mack*   Initials: *JM*   Sign: *T Robbins*   Initials: *TR*   Sign: *Florence Dane*   Initials: *FD*

SITE CODES

A	Abdomen (L)		J	Gluteus (LUQ)
B	Abdomen (R)		K	Gluteus (RUQ)
C	Arm (L)		L	Thigh (L)
D	Arm (R)		M	Thigh (R)
E	Eyes (both)		N	Ventrogluteal (L)
F	Eyes (left)		O	Ventrogluteal (R)
G	Eyes (right)		P	NPO: Lab
H	Deltoid (mid L)		Q	NPO: Surgery
I	Deltoid (mid R)		R	Withheld/See nurse's notes

GENERAL HOSPITAL

Clinical Alert!   Verify pharmacy data on this sheet including dilution instructions. Remember this form is not a *copy* of the original orders. These data have been recopied into the computer.

FIGURE 3-6   Sample medication administration record (MAR).

Acct:						

			MR#:		**M**	**MEDICATION**
Admitted: 10/05/12 1630			DOB: 05-10-60 Sex: F		**A**	**AMINISTRATION**
Att Phys:			HT: 5'7.0" / 170.2 cm		**R**	**RECORD**
Diagnosis: Gastric ulcer			WT: 224 lbs / 101.606 kg			
Allergies: Morphine/Beta-Adrenergic blocking agts						

Start Date/Time	Stop Date/Time	RN/ LPN	Medication	0731-1530	1531-2330	2331-0730
			** ****************** **PRN** ****************** **			
10/05/12 2143	10/12/12 2142		**Promethazine HCL** **(Phenergan Equiv)** **25 mg = 0.5 mL** IV #020 **Q6H PRN** **PRN N/V**			
			When administering IV: **Must be diluted to a** **final concentration of 25 mg/mL.** **IV administration to be at a rate** **not to exceed 25 mg/minute.**			
10/05/12 2100	10/08/12 2059		**Zolpidem Tartrate** **(Ambien)** **10 mg = 2 tablet** Oral #016 **At bedtime PRN for sleep** ****Narcotic sign-out****			Discontinue
10/05/12 2200	10/11/12 2159		**Alum-Mag Hydroxide-Simethicone** **(Maalox Plus/Mylanta Equiv)** **30 mL = 30 mL** Oral #022 **Q4H PRN nausea, flatulence, upset stomach** **Stagger one hr from other meds**			

This is an example of a computer-generated MAR (cMAR) for PRN orders only. There are many similarities to the MAR in Figure 3-6 and also some differences noted: this MAR states the medication unit dose supplied; the medication nurse must enter the exact time the medication was given. In addition to dilution instructions, scheduling instructions are given with the last medication. The site code is different and the dose omission code is amplified. Even if no medication is given to a patient, the MAR must be signed by the nurse responsible for the patient each shift. Medications which are refused, withheld, or mischarted must be circled, timed, and initialed—a standard procedure that may require additional entries on the patient record if the code is not self-explanatory.

Order Date	RN INIT.	Date/Time To Be Given	One Time Orders and Pre-Operatives Medication-Dose-Route	Actual Time Given	Site Codes			Dose Omission Code	
					Arm	LA	RA	A = pt absent	
					Deltoid	LD	RD	H = hold	
					Ventrogluteal	LVG	RVG	M = med absent	
					Gluteal	LG	RG	N = NPO	
					Abdomen	LUQ	RUQ	O = other	
					Abdomen	LLQ	RLQ	R = refused	
								U = unable to tolerate	
					INIT	Signature		INIT	Signature

60321 (8/98)A   CHART

FIGURE 3-7   Computer-generated MAR (cMAR) sample for PRN orders. (From Scottsdale Healthcare, Scottsdale, AZ)

SAMPLE MEDICATION INCIDENT REPORT*

Patient name: _____   Date of incident: _____
                                                   Time of incident: _____

Where incident occurred: Hospital: _____   Unit: _____

Admitting diagnosis: _____

Type of incident: _____   Wrong drug
                                     _____   Wrong time
                                     _____   Wrong dose
Check all that apply: _____   Wrong patient
                                     _____   Wrong route
                                     _____   Other

Medication order: _____

Account of incident and intervention(s) taken: _____
_____
_____
_____

Was the physician notified?_____   Time: _____

What were possible consequences to the patient as a result of this incident?_____
_____
_____

What can be done to prevent this type of incident from occurring again?_____
_____
_____

All persons familiar with incident or involved: _____
_____

_____   _____
Provider signature   Date   Supervisor signature   Date

Incident reports are used to analyze errors and determine error patterns and methods of error prevention. They also assist agency insurers in assessing risk for liability for incidents. Each agency has its own forms and protocols for incidents.

*Also known as Medication Variance or Occurence Reports.

FIGURE 3-8   Example of a medication incident report.

WORKSHEET 3E | Abbreviations, Symbols and Acronyms

Directions: For medication safety, it is important to be very familiar with The Joint Commission "Do Not Use" list (p. 44) and the Institute for Safe Medication Practices (ISMP) Error-Prone Abbreviations list (p. 45). Answer the following questions:

TJC: "Do Not Use" List (p. 44)

1. What are three mistakes that can be made if the abbreviation "U" for units is misread?

2. How can periods and "O" be misread?

3. How can trailing zeros and lack of leading zeros result in a dose error?

4. Which documents must be in compliance with the TJC official "Do Not Use" list?

5. Which is the preferred abbreviation for milliliters? cc, ml, or mL? Why?

ISMP: Dose Designation, Other Information Section, and Symbols Section (p. 45):

6. How can medications ending in the letter "l" cause a major dose error?

7. Why should large doses in the thousands have commas?

8. How should a numerical dose and unit of measure such as "ten milligrams", be spaced to avoid 10 to 100-fold overdoses?

9. How can a slash mark be misread, and what word should be used instead of a slash?

10. How can 3xd be misinterpreted, and how can it be avoided?

WORKSHEET 3F | Interpreting the MAR

Using the MAR in Figure 3-6, briefly answer the following questions.

1. Does the patient have a commonly seen surname? If so, why should the medication nurse take special note of this?   _____

2. Does the patient have any medication allergies? If so, which?   _____

3. This MAR indicates how many days of medication administration?   _____

4. Which drug ordered was withheld or not given as scheduled?   _____

5. By what route is Clotrimazole 1% to be administered?   _____

6. Which order has expired?   _____

7. Which drug was given at 11 PM and in which location?   _____

8. When must the morphine order be discontinued or reordered to continue administration? _____

9. When is the next time Tylenol may be given according to the 24-hour clock? According to traditional time? _____

10. Why do you think this form requires both the initials and the signature of the person giving the medications? _____

Answers on page 353

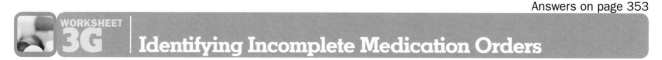

WORKSHEET 3G | Identifying Incomplete Medication Orders

Read the physician order and in a few words state why the order would have to be clarified.

1. Cozaar 25 mg daily in AM

2. Aspirin 2 tablets q4h po prn headache

3. Ampicillin 500 mg q6h × 3 days

▶ 4. Morphine sulfate 5 mg IV for pain

5. Tylenol 2 teaspoons q6h for fever over 100° F

Summary of Safe Medication Administration Practices

Consult hospital policies and The Joint Commission (TJC) policies as well as the Institute for Safe Medication Practices (ISMP) for approved abbreviations and High-Alert Medication list (refer to p. 44; p. 45 p. 335 in the text) as well as the following website: http://www.unchealthcare.org/site/Nursing/servicelines/aircare/additionaldocuments/2009npsg.

Interpretation

- Know the approved and prohibited abbreviations.
- Call the prescriber to clarify unclear orders. Do not guess.
- Be aware of the patient's allergies when reading medication orders.
- Phone orders are only for emergency medication orders and critical laboratory tests.
  Write the phone order on the record and read it back to the prescriber. Repeat numbers and doses by numeral; for example, for 30 mg say, "Three, zero, milligrams."

⊙ CLINICAL ALERT

Beware of confusing similar sounding drugs such as Xanax and Zantac (for anxiety; for gastric reflux and ulcers, respectively), Klonopin and Clonidine (for seizures; hypertension, respectively), and so on. There are many such examples.

Preparation

1. Clean and clear the area. Keep your reading glasses handy. Focus on the task. Try to avoid distractions.
2. Recheck allergies cited on the record. Reconfirm when the medication was last given.

3. If the patient is a transfer or postoperative patient, check receiving information such as operating room, emergency department, recovery room, and nursing home transfer records to see which medications were given and when they were given so that the patient does not receive a double dose, skip a needed medication, or experience an interaction with new orders. (Look for a "medication reconciliation" form.)

4. Assess recent relevant laboratory results.

5. Read label and package inserts, and match the label very carefully to the order. If a medication is liquid, check for dilution instructions.

6. Discard improperly labeled medications according to hospital policy.

If the dose will exceed 1 to 2 capsules or tablets, or 1 to 2 mL injectable, or more than two doses of the drug concentration supplied on the label, recheck the original order and a current pharmacology reference. Give the medication if the dose is appropriate. If there is doubt, contact your instructor, the pharmacy, or the prescriber.

Note: Oral liquid dose concentrations on the label often may exceed 1 to 2 mL, but again, the label concentration (e.g., 250 mg per 5 mL) is a guide to the "usual adult dose" ordered and is used for the calculations for "have on hand."

Check for sediment and presence of discoloration in liquids and for intact seals on controlled substances. Discard according to agency procedures.

Recheck the label three times before returning or discarding medication container. With single dose medications, retain the container at least until the medication has been administered.

⊖ CLINICAL ALERT

Fatal errors have occurred when a nurse miscalculated a dose and gave multiple ampules or multiple pills of a medication instead of looking up safe dose ranges (SDR) and questioning doses that exceed the drug concentration supplied. Remember also that usual doses for adults are very different from usual doses for children, those who are very ill, or adults who are above and below average weight.

Calculations

Learn to do your own dose calculations accurately. Estimate your answers to avoid a major math error before calculating the dose. Have a reliable current pharmacology drug reference on hand to verify safe dose ranges; usual doses for the age, weight, and condition of your patients; required dilutions, recommended frequency of administration, and administration timing techiniques. Call the pharmacy if there are questions.

The drug order, dose, and label must be checked *three times* before administration of the drug.

⊖ CLINICAL ALERT

If hospital policy calls for a second independent nurse check, it is done *before* administration. The second nurse must do an entire check totally independently *before* comparing results (right patient, drug, dose, route, time and safe dose range (SDR) with the first nurse.

remember An independent check by a second nurse means "look for mistakes," (patient, drug, dose, route, time) and this is achieved by going through all the steps (except preparation) separately from the first nurse. In many cases, the preparation may need to be observed after the order and calculations are verified—for example, dilutions and mixes of high-alert drugs.

Administration

The Joint Commission requires that *two* patient identifiers always be used and checked with medications records such as name, hospital identification number, or birthdate. Room or bed numbers are not valid patient identifiers. Wristbands, if used, must be on the patient, not on a table or taped to a bed. Special precautions for children, such as verification with a parent or other nurse, must be used. There is a growing trend to use barcode scanners to scan the two patient identifiers on the patient and the

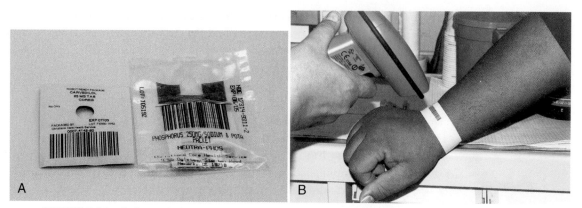

FIGURE 3-12 **A,** Bar coded patient unit-dose medications. **B,** Bar code reader. (From Kee JL, Marshall SM: Clinical calculations: with applications to general and speciality areas, ed. 5, St. Louis, 2009, Saunders.)

medication sent from pharmacy for a match. The scanners reduce the amount of wrong patient/wrong drug errors.

⊘ *CLINICAL ALERT*

Avoid asking, "Are you Mister or Ms X?" A confused or hard-of-hearing patient or a child may mistakenly answer, "Yes."

Medication Reconciliation

Meaures to reduce the high rate of medication errors upon transfers, admissions, and discharges are known as "Medication Reconciliation" or "Medication Remediation." The Joint Commission requires that all agencies that administer medications, including long-term care and home health care, provide evidence of medication reconciliation. The procedure includes checking allergies and all the medications the patient is taking from all providers, as well as over-the-counter (OTC) medications the patient takes at home. The nurse plays a major role in this review, as does the patient, family, pharmacy, and prescribers. Check your agency's policies, forms, and computerized medical data bank, if available.

⊘ *CLINICAL ALERT*

Failure to perform Medication Reconciliation on admission, transfer, and discharge, can result in serious adverse drug events, such as double dosing and other types of wrong doses, missed drugs, incompatible medication reactions with prescription and OTC medications, as well as drugs that have been discontinued but are still being given, to name a few. Agencies have developed their own Medication Reconciliation forms and procedures to meet this challenge. Look for this procedure when you are oriented to each clinical agency. Refer to Appendix A for a Hand-off communication example which illustrates a thorough hand-off report.

The following websites are highly recommended reading for useful medication safety information: http://www.unchealthcare.org/site/Nursing/servicelines/aircare/additionaldocuments/2009npsg http://www.intermedhx.com/

Answers on page 353

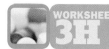 **WORKSHEET 3H** | **Multiple-Choice Practice**

1. When administering a medication at the bedside, which should be the *first* priority?
   a. Make appropriate assessments.
   b. Identify the patient.
   c. Document the administration of the medication.
   d. Recheck the medication label.

2. If a medication-related problem is identified, which should be the *first* measure the nurse takes?
   a. Assess the patient for side effects.
   b. Notify the supervisor.
   c. Call the physician.
   d. Document the problem in detail on an incident report.

3. Which is the *drug concentration* for the medication shown below?
   a. 50 mg/5 mL
   b. 1 pint
   c. 473 mL
   d. 200 mg

Vibramycin®
SYRUP *Calcium*
doxycycline calcium
oral suspension
50 mg/5 ml†
1 PINT (473 ml)
†Each teaspoonful (5 ml) contains
doxycycline calcium equivalent
to 50 mg of doxycycline.
USUAL DOSAGE:
Adults: 200 mg on the first day
(100 mg every 12 hours) followed by
a maintenance dose of 100 mg a day.
Children above eight years of age:
Under 100 lbs.—2 mg/lb. of body
weight daily divided in two doses
on the first day, followed by
1 mg/lb. of body weight on
subsequent days in one or two doses.
Over 100 lbs.—See adult dosage.
doxycycline U.S. Pat. No. 3,200,149
READ ACCOMPANYING
PROFESSIONAL INFORMATION
RECOMMENDED STORAGE
STORE BELOW 86°F. (30°C.)
Dispense in tight, light resistant
containers (USP).
CAUTION: Federal law prohibits
dispensing without prescription.

Pfizer **LABORATORIES**
DIVISION
PFIZER INC.,
NEW YORK, N.Y. 10017

MADE IN U.S.A. 2

Pfizer
NDC 0069-0971-93
6188

Vibramycin®
Calcium
SYRUP
doxycycline calcium
oral suspension

50 mg/5ml†

1 PINT
(473 ml)

RASPBERRY/APPLE
FLAVORED

For oral use
only

SHAKE WELL
BEFORE USING

IMPORTANT:
This closure is
not child-resistant.

4. If a hand-written medication order is illegible or unclear, which would be the best nursing decision?
   a. Check with pharmacy.
   b. Rewrite the order to make it more legible.
   c. Give the usual unit dose and clarify.
   d. Clarify with the physician who wrote it.

5. The nurse gives a medication at 1 PM. The correct equivalent international or military time on the 24-hour clock would be:
   a. 1000
   b. 1300
   c. 1500
   d. 0100

6. Which of the following statements regarding medications is *true*?
   a. Each nurse must be able to perform accurate simple and complex medication calculations.
   b. The unit dose and the total dose in a vial are one and the same.
   c. It is wise to rely on experienced colleagues to calculate drug doses.
   d. Medication errors rarely occur in the hospital setting.

7. The Joint Commission's "Do Not Use" list (p. 44) of abbreviations specifically applies to which documents?
   a. Patient-provided history and medication records brought from home
   b. Laboratory results including x-rays and blood work
   c. All forms in a patient's record that are handwritten
   d. All orders and medication-related documentation that is handwritten or on preprinted forms or free-text computer entry

8. A tablet is ordered for a patient with a nasogastric feeding tube who is NPO. Which is the most appropriate action for the nurse to take?
   a. Crush the tablet, dilute with water, and administer via the tube.
   b. Consult with the charge nurse about the medication routine for NPO patients.
   c. Ask the patient if there have been any problems with swallowing the pill, and then give it by mouth.
   d. Clarify the route with the physician who wrote the order.

9. A physician ordered ceftazidime 1g qh IM at 0800, 1400, and 2400 hours for a patient with an infection. The nurse administered 1 gram of cefapime IM at 0800 hours. Which patient right was violated?
   a. Right drug
   b. Right dose
   c. Right route
   d. Right time

10. An order for morphine sulfate 10 mg IM q4h prn for pain expired after 48 hours, during the previous shift. The patient continues to complain of postoperative pain and requests another pain injection. Which action is an *inappropriate* nursing action?
   a. Attempt alternative measures for pain relief such as repositioning and other comfort measures.
   b. Administer the medication because the patient has had no untoward side effects as the result of any of the prior doses.
   c. Assess the patient for unexplained sources of continued pain.
   d. Explain that the medication order has expired but that you will call for a renewed order.

Critical Thinking Exercises

Analyze the following examples of medication errors with your peers and/or instructor and discuss the issues suggested in the left-side guidelines, using this chapter and pharmacology references. As you study the error, consider which patient rights on pages 41 through 43 have been violated. What suggestions might you have for procedural changes at the hospital to prevent this from happening again? Include those that might involve pharmacy staff, providers, nurses, and patients.

1.	**Ordered:**	Tylenol #2, stat
	Supplied:	Tylenol in patient medication drawer and Tylenol #2 (in locked cabinet)
	Given:	Two Tylenol tablets
	Error(s):	The wrong medication was given. Two tablets of plain Tylenol were given instead of one tablet of Tylenol #2, which contains a narcotic. (If an incident report must be filed, this is the way the incident should be described in the space provided for a description of the incident.)
	Potential injuries:	Lack of comfort and its physiologic and emotional effects; lack of security; need for an alternative medication, perhaps to avoid acetaminophen (Tylenol) overdose.
	Nursing actions:	Report to supervisor and provider. Obtain orders to give additional pain medication. Document on medical record and file incident report per hospital policy. Assess patient periodically for side effects and document the results.

Preventive measures: Familiarize oneself with the medications ordered and commonly used in the unit, as well as with all controlled medications supplied, including those used in emergencies.

If this common medication was known to the giver, and a lack of attention or focus was a contributing cause, techniques to avoid distractions must be addressed. If this medication was not known to the giver, a pharmacology review of commonly used medications is in order. Nurses should always look up unfamiliar medications in current pharmacology references or check with the pharmacy before administering them. Nursing students should check with an instructor or supervisor after the reference check if they are unfamiliar with a medication. It is also wise to inform the patient at the bedside exactly which medications are to be given, because the patient may question the order. An informed patient presents the last line of defense in error prevention.

2. **Ordered:** Aspirin 650 mg PO, two tablets at bedtime

   Supplied: Aspirin 325 mg per tablet

   Given: Aspirin 1300 mg by a nurse the first night; Aspirin 650 mg by another nurse the second night.

   Error(s):

   Potential injuries:

   Nursing actions:

   Preventive measures:

3. **Ordered:** Narcotic for pain q3h prn, last noted on record as given by recovery room nurse at 1445 hours

   Given: Narcotic for pain at 1545 hours by nurse who had just started evening shift and admitted patient to unit

   Error(s):

   Potential injuries:

   Nursing actions:

   Preventive measures:

4. **Ordered:** Prednisone 60 mg daily

   Given: Prednisolone 60 mg daily

   Error(s):

   Potential injuries:

   Nursing actions:

   Preventive measures:

5. **Ordered:** Percocet

   Given: 8/11 Percodan. Recorded on the medical record; patient allergic to aspirin

   Error(s):

   Potential injuries:

   Nursing actions:

   Preventive measures:

Final

1. List the seven patient rights stated in the text.

   a. _____

   b. _____

   c. _____

   d. _____

   e. _____

   f. _____

   g. _____

2. Fill in the recommended term or abbreviation in the space provided.

Term/Abbreviation	Meaning	Term/Abbreviation	Meaning
c		s	
po		npo	
IV		IM	
supp		bid	
tid		q6h	
prn		ad lib	
ac		pc	
subcut		ID	
SL		NG	
stat		top	

3. Write the approved abbreviation in the space provided.

Term	Abbreviation
milligram	
microgram	
gram	
kilogram	
liter	
milliliter	

4. State the comparable times in the space provided.

Traditional Time	24-Hour Clock	24-Hour Clock	Traditional Time
12 Noon (12 pm)		2100 hours	
Midnight (12 am)		1400 hours	
1 pm		0145 hours	
9 am		0030 hours	
5 pm		1645 hours	

5. Study the label and supply the requested information.

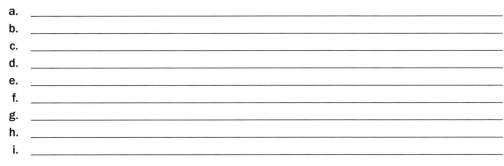

a. Generic name _____

b. Drug form _____

c. Unit dose per capsule _____

d. Single dose or multidose container (circle one)

6. State nine pieces of information that the medication label may contain:

a. _____

b. _____

c. _____

d. _____

e. _____

f. _____

g. _____

h. _____

i. _____

7. How would you write out this order: Aspirin tab 325 mg po q4h prn headache?

8. What is the purpose of The Joint Commission's Do Not Use list?

9. What should the nurse do if an order is unclear?

10. How can decimal points lead to errors in medication orders?

ℯvolve **Refer to the Safety in Medication Administration section on Drug Calculations Companion, version 4 on Evolve for additional information.**

Drug Measurements and Oral Dose Calculations

Objectives
- Convert milligrams, micrograms, grams, and kilograms.
- Memorize milliliter and liter conversions.
- Calculate gram and milligram conversion problems.
- Round medication doses to the nearest measurable amount.
- Identify metric and household liquid equivalents.
- Identify one- and two-step metric conversion problems.
- Distinguish unit and milliequivalent labels.
- Analyze medication errors using critical thinking.

Introduction
Medications are ordered and supplied primarily in the metric system of measurement. This chapter teaches the application of basic mathematics, ratio and proportion, nursing process and critical thinking used in safe medication preparation. Mastery of this chapter will provide the reader with an excellent foundation for all drug dose calculations.

Metric System

The International System of Units (SI), which is commonly known as *the metric system,* is now being used exclusively in the United States Pharmacopeia. SI is the abbreviation for the French *Système International d'Unités.* The metric system is the preferred system for weights, volume, and lengths and is used in computers. It is the preferred system for medication administration.

The basic units are multiplied and divided by a multiple of 10 to form the entire system. Table 4-1 illustrates the relationships and values within the metric system. There are a few equivalents used frequently in medicine. These should be memorized and are as follows:

Weight

1 mg (milligram)   = 1000 mcg (micrograms)
1 g (gram)   = 1000 mg (milligrams)
1 kg (kilogram)   = 1000 g (grams)

Volume

1 L (liter) = 1000 mL (milliliters)

remember   The abbreviation (such as g or mg) always *follows* the amount in the metric system. There is a space between the number and the abbreviation.

Examples   1000 mg
           1 g

Examples

Weight	**Volume**	**Length**
microgram (mcg)	milliliter (mL)	millimeter (mm)
milligram (mg)	deciliter (dL)	centimeter (cm)
kilogram (kg)	liter (L)	meter (m)
		kilometer (km)

⊖ CLINICAL ALERT

The nurse may encounter the symbol mgm for mg (milligram), μg for mcg (microgram), gm for g (gram), lowercase l for L (liter), and cc for mL (milliliter). Use the preferred highlighted symbols. The others have led to medication errors.

Table 4-1 Metric Measurements, Prefixes, and Their Values

Prefix	Numerical Value	Power	Meaning	Example	Meaning
micro (mc)	0.000001	10^{-6}	**Millionth** ($10 \div 10{,}000{,}000$)	microgram	one millionth of a gram
milli (m)	0.001	10^{-3}	**Thousandth** ($10 \div 10{,}000$)	milliliter	one thousandth of a liter
centi (c)	0.01	10^{-2}	**Hundredth** ($10 \div 1000$)	centimeter	one hundredth of a meter
deci (d)	0.1	10^{-1}	**Tenth** ($10 \div 100$)	deciliter	one tenth of a liter
	1	10^{0}	**One** ($10 \div 10$)	gram	one gram
deka (da)	10	10^{1}	**Tens** (1×10)	dekagram	10 grams
hecto (h)	100	10^{2}	**Hundreds** (10×10)	hectogram	100 grams
kilo (k)	1000	10^{3}	**Thousands** ($10 \times 10 \times 10$)	kilogram	1000 grams

Note: The Numerical Value column illustrates that you are moving decimals to the right or the left, either multiplying by 10 or dividing by 10. The amount of decimal movement depends upon the exponent (power). These prefixes can be combined with any metric base unit such as liters, meters, and grams. They can be seen in medication and scientific literature as well as in laboratory reports.

Metric Equivalents

The metric system is a *decimal system*.

remember   1000 mg = 1 g
                1000 mcg = 1 mg

RULE To convert grams (large) to milligrams (small), multiply by 1000.

Examples
5 g = 5.000. mg = 5000 mg

0.2 g = 0.200. mg = 200 mg

0.04 g = 0.040. mg = 40 mg

RULE To convert milligrams (small) to grams (large), divide by 1000.

Examples
250 mg = 0.250. g = 0.25 g

20 mg = 0.020. g = 0.02 g

5 mg = 0.005. g = 0.005 g

RULE To convert milligrams (large) to micrograms (small), multiply by 1000.

Examples
5 mg = 5.000. mcg = 5000 mcg

0.8 mg = 0.800. mcg = 800 mcg

0.05 mg = 0.050. mcg = 50 mcg

RULE To convert micrograms (small) to milligrams (large), divide by 1000. Figure 4-1 illustrates the decimal movement.

Examples
2500 mcg = 2.500. mg = 2.5 mg

400 mcg = 0.400. mg = 0.4 mg

10 mcg = 0.010. mg = 0.01 mg

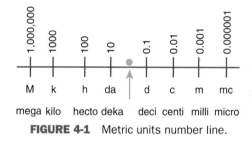

FIGURE 4-1 Metric units number line.

Answers on page 355

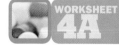

WORKSHEET 4A | Metric Equivalents

Fill in the following equivalents in the space provided:

remember 1 g = 1000 mg.
1 mg = 1000 mcg

1. 1 g = _____ mg

2. 2 g = _____ mg

3. 0.5 g = _____ mg

4. 1.5 g = _____ mg

5. 0.25 g = _____ mg

6. 0.05 mg = _____ mcg

7. 0.05 g = _____ mg   8. 0.1 g = _____ mg

9. 0.3 g = _____ mg   10. 1.1 g = _____ mg

11. 25 mg = _____ g   12. 5 mg = _____ mcg

13. 3000 mg = _____ g   14. 1500 mg = _____ g

15. 15,000 mg = _____ g   16. 10 mg = _____ g

17. 100 mcg = _____ mg   18. 0.5 mg = _____ g

19. 7.5 mg = _____ g   20. 2.5 mg = _____ mcg

⊖ CLINICAL ALERT

The *microgram, milligram,* and *gram* are the most commonly used units of measurement in medication administration.

Medication tablets and capsules are most often supplied in milligrams. Antibiotics can be supplied in grams, milligrams, or units.* Micrograms are used in pediatrics and critical care cases for small doses and/or for powerful drugs, and the need to convert is frequent. You *must* be skilled in the measurement and conversion of all three units.

*Units must be written out. Refer to The Joint Commission's Do Not Use list on p 44.

Rounding Medication Doses

RULE   Round your answers to the nearest *measurable dose* based on the selected equipment available and your patient's condition after you verify that the dose is correct for that patient.

Example   Tablets: *scored*   Round to the nearest $\frac{1}{2}$ tablet
    1.8 tabs   Give 2 tablets
    1.5 tabs   Give 1.5 tablets
    1.2 tabs   Give 1 tablet

Tablets: *unscored*   Do not break unscored tablets. Verify order. Recheck if the dose is more than 1 or 2 tablets. To break a "scored" tablet, use a pillcutter (Fig 4-2).

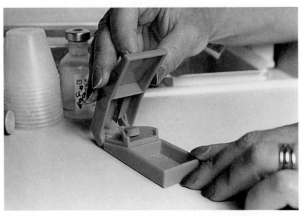

FIGURE 4-2   Pillcutter. (From Perry AG, Potter PA; Clinical nursing skills and techniques, ed 7, St Louis, 2010, Mosby.)

remember Seldom does a patient receive more than one or two multiples of the drug unit dose supplied.

Rounding Milliliters

Examine the equipment you plan to use. On a syringe, the markings might be tenths or hundredths of a milliliter. On a larger syringe, markings might be in 0.2-mL increments.

Rounding to the Nearest Tenth

RULE To round to the **nearest tenth,** examine the *hundredths* column. If it is 0.05 or greater, round up to the next tenth. If it is 0.04 or less, the tenths column remains the same.

Example 1.55 mL or 1.57 mL: Round to 1.6 mL
1.53 mL or 1.54 mL: Round to 1.5 mL

Ordered 1.75 mL. The 3-mL syringe shown below, the most commonly used syringe, is shaded to 1.8 mL, the nearest tenth, the nearest measurable dose.

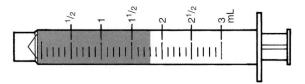

Rounding to the Nearest Hundredth

RULE To round to the **nearest hundredth,** examine the thousandths column. If it is 0.005 or greater, round up to the next hundredth.

Example 0.756: Round to 0.76
0.754: Round to 0.75

The 1-mL syringe is shaded to 0.75 mL because the 1-mL syringe is calibrated in hundredths and permits more exact measurement of small doses.*

---

*For further discussion of syringe calibrations, refer to Figure 5-1.

Drops

- Drops are so small that it is impossible to divide them. Drops are administered to the nearest whole drop.
- If a specially calibrated dropper is provided to give drops of liquid medicines, you must use that calibrated dropper and measure exactly.
- If an oral medication is to be administered, use the calibrated special spoon, prefilled syringe, or dropper provided (Figures 4-3 and 4-4) or draw it up in an appropriate syringe (without the needle) to the exact or nearest measurable amount.

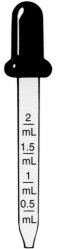

FIGURE 4-3 Medicine dropper. (From Clayton BD, Stock YN, Cooper S: Basic pharmacology for nurses, ed 15, St Louis, 2010, Mosby.)

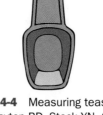

FIGURE 4-4 Measuring teaspoon. (From Clayton BD, Stock YN, Cooper S: Basic pharmacology for nurses, ed 15, St Louis, 2010, Mosby.)

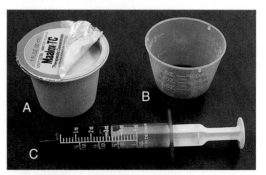

FIGURE 4-5 **A,** Liquid medication in a single-unit-dose package. **B,** Liquid measured in medicine cup. **C,** Oral liquid medicine in syringe. (From Perry AG, Potter PA: Clinical nursing skills and techniques, ed 7, St Louis, 2010, Mosby.)

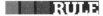 **RULE** Round to the *nearest measurable calibration* on the equipment you are using.

> ⊖ **CLINICAL ALERT**
>
> To avoid overdosing the patient, never round up liquid medications to the nearest whole number. If the answer is 1.7 mL, DO NOT round up to 2 mL. Use a syringe with the appropriate calibrations to measure an exact dose.

One-Step Metric Ratio and Proportion Calculations

Ratio and proportion *is* a provable method of solving medication calculation problems. It can be used to calculate metric equivalents and medication doses with accuracy and logic. There are two types of metric one-step calculations: metric equivalent problems and metric dose problems.

Example   40 mg = ? g (metric equivalent problem)

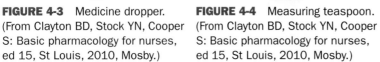 **RULE** Place the known metric *equivalents* from the metric tables on the **left**. Be sure to select the equivalents with the same terms as your problem (e.g., mg to g), and place the unknown on the **right** side of the equation in the same order as shown below.

Follow the same procedures as in Chapter 2 for ratio and proportion. Label all terms and prove your answer.

KNOW   WANT TO KNOW
1000 mg : 1 g :: 40 mg : x g
      (mg : g :: mg : g)

$$\frac{\cancel{1000}}{\cancel{1000}} x \quad \frac{\cancel{40}}{\cancel{1000}}$$

$x = 0.04$ g

PROOF
1000 × 0.04 = 40
1 × 40 = 40

ANSWER
40 mg = 0.04 g

Example   **Ordered:** 50 mg. **Unit dose on label:** 25 mg per tab (medication dose problem)

The second example of common metric one-step ratio and proportion problems is this: *Ordered: 50 mg. Label for the medicine: 25 mg per tab.* Since *both* the order and the label are in the same terms—milligrams—this involves only a *one-step* calculation. It is now easy to estimate if you will be giving more or less than the drug concentration per tablet on hand.

RULE   Place what you have on hand or what you know (the label unit dose) on the **left** and what is ordered (want to have or know) on the **right**. Follow through with your math to verify your estimate as shown in the ratio and proportion examples in Chapter 2.

KNOW   WANT TO KNOW
25 mg : 1 tab :: 50 mg : x tab

$$\frac{\cancel{25}}{\cancel{25}}x = \frac{50}{25} = 2$$

x = 2 tab

PROOF
$25 \times 2 = 50$
$1 \times 50 = 50$

ANSWER
Give 2 tab

⊘ CLINICAL ALERT

Some of these problems can be easily solved without being written. However, it is safer to verify your answer using ratio and proportion. More complex problems will be more easily solved after practice with easier problems.

Answers on page 355

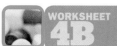

WORKSHEET
4B | **One-Step Metric Equivalents**

Use ratio and proportion to solve the following one-step metric equivalent problems. Prove and label all answers.

remember

1000 mcg	= 1 mg
1000 mg	= 1 g
1000 g	= 1 kg (2.2 lb)
1000 mL	= 1 L (liter)

Change milligrams to grams.

1. 4 mg	**2.** 200 mg	**3.** 350 mg
4. 25 mg	**5.** 15 mg	

Change grams to milligrams.

6. 2.5 g	**7.** 4.6 g	**8.** 0.03 g
9. 0.5 g	**10.** 0.01 g	

Change micrograms to milligrams.

11. 150 mcg	**12.** 500 mcg	**13.** 50 mcg
14. 2500 mcg	**15.** 3000 mcg	

CHAPTER 4 Drug Measurements and Oral Dose Calculations

Change milligrams to micrograms.

16. 20 mg   **17.** 200 mg   **18.** 5 mg

19. 0.1 mg   **20.** 0.04 mg

Change kilograms to grams. (Both of these measurements are used for infant weights.)

21. 5.5 kg   **22.** 12 kg   **23.** 3 kg

24. 1.3 kg   **25.** 0.5 kg

Change liters to milliliters.

26. 0.5 L   **27.** 1.3 L   **28.** 1.5 L

29. 3 L   **30.** 2.8 L

Identifying Units and Milliequivalents in Medication Dosages

The following measurements in addition to micrograms, milligrams, and grams may be seen in medication orders. They may also be seen in laboratory values.

Term	Abbreviation	Meaning
unit*	write out	Is a quantity that represents a laboratory standard of measurement. It is often used as unit of measure for products that have some or all animal or plant contents (e.g., heparin, insulin, antibiotics).
milliunit*	write out	Equals 1/1000 of a unit. Pitocin is an example of a medication ordered this way.
milliequivalent	mEq	Represents the number of grams of solute dissolved in a milliliter of solution. Electrolytes are commonly dissolved in solution and measured in milliequivalents (e.g., sodium, potassium, chlorides).
milliequivalent per liter	mEq per L	Equals one thousandth of 1 g of a specific substance dissolved in a liter of a solution. Electrolytes are frequently supplied in milliequivalents per liter for intravenous infusion (e.g., KCl 40 mEq per L).
milliequivalent per milliliter	mEq per mL	Equals one thousandth of 1 g of a specific substance dissolved in 1 mL. (The 1 is implied when a number is absent in front of mL.) 2 mEq per mL would equal two thousandths of a gram dissolved in 1 mL.

🔅 *CLINICAL ALERT*

"Unit" must be written out to avoid confusion with the zero (0) or the letter "O."

---

*Refer to The Joint Commission's Do Not Use list on p. 44.

Comparing Metric Unit Doses and Orders

As explained earlier in the chapter, a drug may be standardized in a laboratory and measured in "units or International Units" instead of by weight (gram) or other measurement.

A *"unit dose"* on medication labels is a single serving dose of the form supplied. An example is 5 mg per tablet or 5 mg per milliliter (mL) or per 5 milliliters (mL*). The unit dose may be in a single serving package (unit dose packaging) or multiple serving (multidose) container. The unit dose is related to the most commonly ordered safe dose of that drug. An antibiotic may have a recommendation to give 250 to 500 mg four times a day. It would be foolish for the drug manufacturer to provide 1000 mg tablets or 1000 mg per mL if the usual dose is 250 mg or 500 mg.

The trend in clinical agencies is to provide patient medications in unit dose containers (unit dose packaging) to prevent possible overdose errors and to prevent waste.

Drug concentration on labels (ratio of drug to amount of solid or liquid) is the same as in the unit dose provided. The drug concentration is unchanged regardless of the *amount* of medication provided. The unit dose (single serving dose) provided permits the usual doses to be given.

The nurse should read the medication order and then compare it to unit dose on the label.

Drug concentration On label:	Unit dose supplied	Usual doses ordered
1. 100 units per mL	10 units per 0.1 mL	2 to 50 units
2. 50 mg per 2 tablets or 25 mg per tablet	25 mg (per tablet or capsule)	25 to 100 mg
3. 500 mg per 10 mL*	100 mg (per 2 mL)	100 mg to 500 mg

Unit *doses* of liquids often must be dissolved in more than 1 mL to be mixed thoroughly and, with oral drugs, to be more palatable e.g., cough medicine 5 mL [1 tsp], or to be effective (a laxative 15 mL [1/2 ounce]).

The nurse should look at the order, then the unit dose, and *estimate* how much of the unit dose will be needed. The estimate is followed by an exact calculation. Estimates can alert the nurse to major math errors.

_____

*Note that metric units are not pluralized. Write mL not mLs.

Answers on page 358

WORKSHEET 4C | **Comparing Ordered and Available Unit Dose Amounts Practice**

Examine the ordered oral drug amount (first), then read the available unit dose supplied and indicate whether you will give *one serving*, or *more*, or *less* than one serving of the unit dose supplied.

1. Order   a. Rifadin 600 mg   b. Unit dose: 300 mg per tablet   c. Estimate:_____

2. Order   a. prednisone 25 mg   b. Unit dose: 10 mg per tablet   c. Estimate:_____

3. Order   a. Lanoxin 120 mcg   b. Unit dose: 0.125 mg per scored tablet
c. Estimate:_____

4. Order   a. cimetidine 0.8 g   b. Unit dose: 400 mg per tablet   c. Estimate:_____

5. Order   a. fluoxetime hydrochloride sol. 15 mg   b. Unit dose: 20 mg per 5 mL
c. Estimate:_____

6. Order   a. valproic acid syrup 200 mg   b. Unit dose: 250 per 5 mL
c. Estimate:_____

7. Order   **a.** Benaddryl 25 mg   **b.** Unit dose: 12.5 mg per 5 mL   **c.** Estimate:_____

8. Order   **a.** Halcion 125 mcg   **b.** Unit dose: 0.25 mg per scored tablet

c. Estimate:_____

9. Order   **a.** Synthroid 175 mcg   **b.** Unit dose: 0.175 mg per tablet   **c.** Estimate:_____

10. Order   **a.** ampicillin susp. 0.25 g   **b.** Unit dose: 100 mg per 2.5 mL
c. Estimate:_____

Note: Estimates help prevent major math errors.

Answers on page 358

WORKSHEET 4D | One-Step Oral Medication Problems

Use ratio and proportion and metric conversions to solve the following problems, and prove all work.

1. Ordered: Amoxicillin 500 mg po q8h for a patient with a severe bacterial infection. How many *capsules* will you administer?

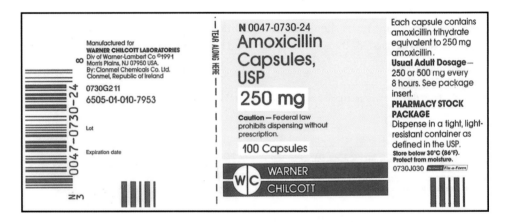

2. Ordered: Synthroid (levothyroxine sodium) 350 mcg daily po for a patient with hypothyroidism. How many *tablets* will you give?

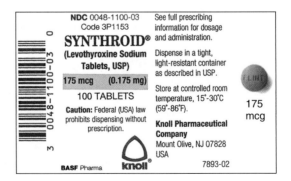

3. Ordered: Lanoxin 0.0625 mg daily po for a patient with heart failure. How many *tablets* will you give?

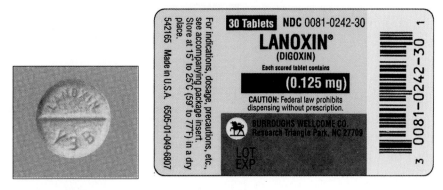

Lanoxin Tablet

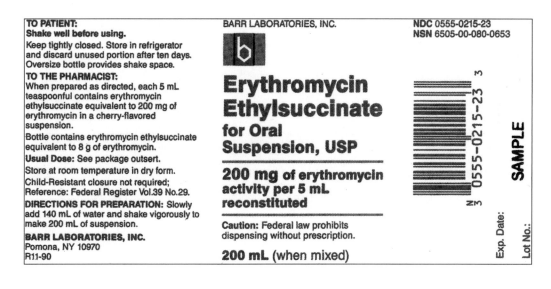

CLINICAL ALERT

If a tablet is scored, that is, has a line cut across it to denote a breaking point, you may break it. Use a pill cutter. Unscored tablets may not be broken because they will not break evenly and because the medication is not distributed evenly in the tablet. Refer to figure 4-2.

4. Ordered: Erythromycin ethylsuccinate suspension 300 mg po tid for a patient with an infection. How many milliliters will you administer?

5. Ordered: Infants' Tylenol (acetaminophen) Concentrated Drops 40 mg q4h po prn for pain/restlessness. How many milliliters will you give?

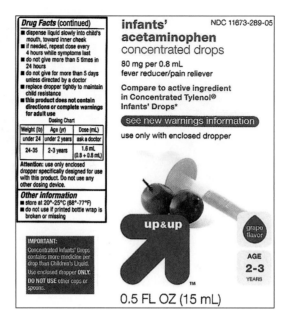

Drug Facts (continued)
- dispense liquid slowly into child's mouth, toward inner cheek
- if needed, repeat dose every 4 hours while symptoms last
- do not give more than 5 times in 24 hours
- do not give for more than 5 days unless directed by a doctor
- replace dropper tightly to maintain child resistance
- this product does not contain directions or complete warnings for adult use

Dosing Chart

Weight (lb)	Age (yr)	Dose (mL)
under 24	under 2 years	ask a doctor
24-35	2-3 years	1.6 mL (0.8 + 0.8 mL)

Attention: use only enclosed dropper specifically designed for use with this product. Do not use any other dosing device.

Other information
- store at 20°-25°C (68°-77°F)
- do not use if printed bottle wrap is broken or missing

IMPORTANT:
Concentrated Infants' Drops contains more medicine per drop than Children's Liquid. Use enclosed dropper ONLY. DO NOT USE other cups or spoons.

infants'
acetaminophen
concentrated drops
NDC 11673-289-05
80 mg per 0.8 mL
fever reducer/pain reliever

Compare to active ingredient in Concentrated Tylenol® Infants' Drops*

see new warnings information

use only with enclosed dropper

up&up

grape flavor

AGE 2-3 YEARS

0.5 FL OZ (15 mL)

CLINICAL ALERT

Distinguish infants' medications from children's medications.

CLINICAL ALERT

Read labels for liquids carefully to determine the unit dose and to see whether the liquid must be diluted, rolled, shaken, or mixed before administration. A "concentrated" medication such as this Infants' Tylenol can cause grave harm if an overdose is administered. This medication includes a calibrated dropper. Do NOT use household equipment.

Answers on page 359

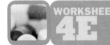

WORKSHEET 4E | **Metric Oral One-Step Practice Problems**

Estimate your answer. Use ratio and proportion to verify your estimate. Label and prove all work.

1. Ordered: Desyrel 75 mg. Label: Desyrel 50 mg scored tablets. How many tablet(s) will you give?

2. Ordered: Phenobarbital 30 mg. Label: 15 mg/tab. How many tablet(s) will you give?

3. Ordered: Theo-Dur 450 mg. Label: 300 mg scored tablets. How many tablet(s) will you give?

4. Ordered: Lanoxin 0.25 mg. Label: 0.125 mg/tab. How many tablet(s) will you give?

5. Ordered: Digitoxin 0.2 mg. Label: 0.1 mg tablets. How many tablet(s) will you give?

6. Ordered: KCl 20 mEq. Label: 8 mEq/5 mL. How many milliliters will you give?

7. Ordered: Synthroid 0.02 mg. Label: 0.01 mg tablets. How many tablet(s) will you give?

8. Ordered: Diazepam 5 mg. Label: Diazepam 10 mg scored tablets. How many tablet(s) will you give?

9. Ordered: Clinoril 800 mg. Label: Clinoril 400 mg tablets. How many tablet(s) will you give?

10. Ordered: Voltaren 450 mg. Label: Voltaren 150 mg tablets. How many tablet(s) will you give?

Two-Step Metric Ratio and Proportion Calculations

When a medication is ordered that is not in the same terms of measurement as the label—for example, grams ordered and milligrams on label, or micrograms ordered and milligrams on label—a two-step calculation must be completed.

Example   Ordered: 100 **mg**. You have 0.05 **g** tablets on hand. How many tablets will you give?

Step 1   Select the correct equivalents.
Have grams on hand. Need to change **mg** to the equivalent **g** on hand.

Equivalency tables: 1000 **mcg** = 1 mg
                           1000 mg = 1 g

KNOW   WANT TO KNOW
1000 mg : 1 g :: 100 mg : x g
        (mg : g :: mg : g)

$\dfrac{\cancel{1000}}{\cancel{1000}} x = \dfrac{\cancel{100}}{\cancel{1000}} = 0.1$

$x = 0.1$ g   My estimate is that I will give 2 tablets.

> PROOF
> $1000 \times 0.1 = 100$
> $1 \times 100 = 100$

Step 2   Insert the equivalent measure from Step 1 into your ratio and proportion now that all terms of measurement are the same.

HAVE   WANT TO HAVE
0.05 g : 1 tab :: 0.1 g : x tab

$\dfrac{\cancel{0.05}}{\cancel{0.05}} x = \dfrac{0.1}{0.05}$ or $0.05\overline{)0.1}$

$x = 2$ tabs

> PROOF
> $0.05 \times 2 = 0.1$
> $1 \times 0.1 = 0.1$

Tips on How to Avoid Errors

1. Analyze your problem. Is it a one-step or two-step calculation? (Are the terms the same or different?)
2. Always place a zero in front of a decimal when the number is less than one. It reminds you that the next figure is a decimal, not a number 1 (0.4).
3. Eliminate trailing zeros at the end of a decimal (0.75$\cancel{0}$).
4. Write neatly; estimate and prove your answer. Ask yourself whether this is a reasonable amount of medication. (Close to unit dose?)
5. If you doubt your math, recalculate without looking at your original work. If still in doubt, check reliable sources.

Answers on page 360

Use ratio and proportion and metric equivalents to change the order to what is on hand for the first step, then use ratio and proportion to determine the correct dose for the second step. Prove all work. Remember to estimate your answer when you set up the second step. Refer to the metric equivalency table, page 72, and the two-step explanation, page 83.

1. Ordered: Procanbid (procainamide HCl) 0.5 g po bid for a patient with an arrhythmia. How many tablets will you give?

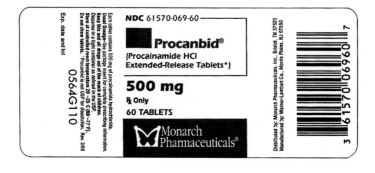

Step 1 **Step 2**

2. Ordered: Dilantin (extended phenytoin sodium) capsules 0.3 g bid po for a patient with seizures. How many capsules will you give?

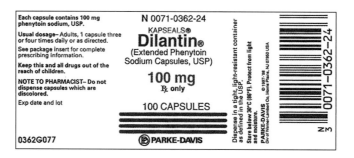

Step 1 **Step 2**

3. Ordered: Glucophage (metformin) 1 g po daily for a patient with type 2 diabetes. How many tablets will you give? (Glucophage is a high risk drug [⚑]).

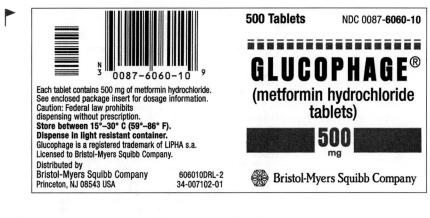

Step 1   Step 2

4. Ordered: Rifadin (rifampin) 0.3 g po b.i.d. for a patient with tuberculosis. How many capsules will you give?

Step 1   Step 2

5. Ordered: Lopid (gemfibrozil) 0.6 g po daily for a patient with high cholesterol levels. How many tablets will you give?

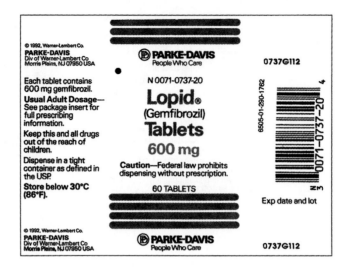

Step 1   Step 2

  CLINICAL ALERT

Document all administered medications carefully and promptly according to hospital policy.

Answers on page 361

WORKSHEET 4G | Metric One-Step and Two-Step Problem Practice

Use ratio and proportion and metric conversions to solve the following problems. Observe the generic and trade names. Prove all work and label answers.

1. Ordered: alprazolam 0.5 mg po at bedtime nightly for a patient with anxiety. How many tablets will you give?

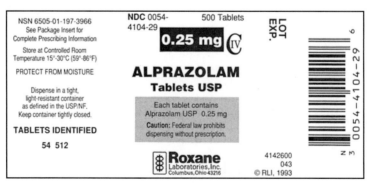

2. Ordered: zidovudine cap 0.2 g po tid for a patient with HIV infection. How many capsules will you give?

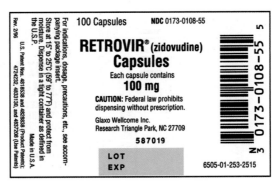

3. Ordered: Zofran 6 mg po 30 minutes before treatment for a patient receiving chemotherapy. How many mL will you give?

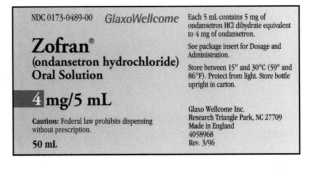

4. Ordered: levofloxacin tab 0.5 g po daily for seven days for a patient with an infection. How many tablets will you give?

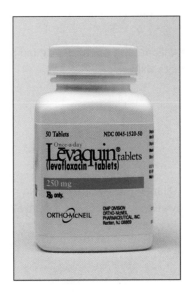

5. Ordered: fluoxetine hydrochloride sol. 25 mg po daily in the morning for a patient with depression. How many mL will you prepare, to the nearest tenth of a mL?

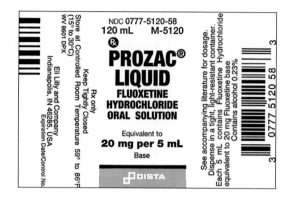

Answers on page 362

WORKSHEET 4H | **Additional Practice in Metric Oral Two-Step Problems**

Solve the following two-step problems using ratio and proportion. First convert the order to the equivalent on hand, then calculate the amount of medication. Prove all work.

1. Ordered: Halcion (triazolam) 125 mcg po at bedtime for a patient with insomnia. Label: 0.125 mg tablets. How many tablets will you give?

   Step 1   **Step 2**

2. Ordered: Valium (diazepam) 0.01 g bid po for a patient with anxiety. Label: 5 mg tablets. How many tablets will you give?

   Step 1   **Step 2**

3. Ordered: Dilantin (phenytoin) 0.2 g bid po for a patient with seizures. Label: 100 mg capsules. How many capsules will you give?

   Step 1   **Step 2**

4. Ordered: Diuril (chlorothiazide) 0.05 g po daily for a patient with hypertension. Label: 25 mg tablets. How many tablets will you give?

Step 1   **Step 2**

5. Ordered: Lanoxin (digoxin) 0.25 mg every other day po for congestive heart failure. Label: 125 mcg tablets. How many tablets will you give?

Step 1   **Step 2**

Answers on page 363

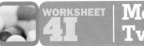

More Practice in Metric Oral Two-Step Problems

1. Ordered: Biaxin (clarithromycin) 0.5 g po q12h for a patient with an infection. How many tablets will you give?

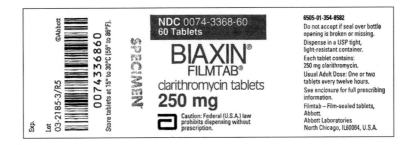

Step 1   **Step 2**

2. Ordered: CellCept (mycophenolate mofetil) 0.5 g po bid for a patient who received a transplant. How many capsules will you give?

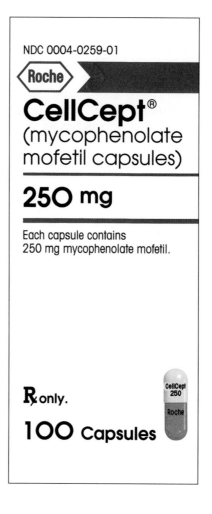

NDC 0004-0259-01

Roche

CellCept®
(mycophenolate
mofetil capsules)

250 mg

Each capsule contains
250 mg mycophenolate mofetil.

℞ only.

100 Capsules

CellCept
250
Roche

Step 1   Step 2

3. Ordered: Depakene (valproic acid) syrup 0.3 g po four times daily for a patient with seizures. How many mL will you give?

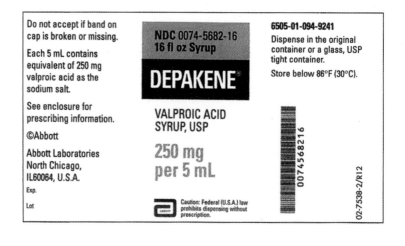

Do not accept if band on cap is broken or missing.

Each 5 mL contains equivalent of 250 mg valproic acid as the sodium salt.

See enclosure for prescribing information.

©Abbott

Abbott Laboratories
North Chicago,
IL60064, U.S.A.

Exp.

Lot

NDC 0074-5682-16
16 fl oz Syrup

DEPAKENE®

VALPROIC ACID
SYRUP, USP

250 mg
per 5 mL

Caution: Federal (U.S.A.) law prohibits dispensing without prescription.

6505-01-094-9241

Dispense in the original container or a glass, USP tight container.

Store below 86°F (30°C).

0074568216

02-7538-2/R12

Step 1   Step 2

4. Ordered: Dynapen (dicloxacillin) 1 g po stat for a patient with an infection. How many capsules will you give?

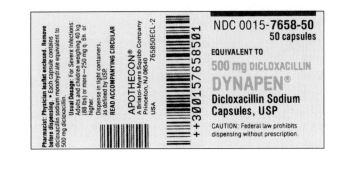

Step 1   **Step 2**

CLINICAL ALERT

Some medications ordered for elderly patients have a potential for adverse effects for physiological reasons, such as impaired renal or liver function.

These effects include high risk for injury due to confusion, sedation, agitation, gastrointestinal problems, hypotension, potassium imbalances, dehydration, elevated and toxic serum levels of the medication, and medication interactions. Dosages for elderly patients often are lower than those for average adults.

If a patient experiences a *new* problem after admission (rash, confusion, constipation, diarrhea, or others from the above list), review the medication orders and drug serum levels, if applicable. Report and document problems promptly.

5. Ordered: Cytotec (misoprostol) 0.2 mg daily with breakfast for a patient with an intermittent history of gastric ulcers. How many tablets will you give?

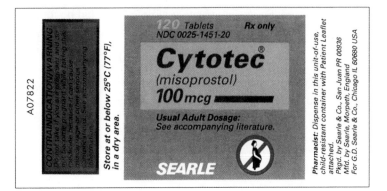

Step 1   **Step 2**

Comparing Metric and Household Measurements

Using metric measurements exclusively for all medication-related records is a recommendation of many national agencies that deal with patient safety. Learning the approximate household equivalents is also important because they may occasionally be seen in an order, particularly tsp, tbsp, ounce, and cup. The major implications are for discharge teaching. Patients must be instructed to use metric calibrated equipment if it is provided with the medication. Household equipment is not calibrated. The capacity of a cup, a teaspoon, or tablespoon varies widely, and if used, they can result in a major under- or over-dose. Refer to Table 4-2.

Table 4-2 Approximate Equivalents of Liquid Metric and Household Measurements

Metric	Household
5 mL*	1 teaspoon (tsp)
15 mL	1 tablespoon (Tbsp)
30 mL	2 tablespoons (Tbsp)
240 mL	1 measuring cup (8 ounces)
500 mL	1 pint
1000 mL (IL)	1 quart

*The abbreviations mL and cc have been used interchangeably in the past. Remember, mL is preferred because cc has been misread and has led to medication errors.

⊜ CLINICAL ALERT

Teaching discharged patients to use calibrated equipment at home, such as measuring spoons and oral syringes and droppers provided with their medications, is a very important nursing responsibility.

Answers on page 364

WORKSHEET 4J | Multiple-Choice Practice

Solve the following problems and circle the correct answer. Use scrap paper, set up your ratio and proportion neatly, and *prove* your work. Remember to focus on whether the calculation is one-step or two-step and *estimate* your answer. If it does not seem right, recalculate the problem without looking at your original work.

1. Ordered: Potassium chloride elixir 20 mEq bid po for a patient with potassium deficiency. Label: 8 mEq/5 mL. How many milliliters will you give?
   a. 12.5   b. 15   c. 32   d. 40

2. Ordered: Quinidine sulfate 0.3 g bid po for a patient with an arrhythmia. Label: 150 mg tablets. How many tablets will you give?
   a. 0.5   b. 1   c. 2   d. 3

3. Ordered: L-Dopa (levodopa) 2 g bid po for a patient with Parkinson's disease. Label: 500 mg tablets. How many tablets will you give?
   a. 2   b. 3   c. 4   d. 5

4. Ordered: AZT (zidovudine) 0.2 g q4h po for symptomatic HIV infection. Label: 100 mg tablets. How many tablets will you give?
   a. 0.5   b. 1   c. 1.5   d. 2

5. Ordered: Lanoxin 0.25 mg daily po for a patient with CHF. Label: 0.125 mg tablets. How many tablets will you give?
   a. 0.5   b. 1   c. 1.5   d. 2

6. Ordered: Furadantin 250 mg qid po with food for a patient with a urinary tract infection. Label: 0.5 g scored tablets. How many tablets will you give?
   a. $\frac{1}{4}$ b. $\frac{1}{2}$ c. 1   d. 2

7. Ordered: Halcion (triazolam) 0.25 mg HS for sedation. Label: 0.125 mg scored tablets. How many tablets will you give?

   a. $\frac{1}{2}$ b. 1   c. 2   d. 3

8. Ordered: Azulfidine (sulfasalazine) 1g q8h po with food for a patient with rheumatoid arthritis. Label: 500 mg per tablet. How many tablets will you give?

   a. 1   b. 2   c. 3   d. 4

9. Ordered: Cipro (ciprofloxacin HCl) 0.75 g q12h for eight weeks for a patient with a severe joint infection. Label: 250 mg tablets. How many tablets will you give?

   a. 1   b. 2   c. 3   d. 4

10. Ordered: Verelan 0.12 g cap for a patient with hypertension. Label: 120 mg per S-R capsule. How many capsules will you give?

    a. 1   b. 2   c. 3   d. 4

Critical Thinking Exercises

Analyze and discuss the following scenarios with a classmate.*

1. Mr. R. is an alert, anxious-appearing, frail gentleman, 76 years old, weighing 65 kilograms. He was admitted two days before with complaints of chest pain. His medication orders included Lanoxin 0.125 mg daily every morning. This was the only medication ordered for the morning. On hand was digoxin 0.25 mg/tablet (scored).

   After you provided care for him on the evening shift, he mentioned that his doctor must have changed his orders because for two days he had been taking only a half of a tablet in the morning, and yesterday and today, his new nurse had given him two tablets each day. His wife agreed. He wanted to know if this meant that his heart problem was getting worse.

Ordered:

Supplied:

Given:

Error(s):

Potential injuries:

Nursing actions:

Preventive measures: How could this have been avoided? If you were on a hospital committee that studies incidents, what sort of recommendations would you make for this specific incident, the nurse involved, and the pharmacy department, keeping in mind that you would not want to discourage the reporting of medication errors?

*Critical Thinking Exercises provide math and medication safety issues for student discussion. Answers are not provided.

2. Mrs. D is a housewife who has been admitted to the hospital for surgery for a throat tumor. She has been taking fluoxetine (Prozac) tablets for the past year for depression. The prescriber changed her prescription to Prozac oral solution 60 mg daily because of postoperative throat discomfort. The nurse administered 60 mL (2 oz) of Prozac.

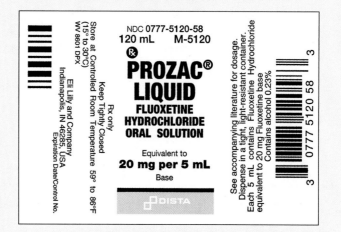

Ordered:

Supplied:

Given:

Error(s):

Potential injuries:

Nursing actions:

Preventive measures (refer to the questions in the prior exercise):

3. Mr. Z, a 70-year-old nursing home patient who has seizures, has an order for an antiseizure drug daily. The nurse notices he complains of being very tired, sleeps most of the day, and is unwilling to walk since he has been on the new medication. The doctor reduces the order from 0.5 mg po daily at bedtime to 0.1 mg. The 0.1 mg dose has not yet been delivered. The nurse reads the new order and gives two 0.5 mg tablets to the patient. (Read the adverse affects of any antiseizure medications.)

Errors:

What is the amount of the error compared to the new order? And compared to the original order?

Potential injury to the patient:

Nursing actions:

What would you recommend to the Patient Safety Committee?

Use ratio and proportion and your knowledge of conversion tables to solve these problems. Focus on whether you should use a one-step or a two-step calculation. *Estimate* and *prove* all work. Label your answers.

1. Ordered: Geodon 80 mg po bid for a patient with bipolar disorder. How many capsules will you give?

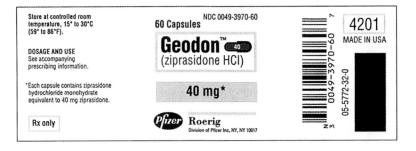

2. Ordered: Klonopin 1 mg tid po for a patient with panic disorder. How many tablets will you give?

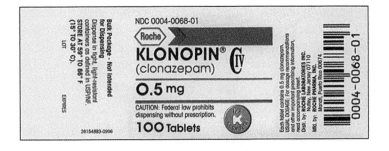

3. Ordered: Cipro 0.75 g po tab q12h for 10 days for a patient with an infection. How many tablets will you give?

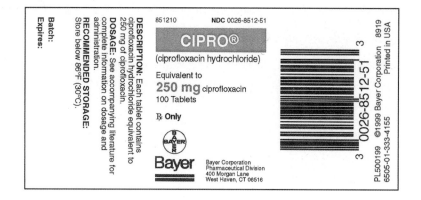

4. Ordered: Zyloprim 0.2 g po daily in AM for a patient with gout. How many tablets will you give?

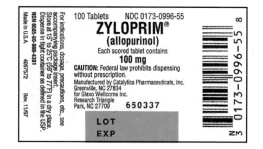

5. Ordered: Cytotec 0.1 mg po four times daily with meals and at bedtime for a patient with a history of gastric ulcers. How many tablets will you give?

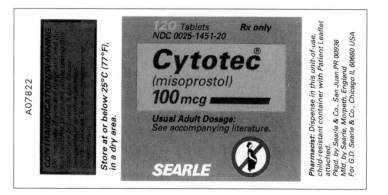

6. Ordered: fluoxetine oral solution 50 mg po daily in AM for a patient with obsessive-compulsive disorder (OCD) and anxiety. How many mL will you give?

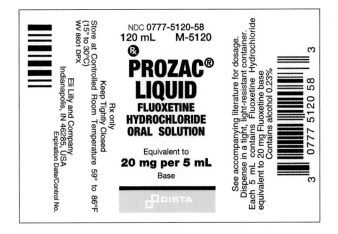

7. Ordered: zidovudine syrup 200 mg po bid for a patient who is HIV positive. How many mL will you prepare to the nearest tenth of a milliliter?

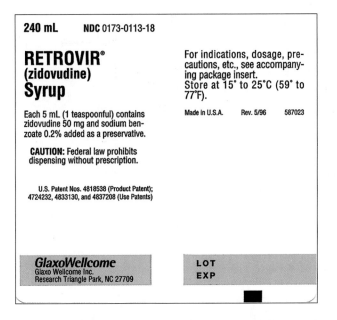

Note: 5 mL = 1 calibrated medication teaspoon (not a household teaspoon).

8. Ordered: isoniazid 0.3 g daily po as preventive therapy for a patient at high risk for tuberculosis. How many tablets will you give?

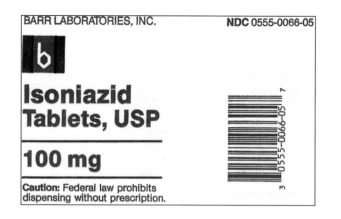

9. Ordered: cimetidine 0.8 g bid po for a patient with an ulcer. How many tablets will you give?

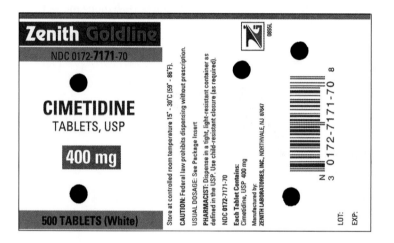

10. Ordered: minoxidil 0.04 g once a day for hypertension. How many tablets will you give?

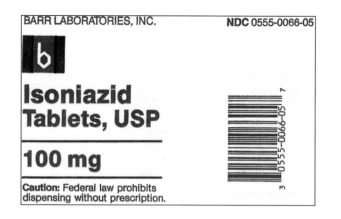

evolve **Refer to the Drug Measures section of Drug Calculations Companion, verison 4 on Evolve, for additional information.**

Injectable Medication Calculations

Objectives

- Read and indicate measurable doses on syringes.
- Calculate injectable doses.
- Calculate and combine doses for two medications to be mixed in one syringe.
- Identify safety hazards of injectable medications.

Introduction

Medications may be ordered to be given by a parenteral route—a route outside of the gastrointestinal tract. This chapter covers injectable medications that may be ordered for the intradermal, subcutaneous, or intramuscular route. Related safety issues are discussed. The dose calculations for mL using the ratio and proportion method have already been covered in Chapter 4 and will be used also in this chapter.

Measuring and Reading Amounts in a Syringe

The best way to learn to read the measurements on a syringe is to examine some unfilled syringes while you read this (Figure 5-1). Then examine some filled syringes, and verify the amounts with your instructor or lab partner.

Steps for Measuring and Reading Amounts in a Syringe

1. Examine the *total amount* the syringe contains first. The 3 mL hypodermic syringe is most commonly used for intramuscular injections and also for subcutaneous injections. The 1 mL tuberculin syringe is used mainly for skin tests.
2. Locate the 1 mL markings on each syringe.
3. Examine the calibrations in 1 mL, 0.2 mL, 0.1 mL, or 0.01 mL, depending on the size of the syringe. The larger the syringe, the larger the calibration.

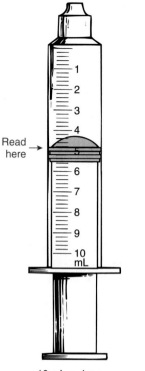

Read here →

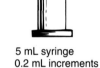

→

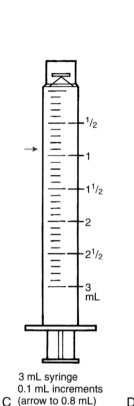

→

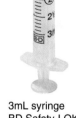

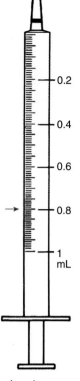

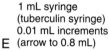
→

A 10 mL syringe
0.2 mL increments
(arrow to 4.8 mL)

B 5 mL syringe
0.2 mL increments
(arrow to 0.8 mL)

C 3 mL syringe
0.1 mL increments
(arrow to 0.8 mL)

D 3mL syringe
BD Safety-LOK
syringe

E 1 mL syringe
(tuberculin syringe)
0.01 mL increments
(arrow to 0.8 mL)

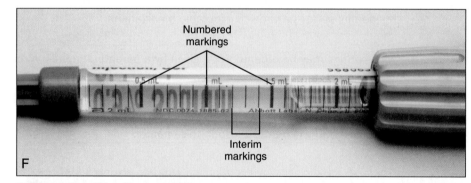

Prefilled syringe with calibration markings.

FIGURE 5-1 Comparison of syringe sizes and calibrations. Note the red arrows where the dose is measured. There are two black rings on the plunger and a rounded or pointed tip. Ignore the rounded/pointed tip and read the uppermost ring, as shown in **A.** The rings are not shown in **C** and **E** so the dose and calibrations can be better visualized. **E,** 1 mL tuberculin syringe. **F,** Prefilled syringe with calibration markings. (**D,** From Becton, Dickinson, and Company, Franklin Lakes, NJ. **F,** From Macklin D, Chernecky C, Infortuna H: Math for clinical practice, ed 2, St Louis, 2011, Mosby.)

WORKSHEET 5A | Reading Syringe Measurements

Examine the following syringes. Note the total capacity and the 1 mL markings. Indicate the filled-in dose measurements in the space provided.

1. Total capacity: _____ mL   Smallest measurable dose:_____ mL
   Indicated dose: _____

2. Total capacity: _____ mL   Smallest measurable dose:_____ mL
   Indicated dose: _____

3. Total capacity: _____ mL   Smallest measurable dose:_____ mL
   Indicated dose: _____

4. Total capacity: _____ mL   Smallest measurable dose:_____ mL
   Indicated dose: _____

5. Total capacity: _____ mL   Smallest measurable dose:_____ mL
   Indicated dose: _____

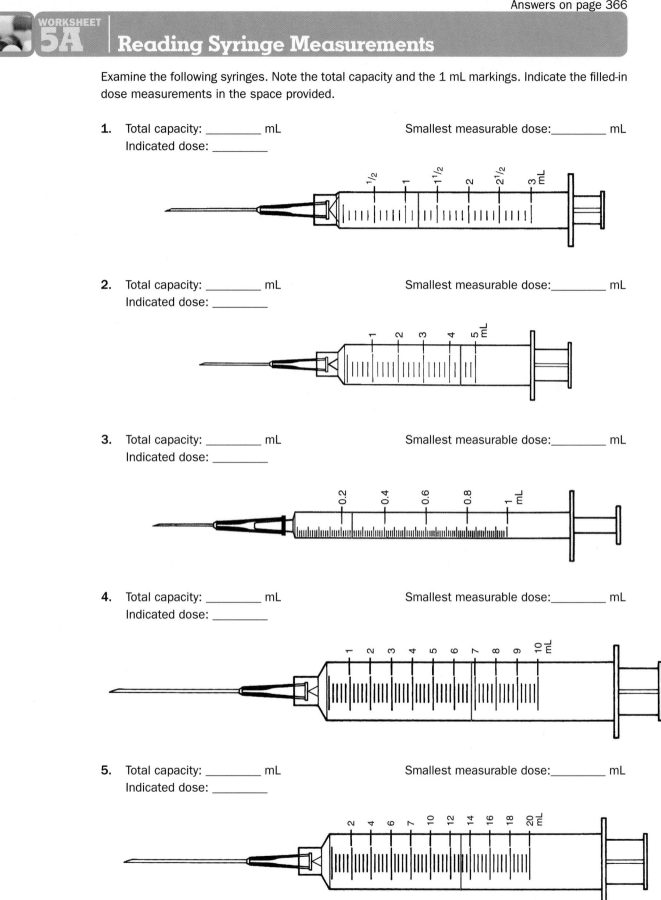

Answers on page 367

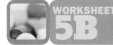

WORKSHEET 5B | Syringe Volume Practice

Examine the following syringes. Note the total capacity and the 1 mL and 0.5 mL markings. Fill in the blanks and shade the syringe to the volume requested. If possible, practice with real syringes.

1. Total capacity: _____ mL. Calibrated in tenths or hundredths of a milliliter? (Circle one)
   Indicate 1.6 mL.

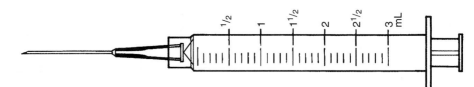

2. Total capacity: _____ mL. Calibrated in 0.1, 0.2, or 0.01 mL increments? (Circle one)
   Indicate 4.6 mL.

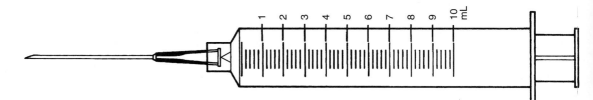

3. Total capacity: _____ mL. Calibrated in 0.1, 0.2, or 0.01 mL increments? (Circle one)
   Indicate 3.4 mL.

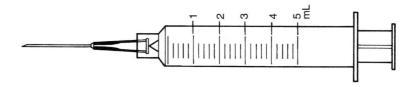

4. Total capacity: _____ mL. Calibrated in tenths or hundredths of a milliliter? (Circle one)
   Indicate 2.5 mL.

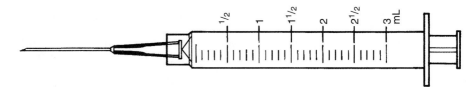

5. Total capacity: _____ mL. Calibrated in tenths or hundredths of a milliliter? (Circle one)
   Indicate 0.75 mL.

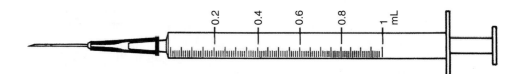

Parenteral Routes

Injectable medications routes known as parenteral (outside the gastrointestinal [GI] tract) include the routes mentioned below as well as intravenous route, which is taught in a later chapter. All equipment and sites are based upon patient size and condition, the type of medication, and the route. Refer to clinical skills manuals for injection techniques.

Many injectables are provided in ampules and vials and prefilled syringes (Figure 5-2 and 5-3).

Intradermal (ID) Injections

These are small-volume injections usually administered as skin tests. The usual dose for a skin test administered with a 1-mL syringe and a 25- to 30- gauge needle is 0.1 mL (Figure 5-4).

Subcutaneous (subcut) Injections

Nonirritating substances up to 1 mL may be injected into subcutaneous fatty tissue sites usually with a 25 to 30 gauge needle. Insulin and anticoagulants are examples of medications that may be delivered by this route. The most common sites for subcutaneous injections are noted in Figure 5-5.

Intramuscular (IM) Injections

Intramuscular (IM) injections are selected to deliver medications for faster absorption. They tolerate more concentrated substances than subcutaneous sites. Doses up to 3 mL may be injected into a single site depending on the patient's skin integrity and muscle size. The most common sites are noted in Figure 5-6. A two inch zone around the umbilicus is to be avoided when giving abdominal subcutaneous injections (Figure 5-5).

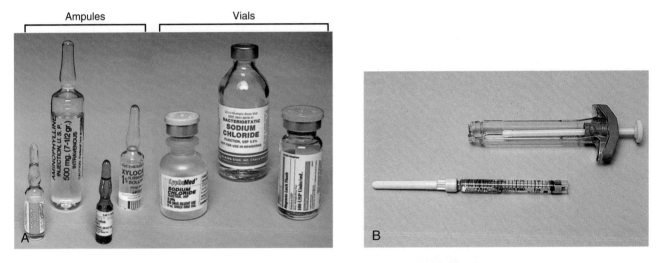

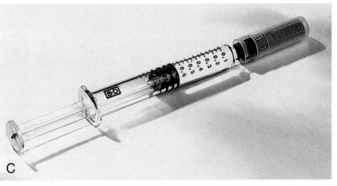

FIGURE 5-2 **A,** Assorted ampules and vials. **B,** Carpuject syringe and prefilled sterile cartridge with needle. **C,** BD-Hypak prefilled syringe. (**A** and **B,** From Perry AG, Potter PA: Clinical nursing skills and techniques, ed 7, St Louis, 2010, Mosby. **C,** From Becton, Dickinson, and Company, Franklin Lakes, NJ.)

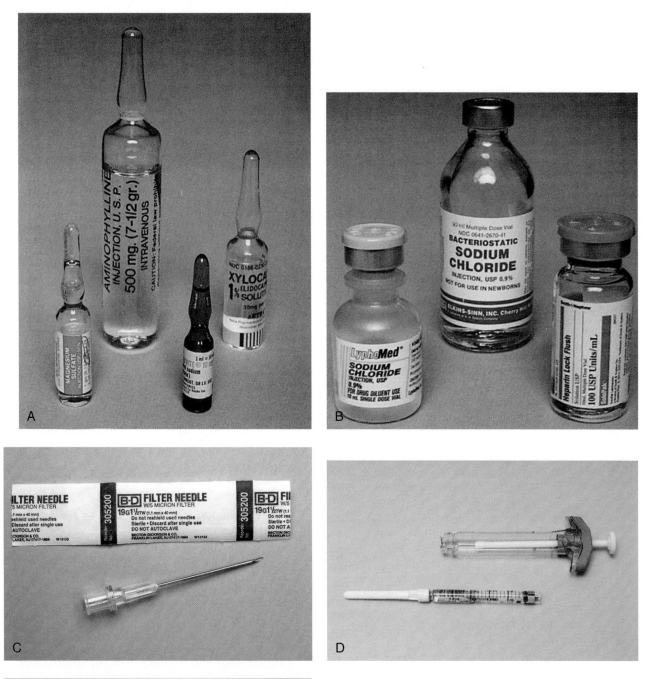

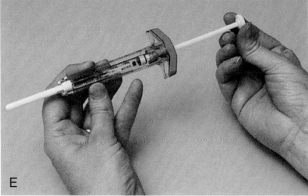

FIGURE 5-3 **A,** Injectable liquid supplied in ampules. **B,** Injectable liquid supplied in vials. **C,** Filter Needle (Bectone Dickinson). **D, E** Carpuject syringe and prefilled sterile cartridge with needle. A, B, D, and E (From Perry AG, Potter PA: Clinical nursing skills and techniques, ed 7, St Louis, 2010, Mosby. C, In Lilley LL, Collins SR, Harrington S, Snyder JS: Pharmacology and the nursing process, ed 6, 2011, Mosby. From Rick Brady, Riva, MD.)

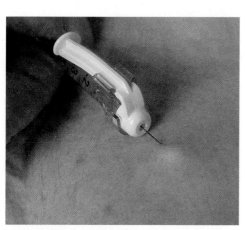

FIGURE 5-4 During intradermal injection, note formation of small bleb on the skin's surface. (From Perry AG, Potter PA: Clinical nursing skills and techniques, ed 7, St Louis, 2010, Mosby.)

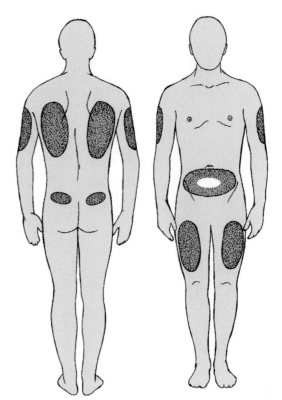

FIGURE 5-5 Sites recommended for subcutaneous injections. (From Perry AG, Potter PA: Clinical nursing skills and techniques, ed 7, St Louis, 2010, Mosby.)

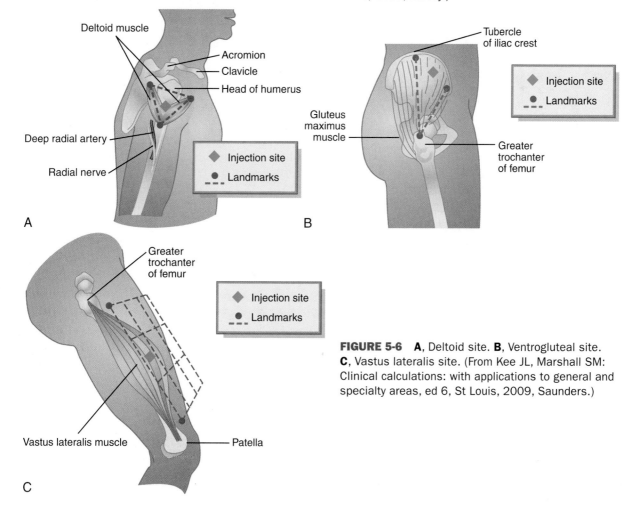

A

Deltoid muscle

Acromion
Clavicle
Head of humerus

Deep radial artery
Radial nerve

◆ Injection site
•--- Landmarks

B

Tubercle of iliac crest

◆ Injection site
•--- Landmarks

Gluteus maximus muscle

Greater trochanter of femur

C

Greater trochanter of femur

◆ Injection site
•--- Landmarks

Vastus lateralis muscle

Patella

FIGURE 5-6 **A,** Deltoid site. **B,** Ventrogluteal site. **C,** Vastus lateralis site. (From Kee JL, Marshall SM: Clinical calculations: with applications to general and specialty areas, ed 6, St Louis, 2009, Saunders.)

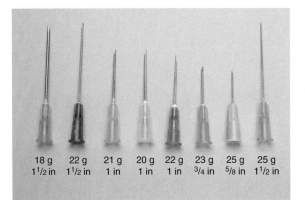

FIGURE 5-7 Needles of various gauges and lengths. (In Lilley LL, Collins SR, Harrington S, Snyder JS: Pharmacology and the nursing process, ed 6, 2011, Mosby. From Rick Brady, Riva, MD.)

| 18 g | 22 g | 21 g | 20 g | 22 g | 23 g | 25 g | 25 g |
| 1½ in | 1½ in | 1 in | 1 in | 1 in | ¾ in | ⅝ in | 1½ in |

> ⊖ **CLINICAL ALERT**
>
> The dorsogluteal area is not recommended for child or adult injections because of potential nerve and vessel damage.

Needle Sizes

Needle sizes refer to length and gauge. They are selected based on the type of medication and size and condition of the patient, as well as area to be injected (Figure 5-7). The larger the gauge, the smaller the diameter of the needle; for example, a 25-gauge needle is "finer" and has a smaller diameter than an 18-gauge needle.

Approximate needle lengths for routes are as follows:

- Intradermal: ⅜ to ½ inch
- Subcutaneous: ⅜ to ⅝ inch
- Intramuscular: ⅝ to 2 inches

Safety Issues

The trend is to use safety syringes to prevent needlestick injuries (Figure 5-8).

> ⊖ **CLINICAL ALERT**
>
> All contaminated syringes and needles must be disposed of promptly in a hazardous waste container. Check agency policies for safe disposal (Figure 5-9).

> ⊖ **CLINICAL ALERT**
>
> Hepatitis B and C and HIV (AIDS) are examples of diseases that can be contracted from a contaminated needle stick. Never attempt to recap a used needle.

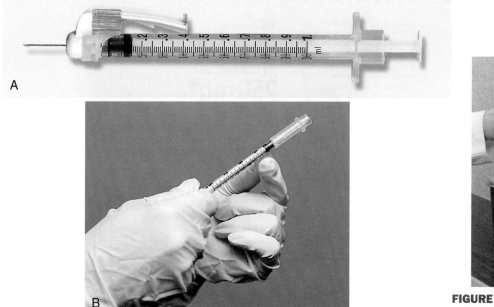

A

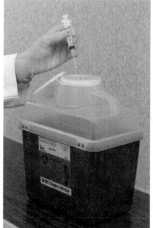

FIGURE 5-9 Sharps container. (In Lilley LL, Collins SR, Harrington S, Snyder JS: Pharmacology and the nursing process, ed 6, 2011, Mosby. From Rick Brady, Riva, MD.)

FIGURE 5-8 **A**, BD SafetyGlide™ tuberculin syringe. **B**, syringe with plastic needle guard. (**A**, From Becton, Dickinson, and Company, Franklin Lakes, NJ. **B**, From Perry AG, Potter PA: Clinical nursing skills and techniques, ed 7, St Louis, 2010, Mosby.)

Answers on page 368

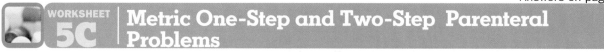

WORKSHEET 5C | **Metric One-Step and Two-Step Parenteral Problems**

Examine the orders and labels below. Is the problem *one-step* or *two-step?* Before you perform the *final calculation*, estimate whether you will give *more* or *less* of what you have on hand. Calculate the dose (to the nearest tenth of a milliliter if applicable). Prove your answers.

1. Ordered: Cleocin phosphate 0.2 g IM stat. (One-step or two-step?)

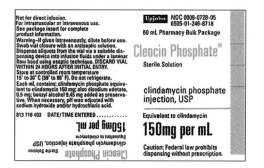

2. Ordered: lorezepam 3 mg IM stat.

   Available: lorezepam 4 mg per mL. (One step or two step?)

3. Ordered: Solu-Cortef 0.2 g IM daily in AM for 3 days. (One-step or two-step?)

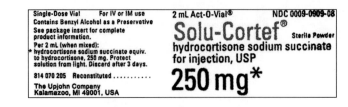

4. Ordered: Solu-Medrol 75 mg IM stat. (One-step or two-step?)

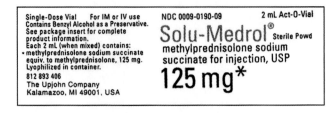

5. Ordered: cyanocobalamin 500 mg IM once a week.

Available: Cyanocobalamin 1000 mcg per mL (One-step or two-step?)

6. Ordered: heparin sodium 4000 units subcut stat.

Available: heparin sodium 5000 units per mL (One-step or two-step?)

7. Ordered: Lincocin 250 mg IM daily. (One-step or two-step?)

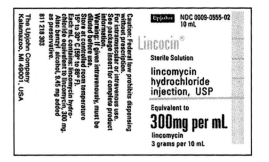

8. Ordered: Depo-Provera 0.3 g IM stat. (One-step or two-step?)

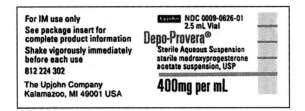

9. Ordered: Penicillin G 400,000 units IM stat.

Available: Penicillin G 500,000 units per 2.5 mL. (One-step or two-step?)

10. Ordered: Magnesium Chloride 50% sol, 1 g (8 mEq) IM stat.

Available: Magnesium Chloride 50% injection single dose vial: 2.5 g per 5 mL (1 mEq per mL) (One-step or two-step?)

WORKSHEET 5D | Metric Parenteral Mixes

Combinations of the following narcotics and antiemetics, antihistamines, or anticholinergics are commonly ordered.

Calculate the amount to be given in milliliters *to the nearest tenth* for each of the two drugs ordered using the labels provided. Then *add* the results to find the total volume to be combined and administered in one syringe.* Estimate your answer. Round to the nearest tenth of a milliliter. Prove all work. Does your estimate match your answer? Shade in the total combined amount on the 3 mL syringe illustration.

1. Ordered: Dilaudid 2 mg
   Prochlorperazine 2.5 mg } IM stat for pain and nausea

   a. How many mg/mL of hydromorphone are available? (label)
   b. How many milliliters of hydromorphone will you prepare?
   c. How many mL of Compazine will you prepare?
   d. Total volume in syringe? (Shade in syringe below.)

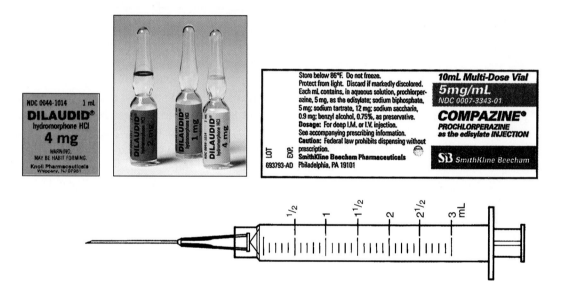

🕑 CLINICAL ALERT

Always consult a current, reliable compatibility reference before mixing parenteral medications. Consult a pharmacist if a reference is unavailable.

*Orders for mixes are usually bracketed in the medication administration record (MAR).

🕑 CLINICAL ALERT

To prepare the correct total volume, it is safer to prepare and verify the total for *each* medication in a seperate syringe and then combine the two in one syringe.

CHAPTER 5 Injectable Medication Calculations

2. Ordered: Morphine 6 mg

Promethazine HCl 25 mg $\Big\}$ IM q4h prn for pain

    a. How many mg/mL of morphine are available? (label)

    b. How many milliliters of morphine will you prepare?

    c. How many mg/mL of promethazine are available? (label)

    d. How many milliliters of promethazine will you prepare?

    e. Total volume in syringe (to nearest tenth)? (Shade in syringe below.)

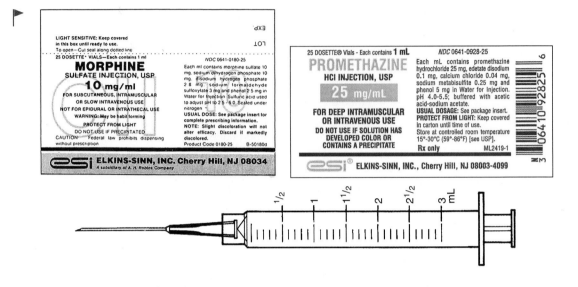

Controlled (scheduled) drugs such as narcotics, opiates and some non-narcotic drugs such as tranquilizers and anti-anxiety agents, have special locked storage, dispensing, disposal and documentation requirements because of potential risk for abuse. They are placed in **Schedules** by the Federal Drug Administation (DEA). Schedule C-1 (Control 1) refers to the highest risk for abuse drugs such as crack cocaine, heroin, etc., Schedules CII through CV drugs which are prescribed for medical purposes, are labeled as such with CV having least potential for abuse. Note the CII classification for Morphine on the label below. Check your agency storage, disposal, and documentation policies for these medications.

3. Ordered: Duramorph 4 mg
   Atropine sulfate 0.6 mg } IM preoperatively on call from OR
   a. How many mg/mL of doramorph are available? (label)
   b. How many milliliters of doramorph will you prepare?
   c. How many mg/mL of atropine are available? (label)
   d. How many milliliters of atropine will you prepare?
   e. Total volume in syringe? (Shade in syringe.)

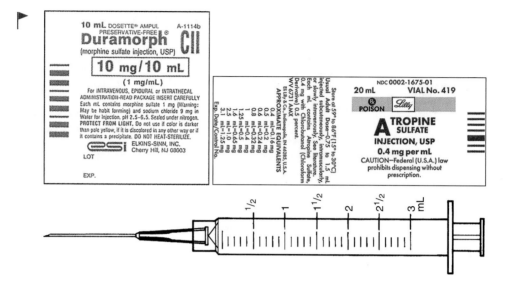

4. Ordered: Morphine 10 mg
   Vistaril 35 mg } IM q4-6h prn for pain
   a. How many milliliters of morphine will you prepare?
   b. How many milliliters of hydroxyzine will you prepare?
   c. Total volume in syringe? (Shade in syringe below.)

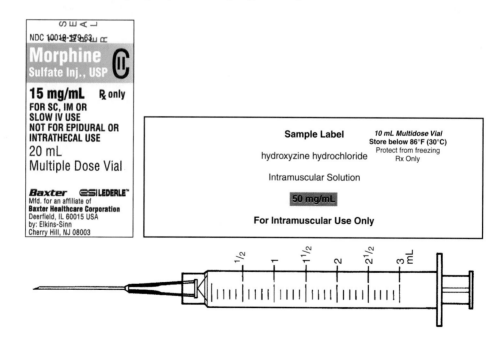

Beginning practitioners who prepare a mix using only one syringe risk making dose and vial contamination errors.

5. Ordered: Morphine sulfate 8 mg } IM stat postoperatively for pain and nausea.
Hydroxyzine 25 mg

    a. How many milliliters of morphine will you prepare?

    b. How many milliliters of hydroxyzine will you prepare?

    c. Total volume in syringe? (Shade in syringe below.)

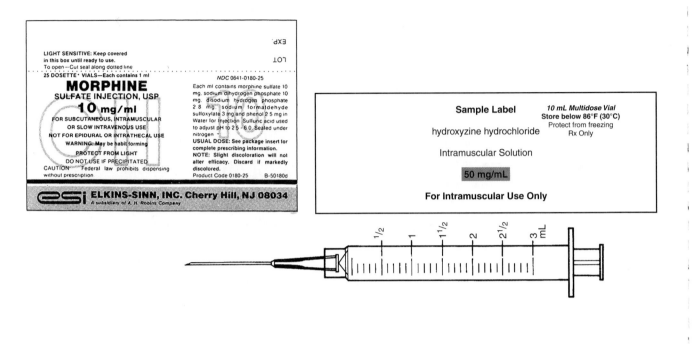

Answers on page 371

WORKSHEET 5E | Multiple-Choice Practice

Solve the following problems and circle the correct answer. For amounts less than 1 mL, calculate to the *nearest hundredth*. For amounts equal to or more than 1 mL, calculate the *nearest tenth*. Use scrap paper, set up your ratio and proportion neatly, and prove your work. Remember to focus on whether it's a one-step or two-step problem and estimate your answer. If your solution does not seem right, recalculate the problem without looking at your original work.

1. Ordered: Stadol 1.8 mg IM stat postoperatively. Label: 2 mg/mL. How many milliliters will you give, to the nearest tenth of a mL?

    a. 0.5 mL   **b.** 0.6 mL   **c.** 0.7 mL   **d.** 0.9 mL

2. Ordered: Compazine (prochlorperazine maleate) 25 mg q4h IM prn for nausea. Label: 10 mg/mL. How many milliliters will you give?

    a. 1.5 mL   **b.** 2.5 mL   **c.** 3 mL   **d.** 3.5 mL

3. Ordered: Potassium chloride elixir 20 mEq bid po for a patient with potassium deficiency. Label: 8 mEq/5 mL. How many milliliters will you give?

    a. 12.5 mL   **b.** 15 mL   **c.** 32 mL   **d.** 40 mL

4. Ordered: Atropine 0.4 mg IM stat. Label: 0.3 mg/0.5 mL. How many milliliters will you give?

    a. 1.2 mL   **b.** 0.7 mL   **c.** 0.66 mL   **d.** 0.67 mL

5. Ordered: Vitamin B$_{12}$ 1000 mcg deep IM once a month for a patient who has had a gastrectomy. Label: 0.5 mg/mL. How many milliliters will you give?

   a. 1 mL   **b.** 1.5 mL   **c.** 2 mL   **d.** 2.5 mL

6. Ordered: Benztropine mesylate (Cogentin) 0.5 mg, IM initial dose for a frail patient with tremors. Label: 2 mg per 2 mL. How many mL will you give?

   a. 0.5 mL   **b.** 1 mL   **c.** 1.5 mL   **d.** 5 mL

7. Ordered: Dexamethasone 0.05 g IM stat for a patient with an allergic reaction. Label: 24 mg per mL. How many mL will you give?

   a. 0.5 mL   **b.** 0.8 mL   **c.** 2.1 mL   **d.** 2.8 mL

8. Ordered: Digoxin 0.1 mg IM daily for a patient with heart failure. Label: 50 mcg per mL. How many mL will you give?

   a. 0.5 mL   **b.** 1 mL   **c.** 1.5 mL   **d.** 2 mL

9. Ordered: Morphine 4 mg IV for a patient with severe pain. Label: Morphine sulfate 5 mg per mL. How many mL will you give?

   a. 0.6 mL   **b.** 0.8 mL   **c.** 1.2 mL   **d.** 1.5 mL

10. Ordered: Flu vaccine 0.5 mL, the standard dose for an adult. Available: A multidose vial with 10 doses of the standard dose. How many mL are in the vial?

   a. 1 mL   **b.** 5 mL   **c.** 10 mL   **d.** 50 mL

Critical Thinking Exercises

1. Ordered: Promethazine 25 mg IM stat for a patient who has nausea.

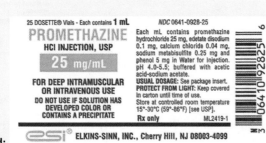

On hand:

Given: Promethazine 25 mg IM using a 1-inch needle in a patient weighing 109.1 kg (240 lb).

Error:

Potential problem for patient:

Recommendations for the Patient Safety Committee for this nurse:

2. Ordered: Robinul 0.2 mg IM stat preop for an operative patient to reduce secretions during surgery.

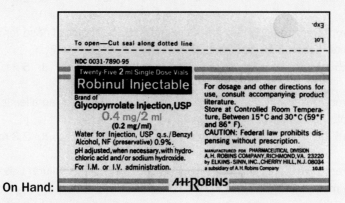

On Hand:

Given: Robinul 2 mL

Error:

Potential injury to patient:

Recommendations for the Patient Safety Committee for this nurse:

3. Ordered: Cyanobalabin (Vitamin Plus B-12) 0.5 mg IM for a patient with vitamin B-12 deficiency.

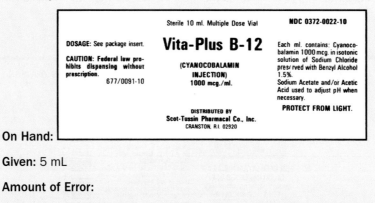

On Hand:

Given: 5 mL

Amount of Error:

Recommendations for the Patient Safety Committee for this nurse:

CHAPTER 5

Final

1. Ordered: codeine 10 mg IM stat for a patient experiencing pain. How many mL will you give? Indicate the nearest measurable dose on the syringe shown.

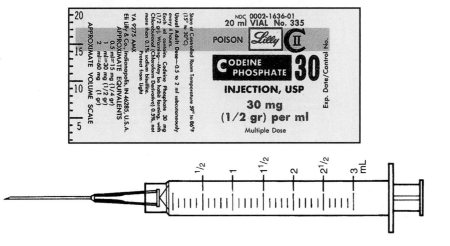

2. Ordered: Amikin 0.3 g IM q12h for a patient with an infection. How many mL will you give? Indicate the nearest measurable dose on the syringe shown.

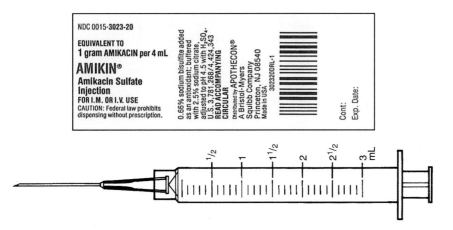

3. Ordered: Ativan 2 mg IM for a patient with agitation. How many mL will you give? Indicate the nearest measurable dose on the syringe shown.

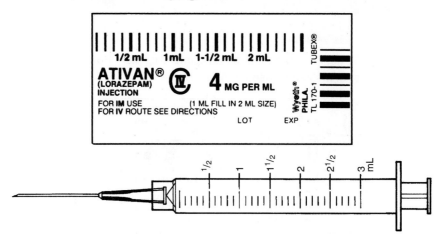

4. Ordered: morphine sulfate 7 mg and atropine sulfate 0.3 mg IM preoperatively.
   a. How many milliliters (to the nearest tenth) each will you prepare of morphine and atropine?
   b. What is the combined dose in mL?

   Indicate the dose on the syringe provided.

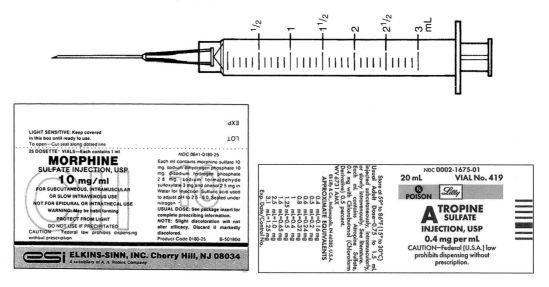

5. Ordered: Lanoxin (digoxin) 125 mcg IM daily.
   a. Safe Dose Range (SDR) is 0.125 to 0.5 mg daily for adults. Is the order safe?
   b. How many milliliters will you give?

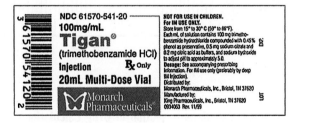

LANOXIN® 2mL
(digoxin) Injection
500 µg (0.5 mg) in 2 mL
(250 µg [0.25 mg] per mL)
Store at 15° to 25°C (59° to 77°F).
PROTECT FROM LIGHT.
Glaxo Wellcome Inc.
Research Triangle Park, NC 27709
Rev. 1/96

542308

LOT
EXP

6. Ordered: Tigan 0.25 g IM q6h prn for nausea.
   a. Estimate: Will you give more or less than the unit dose?
   b. How many mL will you prepare?

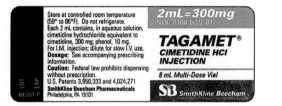

NDC 61570-541-20
100mg/mL
Tigan®
(trimethobenzamide HCl)
Injection   R℞ Only
20mL Multi-Dose Vial
Monarch
Pharmaceuticals®

NOT FOR USE IN CHILDREN.
For IM USE ONLY.
Store from 15° to 30° C (59° to 86°F).
Each mL of solution contains 100 mg trimetho-
benzamide hydrochloride compounded with 0.45%
phenol as preservative, 0.5 mg sodium citrate and
0.2 mg citric acid as buffers, and sodium hydroxide
to adjust pH to approximately 5.0.
Dosage: See accompanying prescribing
information. For IM use only (preferably by deep
IM injection).
Distributed by:
Monarch Pharmaceuticals, Inc., Bristol, TN 37620
Manufactured by:
King Pharmaceuticals, Inc., Bristol, TN 37620
0934063 Rev. 11/99

7. Ordered: Tagamet injection 0.45 g IM for a patient with an ulcer.
   a. What is the unit dose shown on the label?
   b. Will you give more or less than the unit dose?
   c. How many mL will you prepare?

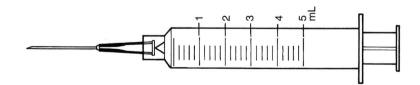

Store at controlled room temperature
(59° to 86°F). Do not refrigerate.
Each 2 mL contains, in aqueous solution,
cimetidine hydrochloride equivalent to
cimetidine, 300 mg; phenol, 10 mg.
For I.M. injection; dilute for slow I.V. use.
Dosage: See accompanying prescribing
information.
Caution: Federal law prohibits dispensing
without prescription.
U.S. Patents 3,950,333 and 4,024,271
SmithKline Beecham Pharmaceuticals
Philadelphia, PA 19101
693957-P

2mL=300mg
NDC 0108 5022 01
TAGAMET®
CIMETIDINE HCl
INJECTION
8 mL Multi-Dose Vial
SB SmithKline Beecham

Indicate the dose on the syringe provided.

8. Read the dose: _____ mL

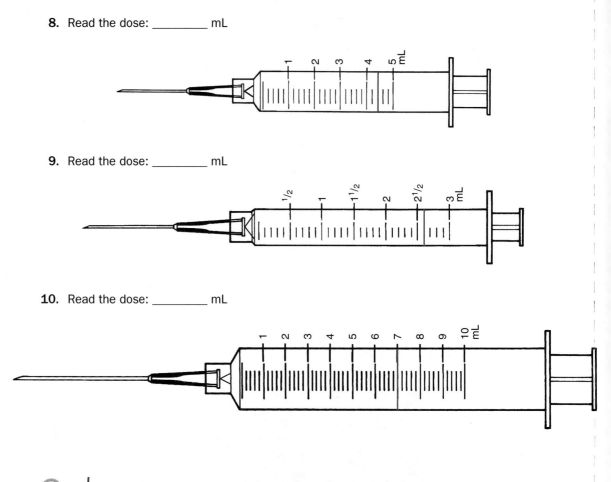

9. Read the dose: _____ mL

10. Read the dose: _____ mL

evolve Refer to the Basic Calculations section of Drug Calculations Companion, version 4 on Evolve for additional practice problems.

Medications from Powders and Crystals: Oral and Intramuscular

6

Objectives
- Read reconstitution labels to determine specific diluents, diluent amounts, specific doses, conditions for storage, and expiration dates.
- State the importance of initialing and writing the date and time of reconstitution on the medication vial or bottle.
- Determine the best dilution strength to use for multiple-dosage strength vials.
- Calculate doses in milligrams, grams, and milliliters for oral and parenteral routes.
- Reconstitute and measure liquid medications.
- Reconstitute medications from powders and crystals.

Introduction
Preparation of reconstituted medications, mostly antibiotics, from powders and crystals is usually the nurse's responsibility. The medications are reconstituted by adding a diluent (liquid) recommended by the manufacturer as the vehicle for administration. The shelf life of reconstituted medications is usually short; therefore, careful consideration must be given to how they are stored, the date and time of reconstitution (initialed by the nurse), the expiration date, and the route of administration. This chapter teaches the steps for safely preparing medications from powders and crystals. The measurement of units will be spelled out in the physician's orders and is used in the problem setups.

Measuring Liquid Medications

When measuring a liquid medication, hold the transparent measuring device at eye level. The curved surface of the liquid is called *the meniscus* (Figure 6-1). All liquid medication is measured at the meniscus level.

Medications can be measured in a medicine cup and transferred to an oral syringe for ease in administration and accuracy (Figure 6-2).

However, liquid medications can be measured more accurately in a syringe than in a medicine cup (Figure 6-3).

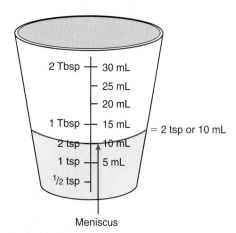

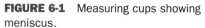

2 Tbsp — 30 mL

— 25 mL

— 20 mL

1 Tbsp — 15 mL = 2 tsp or 10 mL

2 tsp — 10 mL

1 tsp — 5 mL

½ tsp —

Meniscus

FIGURE 6-1 Measuring cups showing meniscus.

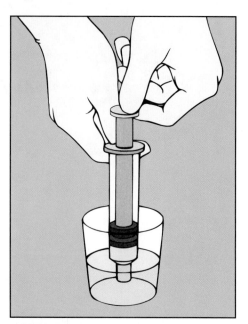

FIGURE 6-2 Filling a syringe directly from medicine cup. (From Clayton BD, Stock YN, Cooper S: Basic pharmacology for nurses, ed 15, St Louis, 2010, Mosby.)

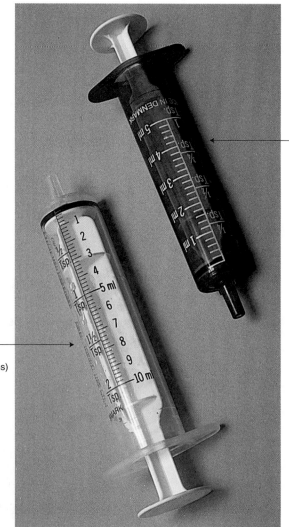

5 mL calibrated in 0.2 mL (two tenths)

10 mL calibrated in 0.2 mL (tenths)

FIGURE 6-3 Oral syringes. Oral syringes are not sterile and are used only for oral medications. (From Clayton BD, Stock YN, Cooper S: Basic pharmacology for nurses, ed 15, St Louis, 2010, Mosby. Courtesy of Chuck Dresner.)

Reconstitution: Medication Labels

Labels for medications that require reconstitution contain information about the amount of diluent to use and the resulting concentration. The important information is as follows:

- Strength-reconstitution directions
- Usual dose
- Route
- Name—generic and proprietary
- Expiration date
- Storage conditions/shelf life

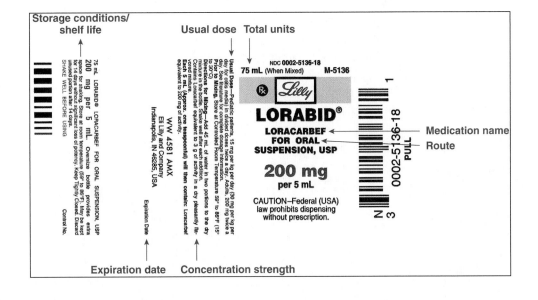

CLINICAL ALERT

If the vial is a multiple-dose vial, the nurse must note on the label the date, time, amount of diluent used, and his or her initials.

Many solutions are unstable after being reconstituted. Read labels carefully for directions on storing the solution in the refrigerator or in a dark place. There is usually a time limit or expiration date on the vial. It is important to date, label, and initial all reconstituted medications.

Answers on page 374

WORKSHEET 6A | **Practice in Reconstituting, Administering, and Measuring Liquid Medications**

Show your calculations and proofs in the following problems. Shade in the correct dose on the medicine cup.

1. Ordered: Lorabid 150 mg po bid.

   Follow mixing directions on the label.
   a. How many total milliliters of water are needed?
   b. How many total milligrams of Lorabid are in the bottle?
   c. How many milliliters will provide 150 mg of Lorabid? Draw the amount you will give on the medicine cup.
   d. How many doses are in the bottle?

2. Ordered: Dynapen (Dicloxacillin sodium) 150 mg po stat, then 62.5 mg every 6 hours.
   a. How many milliliters of water will you add?
   b. How many milliliters will you administer?
   c. How many doses are remaining after administering the stat dose?

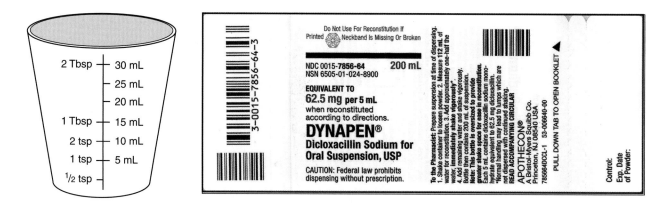

3. Ordered: 500 mg of Vancocin suspension b.i.d. po.
   a. How many milligrams are in the bottle?
   b. How many milliliters will you administer? Draw the amount you will give on the medicine cup.

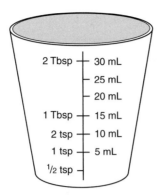

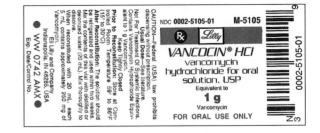

4. Ordered: Augmentin suspension 200 mg po q8h.
   a. How many milliliters of water will you add?
   b. How many total milliliters are in the bottle?
   c. How many milliliters of Augmentin will you administer? Draw the amount you will give on the medicine cup.

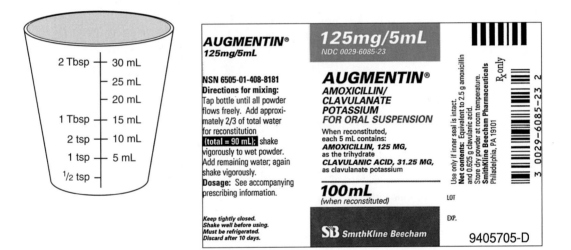

5. Ordered: Lorabid 400 mg po q12h × 14 days 1 hour ac for pneumonia.

   Follow mixing directions on the label.
   a. How many total milliliters of water are needed?
   b. How many total milligrams of Lorabid are in the bottle?
   c. How many milliliters will provide 400 mg? Draw the amount you will give on the medicine cup.
   d. How many doses are in the bottle?

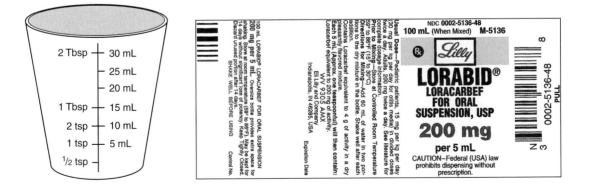

6. Ordered: 40 mg Pepcid po four times a day.
   a. How many milliliters of diluents will you add?
   b. How many total milliliters of Pepcid are in the bottle?
   c. How many milliliters will you administer?
   d. How many doses are in the bottle?

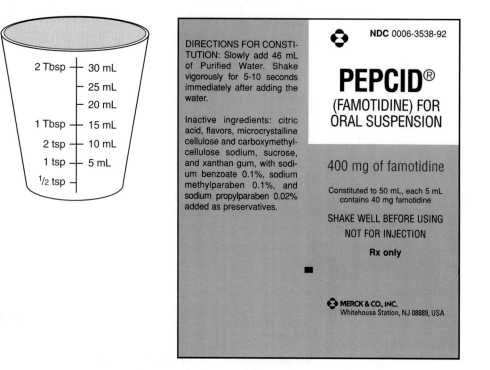

DIRECTIONS FOR CONSTITUTION: Slowly add 46 mL of Purified Water. Shake vigorously for 5-10 seconds immediately after adding the water.

Inactive ingredients: citric acid, flavors, microcrystalline cellulose and carboxymethyl-cellulose sodium, sucrose, and xanthan gum, with sodium benzoate 0.1%, sodium methylparaben 0.1%, and sodium propylparaben 0.02% added as preservatives.

NDC 0006-3538-92

PEPCID®
(FAMOTIDINE) FOR ORAL SUSPENSION

400 mg of famotidine

Constituted to 50 mL, each 5 mL contains 40 mg famotidine

SHAKE WELL BEFORE USING
NOT FOR INJECTION

Rx only

MERCK & CO., INC.
Whitehouse Station, NJ 08889, USA

7. Ordered: Vancocin HCl 300 mg po bid for colitis.

   Follow mixing directions on the label.
   a. How many milliliters of distilled water are needed?
   b. How many total milligrams of Vancocin are in the bottle?
   c. How many milliliters of Vancocin HCl will provide 300 mg? Draw the amount you will give on the medicine cup.

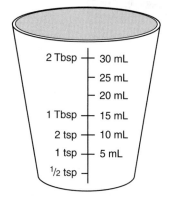

NDC 0002-5105-01   M-5105

VANCOCIN® HCl
vancomycin
hydrochloride for oral
solution, USP
Equivalent to
1 g
Vancomycin
FOR ORAL USE ONLY

8. Ordered: Amoxil (amoxicillin) 500 mg po q8h for endocarditis prophylaxis.
   a. How many milliliters of diluent will you add?
   b. How many total milligrams are in the bottle?
   c. How many milliliters will you administer per dose? Draw the amount you will give on the medicine cup.
   d. How many doses are in the bottle?

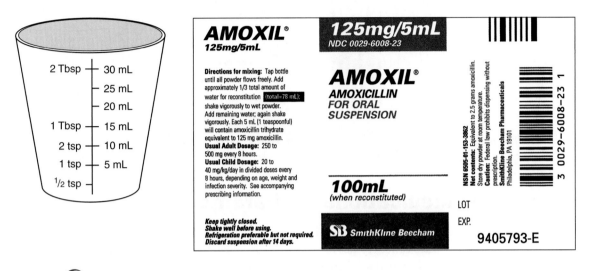

CLINICAL ALERT

For accuracy, read the medication's level at the meniscus.

9. Ordered: Fluconazole 50 mg po twice a day.
   a. How many mL of sterile water will be added to the powder?
   b. How many mL will you administer?
   c. How many 50 mg doses are in the bottle?

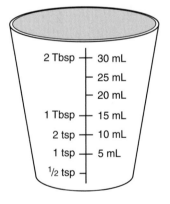

10. Ordered: 200 mg of Biaxin po two times a day.

   a. How many mL of water should be added?

   b. How many mL will you administer?

   c. How many doses are in the bottle?

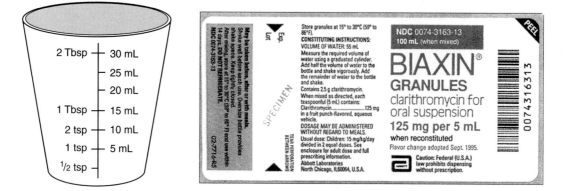

Reconstituting Medications for Parenteral Use

Reconstituting medications is much like making a cup of soup out of dried soup mix from a package or using freeze-dried coffee crystals to make a cup of coffee. The concept is the same. When a lot of liquid, or diluent, as it is referred to when mixing medications, is used, the soup or coffee becomes weaker. The less liquid or diluent used, the stronger the soup or coffee. For some medications that must be reconstituted, various amounts of diluent or liquid can be added to produce various strengths of the medicine. As an example, if you add 16 oz, or 1 quart, of water to 1 Tbsp of instant coffee, you will have very weak coffee. If you add 8 oz of water to 1 Tbsp of instant coffee, you will have stronger coffee and less total volume. The main point is that the amount of instant coffee remains constant; only the amount of liquid (diluent) changes to make stronger or weaker coffee. Reconstituting medications works in the same manner. There is always a certain amount of powder or crystals in the container before the diluent is added. The drug manufacturer tells you what the displacement factor is. This amount is added to the amount of diluent to give the total number of milliliters. The label on the medication vial states the strength (amount) of medication in the vial. That amount never changes. The only thing that can change is the amount of diluent (liquid) that is added.

Most reconstituted medications come in single-dose vials rather than multiple-dose vials, and various amounts of diluent can be added to make varying strengths of medication.

Types of Diluents

► **It is important to use the type of diluent described in the directions for reconstitution.** The diluents used to reconstitute powders vary based on the chemical properties of the powder. For example, erythromycin must be reconstituted with sterile water. If normal saline (NS) is used, the powder clumps and will not go into solution. The bacteriostatic agent used in bacteriostatic water is benzyl alcohol. If sterile water is used instead of bacteriostatic water, it may cause some products to clump instead of going into solution. The choice of diluent is based on the pH and the physical properties of the product (medication).

Dibasic sodium is added to some powders to correct the final pH of the product.

Lidocaine is added to ease pain during IM administration. The amount of lidocaine added to the medication would not affect vasoconstriction.

⊖ CLINICAL ALERT

Always use the diluent recommended for reconstitution.

Diluting Powders or Crystals in Vials

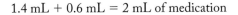

Directions for dissolving medications in vials can be found in the accompanying literature. What will be given is the volume of the powder after it is dissolved in the diluent. For instance, the directions may read: *Add 1.4 mL NS to make 2 mL of reconstituted solution.* These directions tell the user that the powder takes up to 0.6 mL of space. The displacement factor is 0.6 mL.

1.4 mL + 0.6 mL = 2 mL of medication

Example Read the medication label to find out how many units, grams, milligrams, or micrograms are in each milliliter of the reconstituted drug.

Begin by adding 2.7 mL of air to the sterile water for injection (diluent) vial, and then invert the vial to withdraw the 2.7 mL of diluent. Add the 2.7 mL of diluent to the oxacillin sodium vial to make 500 mg of medication in 3 mL (Figure 6-4).

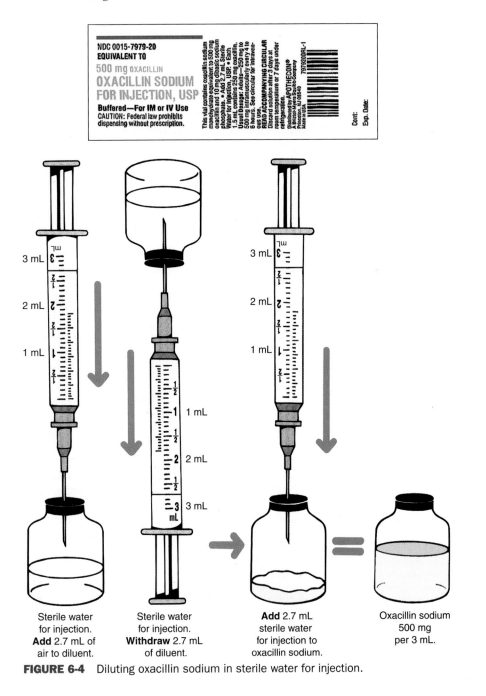

| Sterile water for injection. **Add** 2.7 mL of air to diluent. | Sterile water for injection. **Withdraw** 2.7 mL of diluent. | **Add** 2.7 mL sterile water for injection to oxacillin sodium. | Oxacillin sodium 500 mg per 3 mL. |

FIGURE 6-4 Diluting oxacillin sodium in sterile water for injection.

Ordered: 250 mg oxacillin sodium IM q6h.

KNOW   WANT TO KNOW

3 mL : 500 mg :: *x* mL : 250 mg

500*x* = 3 × 250 = 750

    x = 1.5 mL

PROOF

500 × 1.5 = 750

3 × 250 = 750

Give 1.5 mL of reconstituted solution for each 250 mg.

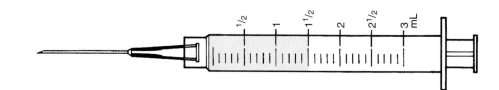

⊝ CLINICAL ALERT

When giving intramuscular injections, always aspirate before injecting. If blood is returned, discard the dose.

When medications to be reconstituted are packaged with the diluent attached, the sterility and accuracy of the reconstituted powder are ensured (Figure 6-5). Some medications are reconstituted by the manufacturer and are delivered in prefilled cartridges or syringes (Figure 6-6).

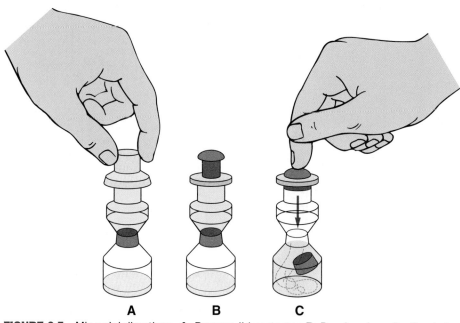

A   **B**   **C**

FIGURE 6-5   Mix-o-vial directions. **A,** Remove lid protector. **B,** Powdered medication is in lower half; diluent is in upper half. **C,** Push firmly on the diaphragm-plunger. Downward pressure dislodges the divider between the two chambers. (From Clayton BD, Stock YN, Cooper S: Basic pharmacology for nurses, ed 15, St Louis, 2010, Mosby. Courtesy of Chuck Dresner.)

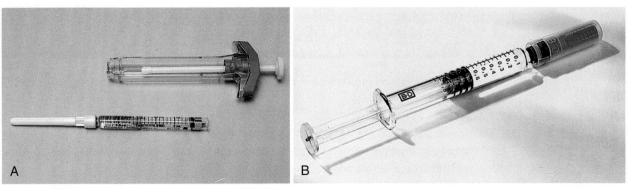

FIGURE 6-6 **A,** Carpuject syringe and prefilled sterile cartridge with needle. **B,** BD-Hypak prefilled syringe. *(A, From Perry AG, Potter PA: Clinical nursing skills and techniques, ed 7, St Louis, 2010, Mosby. B, From Becton, Dickinson, and Company, Franklin Lakes, NJ.)*

Figure 6-7 is a pharmacy generated MAR for 24 hours stated in military time for 8-hour shifts beginning at 0700. At the top, the orders must be signed by an RN indicating that the original order has been verified and is correct and allergies have been noted. SCH is a regularly scheduled medication. The start and stop dates are printed. PRN orders and One Time Only Meds are written in a separate space. Narcotic orders must be rewritten q48h. Discontinued orders are highlighted according to hospital policy and must be renewed if it is necessary to continue them. Site codes are in alpha order. Withheld meds use the code R circled with a nurse's note on the chart. The nurses giving the meds must initial each dose and sign the bottom of the MAR to identify their initials.

Doe, John
ID# 45764304
Age: 50 Sex: M Rm: 406A
Dr. Marin, Cruz

ALLERGIES: DRUGS: _Codeine_
FOODS: _none_

RN Verification: _Mary Smith_

Date: *11-09-12* **(Beg)**
11-13-12 **(End)**

MEDICATION: Dose Route Freq

Time of Administration, Site, and Initials

	START	STOP	0700 TO 1459	1500 TO 2259	2300 TO 0659
SCH	*11-09-12 Kefzol*	*11-13-12*	*0700*	*1500*	*2300*
	300 mg IM q8h		*N MS*	*O IB*	*N JB*

Each health care agency will have a protocol for charting injection sites. This is one example

---

ONE TIME ONLY AND PRN MEDS

Start	Stop	Time	Initials	Full name/title
Lasix 11-16-12		*2000*	*IB*	*Irene Butler, RN*
40 mg IV STAT				

Sign: *Mary Smith*   Initials: *MS*   Sign: *Irene Butler*   Initials: *IB*   Sign: *Jill Beck*   Initials: *JB*

SITE CODES   **GENERAL HOSPITAL**

A	Abdomen (L)	J	Gluteus (LUQ)
B	Abdomen (R)	K	Gluteus (RUQ)
C	Arm (L)	L	Thigh (L)
D	Arm (R)	M	Thigh (R)
E	Eyes (both)	N	Ventrogluteal (L)
F	Eyes (left)	O	Ventrogluteal (R)
G	Eyes (right)	P	NPO: Lab
H	Deltoid (mid L)	Q	NPO: Surgery
I	Deltoid (mid R)	R	Withheld/see nurse's notes

FIGURE 6-7 Medication administration record (MAR).

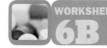

WORKSHEET 6B | **Practice in Reconstituting Parenteral Dosages with Multiple-Strength Decisions**

Show your calculations and proofs in the following problems. Shade in the correct doses on the syringes.

1. Ordered: Cefobid 1000 mg IM q12h. Available: Cefobid 1 g. Reconstitute IM doses with 2.2 mL of bacteriostatic water for injection (taken from insert). The powder displaces 0.4 mL. How many milliliters will be administered?

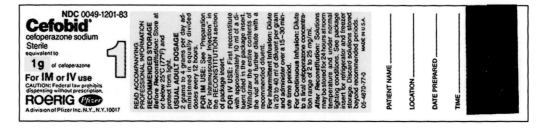

2. Ordered: Nafcillin sodium 0.5 g IM q4h.
   a. How many milliliters of diluent will you add?
   b. How many milligrams per milliliters will this make?
   c. How many milliliters will you administer?
   d. How many doses are in the vial?

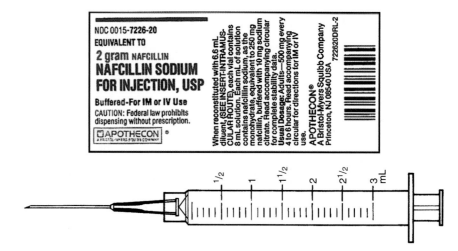

3. Ordered: Ampicillin 1000 mg q6h IM. Available: Ampicillin 1 g.
   a. How many milliliters will you administer?
   b. How many milliliters will you give in each site?

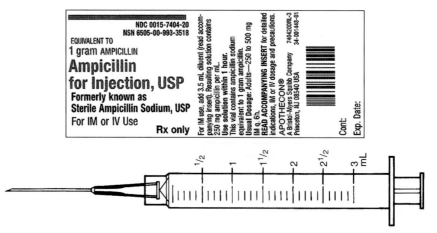

⊘ CLINICAL ALERT

The maximum single injection for adults is 3 mL. Not all patients can tolerate a 3 mL injection. Assess the patient for adequate muscle mass at the site of injection to determine the ability for absorption, which aids in patient comfort as well as therapeutic value.

4. Ordered: Oxacillin sodium 500 mg IV stat. Available: A multidose vial.
   a. How many mL of diluent will you add?
   b. How many mL of oxacillin will you administer?

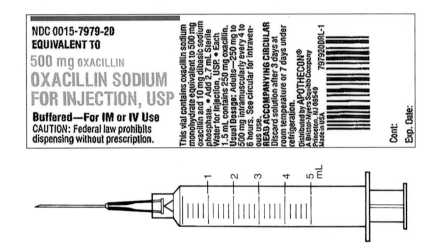

5. Ordered: Pfizerpen (penicillin G potassium) 300,000 units IM bid. Available: 1 million units. Calculate the strength closest to the ordered amount.
   a. How many milliliters of diluent will you add?
   b. How many milliliters will you administer?
   c. How many doses are in the multidose vial?

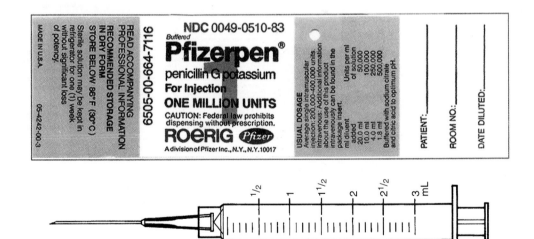

6. Ordered: Penicillin G potassium 300,000 units IM q4h. Available: A multidose vial containing 1 million units.

Select the most appropriate dilution for the ordered dose. Work out all concentrations to determine the appropriate dose for the patient.

   a. Which dilution will you make and label?

   b. What amount will you administer?

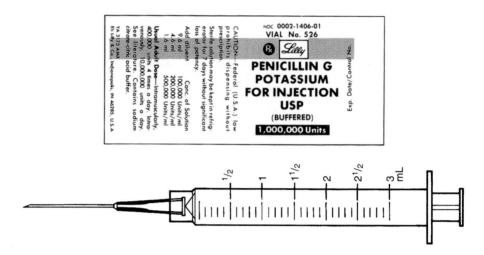

7. Ordered: Tazicef 250 mg IM q8h.

Available: Tazicef 1 g for IM or IV use.

Follow insert directions for reconstitution directions.

   a. How many mL of diluent will be added to the powder?

   b. How many mg/mL will this make?

   c. How many mL will you administer IM?

RECONSTITUTION

Single Dose Vials:

For I.M. injection, I.V. direct (bolus) injection, or I.V. infusion, reconstitute with Sterile Water for injection according to the following table. The vacuum may assist entry of the diluent. SHAKE WELL.

Table 5

Vial Size	Diluent to Be Added	Approx. Avail. Volume	Approx. Avg. Concentration
Intramuscular or Intravenous Direct (bolus) Injection			
1 gram	3.0 ml.	3.6 ml.	280 mg./ml.
Intravenous Infusion			
1 gram	10 ml.	10.6 ml.	95 mg./ml.
2 gram	10 ml.	11.2 ml.	180 mg./ml.

Withdraw the total volume of solution into the syringe (the pressure in the vial may aid withdrawal). The withdrawn solution may contain some bubbles of carbon dioxide.

NOTE: As with the administration of all parenteral products, accumulated gases should be expressed from the syringe immediately before injection of 'Tazicef'.

These solutions of 'Tazicef' are stable for 18 hours at room temperature or seven days if refrigerated (5°C.). Slight yellowing does not affect potency.

For I.V. infusion, dilute reconstituted solution in 50 to 100 ml. of one of the parenteral fluids listed under COMPATIBILITY AND STABILITY.

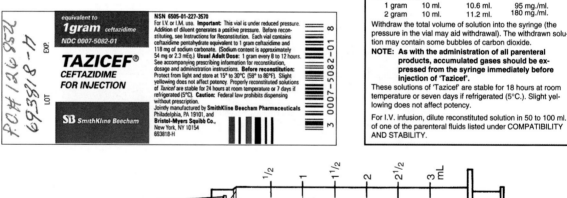

8. Ordered: 100 mg ampicillin IM q12h.
   a. How many milliliters of diluent will be added?
   b. What is the shelf life after reconstitution?
   c. What is the total amount of medication in the vial?
   d. How many milliliters of ampicillin will you administer?

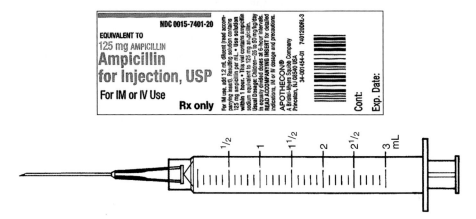

9. Ordered: Cefadyl 700 mg IM q6h. Available: Cefadyl 1 g. Follow directions on label.
   a. How many milliliters will you administer per injection?
   b. How many milligrams will the patient receive in 24 hours?
   c. How many vials will you need for a 24-hour period?

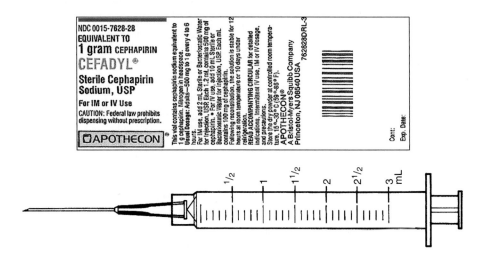

⊖ CLINICAL ALERT

Do not confuse units of medication with milligrams.

10. Ordered: Cefobid 2 g IM q12h. Available: Cefobid 2 g vial. Reconstitution for IM use is found on the package insert. Directions read: Add 3.4 mL of sterile water for injection. The Cefobid powder displaces 0.6 mL. Administer the entire dose.

   a. How many milliliters will you give for the first dose?
   b. How many injections will you administer?
   c. What sites will you select?

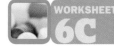

WORKSHEET 6C | Additional Practice in Reconstituting Parenteral Dosages with Multiple-Strength Decisions

Answer the questions in the following problems. Show your calculations and proofs; then shade in the correct dose on the syringes.

1. Ordered: Rocephin 500 mg IM bid

   Directions: For IM use, add sterile water for injection according to directions. Withdraw entire contents to yield 500 mg. Give deep in a large muscle. Aspirate before giving. Calculate both dosages to determine which amount is appropriate for your patient.

Vial Dose Size	Amount of Diluent to Be Added
	1.8 mL ———— 250 mg/mL
500 mg	1 mL ———— 350 mg/mL

Which concentration did you choose? Measure it on the syringe.

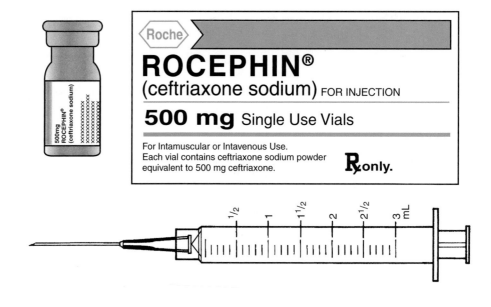

2. Ordered: Cefadyl (cephapirin) 500 mg IM q6h.
   a. How many milliliters of sterile water will you add?
   b. How many mg/per 1.2 mL will you have?
   c. How many milliliters will you administer?

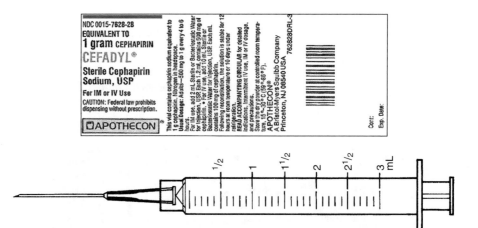

3. Ordered: 500 mg of Monocid IM q12h.
   a. How many milliliters of diluent will be added to the vial?
   b. How many milliliters will you administer?
   c. How many vials of medication will you need for a 24-hour period?

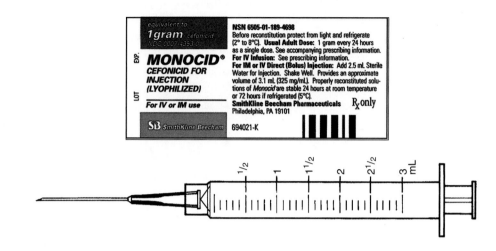

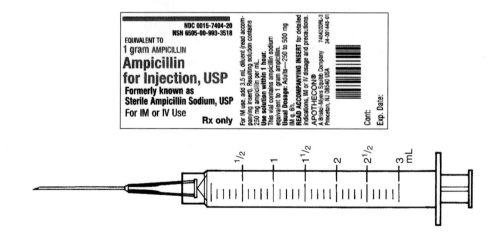

4. Ordered: Ampicillin 500 mg IM q6h.
   a. How many milliliters of diluent are needed to reconstitute the medication?
   b. How many mg/mL will it make?
   c. What is the shelf life of the medication?
   d. How many milliliters will you administer?

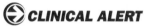

5. Ordered: methylprednisolone 125 mg IM q6h.
   a. How many milliliters of diluent will you add?
   b. How many milligrams per milliliters will this make?
   c. How many milliliters will you give?
   d. How many doses are in the vial?
   e. The medication has to be used within how many hours after reconstituting?
   f. Will all of the doses for this order be given within the recommended time frame?

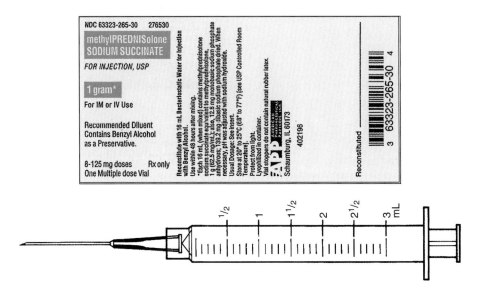

6. Ordered: Pfizerpen 400,000 units IM q12h.
   a. Calculate all three strengths to decide the best dose amount for your patient.
   b. Fill in the amount you will administer on the syringe.

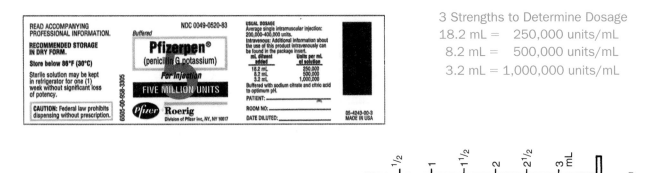

3 Strengths to Determine Dosage
18.2 mL =   250,000 units/mL
 8.2 mL =   500,000 units/mL
 3.2 mL = 1,000,000 units/mL

7. Ordered: Ticar 750 mg IM q8h.
   a. How many milliliters of diluent will be added?
   b. 2.6 mL of Ticar contains how many grams?
   c. What is the shelf life of the medication?
   d. What is the total amount of medication in the vial?
   e. How many milliliters will you administer?

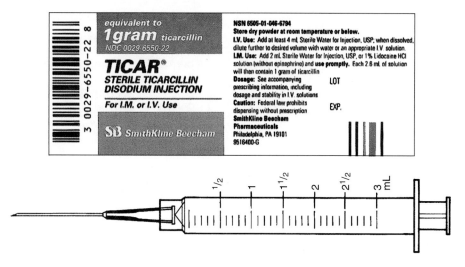

8. Ordered: Penicillin G potassium 750,000 units IM q8h. Select the most appropriate dilution for the ordered dose. The directions read: *Sterile solution may be kept in refrigerator for 7 days without significant loss of potency. Add diluent 9.6 mL for 100,000 units/mL for concentration of solution; add diluent 4.6 mL for 200,000 units/mL; add diluent 1.6 mL for 500,000 units/mL.*
   a. Which strength will you use?
   b. How many milliliters of diluent will be used?
   c. How many milliliters of medication will you administer?
   d. What is the shelf life of the medication after reconstitution?

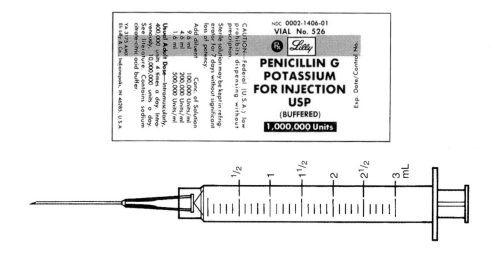

9. Ordered: 400,000 units Pfizerpen IM q6h.

Available: Pfizerpen 1 million units with mixing options.

Choose between adding 4 mL and adding 1.5 mL of diluent.

a. How many units/mL will you administer if you use 4 mL of diluent? Mark the syringe.

b. How many units/mL will you administer if you use 1.5 mL of diluent? Mark the syringe.

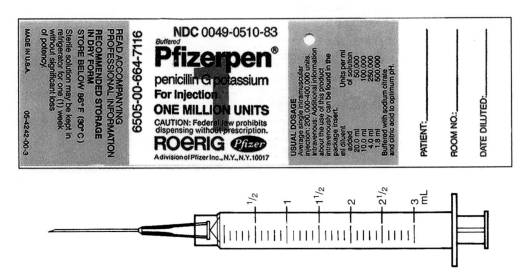

10. Ordered: Oxacillin sodium 450 mg IM q6h.

a. How many milliliters of sterile water will be used for reconstitution?

b. How many mg/mL will it make?

c. What is the shelf life of the medication after reconstitution?

d. What is the total amount of medication in the vial?

e. How many milliliters will you administer?

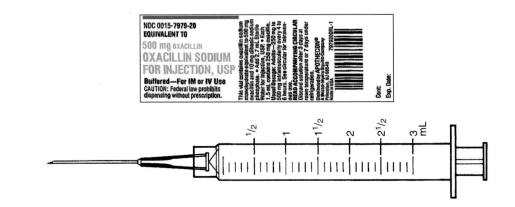

⊖ **CLINICAL ALERT**

Always make sure that the patient's body mass is adequate for the amount of medication that will be given intramuscularly.

1. Ordered: Cefobid 1g IM q12h.
   Available: Cefobid 2 g vial.
   Directions for IM use read: Add 3.4 mL of sterile water for injection. Each 4 mL yields 2 g.
   How many milliliters will you administer?
   a. 3.5 mL   **b.** 4 mL   **c.** 2 mL   **d.** 2.5 mL

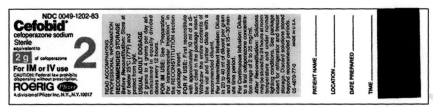

2. Ordered: Ampicillin 250 mg IM q12h.
   Available: Ampicillin 125 mg.
   How many milliliters of diluent will you add?
   a. 2 mL   **b.** 1.2 mL   **c.** 3 mL   **d.** 1.5 mL

   How many vials will you need in 24 hours?
   a. 1 vial   **b.** 2 vials   **c.** 3 vials   **d.** 4 vials

3. Ordered: Oxacillin sodium 500 mg IM q6h.
   Available: Oxacillin 1 gram
   How many milliliters of sterile water will you add?
   a. 3.7 mL   **b.** 5 mL   **c.** 3.1 mL   **d.** 5.7 mL

   How many milliliters will you administer?
   a. 1.5 mL   **b.** 3 mL   **c.** 2.5 mL   **d.** 2 mL

4. Ordered: Cefobid 1.5 g IM q12h.

Available: Cefobid 1 g vial.

Directions read: Add 1.4 mL of sterile water for injection. Each 2 mL yields 1 g.

How many milliliters will you administer?

  a. 2.5 mL   **b.** 3 mL   **c.** 2 mL   **d.** 1.5 mL

How many vials will you need for 24 hours?

  a. 2 vials   **b.** 2.5 vials   **c.** 3.5 vials   **d.** 3 vials

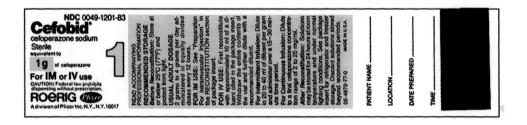

5. Ordered: Levothyroxine 60 mcg IM.

How many milliliters will you administer?

  a. 2 mL   **b.** 1.5 mL   **c.** 2.2 mL   **d.** 2.5 mL

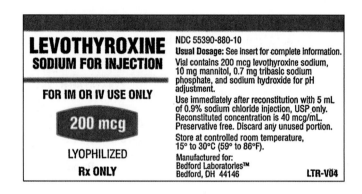

6. Ordered: Ticar 500 mg IM tid.

Available: Ticar 1 gram.

Directions read: Add 2 mL of sterile water for injection.

How many milliliters will you administer?

  a. 2.6 mL   **b.** 2 mL   **c.** 1.3 mL   **d.** 3 mL

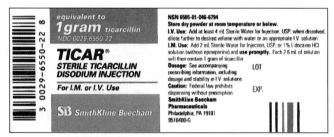

7. Refer to question 6.

   How many vials of Ticar will be needed in 24 hours?

   a. 3 vials   **b.** 4 vials   **c.** 2 vials   **d.** 5 vials

8. Ordered: Pfizerpen 400,000 units IM bid.

   Available: Pfizerpen (penicillin G potassium) 1 million units.

   How many milliliters of diluent will you add?

   a. 5 mL   **b.** 10 mL   **c.** 1.5 mL   **d.** 20 mL

   How many milliliters will you administer?

   a. 2 mL   **b.** 2.5 mL   **c.** 1.6 mL   **d.** 0.8 mL

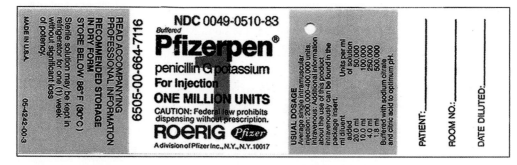

9. Ordered: Streptomycin 500 mg IM bid.

   Available: Streptomycin sulfate 5 g.

   What is the concentration after dilution?

   a. 500 mg/mL   **b.** 1 g/mL   **c.** 400 mg/mL   **d.** 0.5 g/mL

   How many milliliters will you administer?

   a. 1.3 mL   **b.** 1 mL   **c.** 2.2 mL   **d.** 1.8 mL

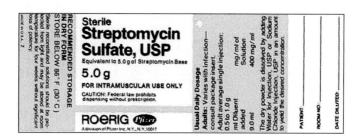

10. Ordered: Ancef 250 mg IM q6h.

    Available: Ancef 1 gram for reconstitution.

    How many mL will you administer?

    a. 2 mL   **b.** 0.5 mL   **c.** 0.8 mL   **d.** 4.5 mL

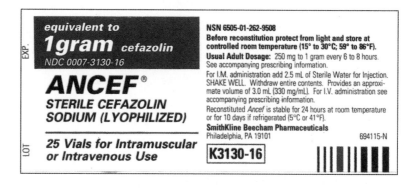

Analyze the following scenarios.

1. A 1 million unit multiple-dose vial of penicillin G potassium has these directions for reconstitution:

Add Diluent	Concentration of Solution
9.6 mL	100,000 units/mL
4.6 mL	200,000 units/mL
1.6 mL	500,000 units/mL

The medication was reconstituted with 9.6 mL of diluent and 200,000 units per mL circled.

Ordered: Penicillin G potassium 200,000 units IM q6h

Given: Penicillin G potassium 1 mL IM q6h

Error(s):

Potential injuries:

Discussion

How many units of penicillin G potassium were given?

What were the potential injuries?

Which concentration would have provided the ordered amount in 1 mL?

How could this error have been prevented?

2. Ordered: Cefadyl 250 mg IM every 12 hours times 4 doses.

```
NDC 0015-7628-28
EQUIVALENT TO
1 gram CEPHAPIRIN
CEFADYL®
Sterile Cephapirin
Sodium, USP
For IM or IV Use
CAUTION: Federal law prohibits
dispensing without prescription.
☐APOTHECON®
```

The Cefadyl (cephapirin) vial was reconstituted with 2 mL of sterile water for injection. The vial was labeled with the date, time, amount of diluent (2 mL of sterile water) circled, and the nurse's initials. The nurse gave the first injection (0.6 mL) of Cefadyl IM at 0800 hours. The next nurse gave the 250 mg dose (0.3 mL) at 2000 hours. The next dose of 250 mg (0.3 mL) was given at 0800 hours. The nurse noted that the vial was empty and discarded it.

How many doses of 250 mg were in the 1 gram vial?

How many doses were given?

What should you do if you found that a medication error had been made by another nurse?

Was the patient's safety jeopardized in any way?

How could this error have been prevented?

3. Multiple-dose vials have various reconstitution directions for both IM and IV administration along with different shelf life and storage requirements.

Discuss how each of these steps for reconstitution of drugs could cause potential harm to a patient if not followed properly.

a. Adding the wrong diluent

b. Adding the wrong amount of diluent

c. Administering the wrong amount of reconstituted medication

d. Administering via the wrong route

e. Storing the medication in the wrong place after reconstitution

f. Keeping the medication longer than the recommended shelf life

g. Not labeling the date and time and initialing the label

CHAPTER 6

Final

1. Ordered: Biaxin 150 mg po twice a day.
   Shade in medicine cup to the appropriate measurement.
   a. How much diluent will you add?
   b. When reconstituted, how many milligrams per milliliter will be in the bottle?
   c. How many milliliters will you administer?

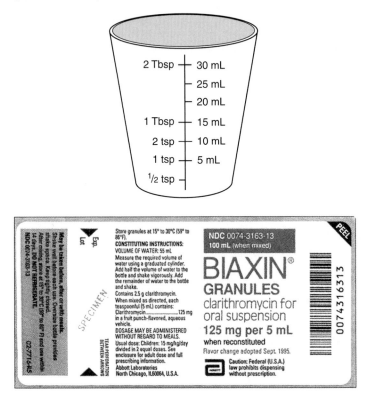

2. Ordered: Carbenicillin 200,000 units IM q6h.
   Available: a vial containing 500,000 units of carbenicillin. The directions read: *Add 4.8 mL of distilled water to make 5 mL of carbenicillin.* Each milliliter will contain 100,000 units. How many milliliters will you administer?

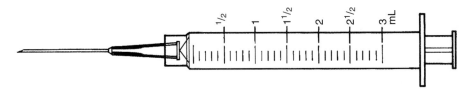

3. Ordered: Ampicillin 250 mg IM q4h for endocarditis prophylaxis.
   a. How much diluent will you add?
   b. How many milliliters will you administer? Shade in the amount on the syringe.

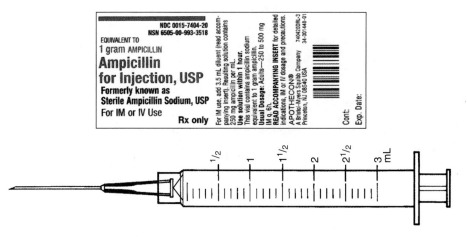

4. Ordered: Ticar 0.5 g IM q6h for salpingitis.
   a. How much diluent will you add?
   b. How many milliliters will you administer? Shade in the amount on the syringe.

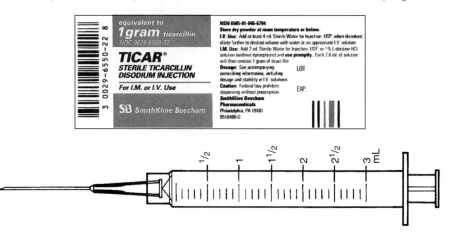

5. Ordered: Pfizerpen 300,000 units IM q12h.
   Available: Pfizerpen 5 million units.
   If you add 18.2 mL of diluent to the Pfizerpen:
   a. How many units/mL will this yield?
   b. How many milliliters will you administer?
   c. How many doses are in the multidose vial?

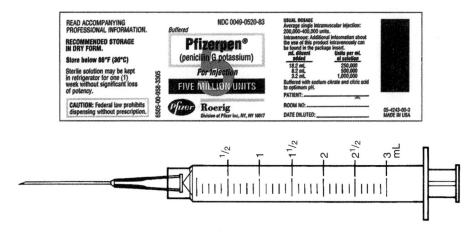

6. Ordered: Carbenicillin 750 mg IM q8h.
   Available: Geopen (carbenicillin) 5 gram for reconstitution.
   a. How many mL of diluent will you add?
   b. How many mL will you administer? Shade in the syringe.

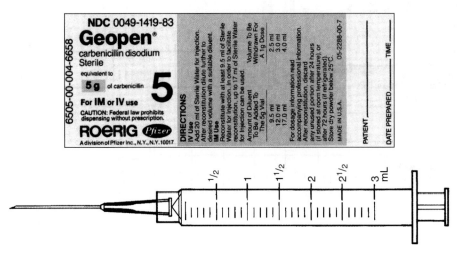

7. Ordered: Monocid 500 mg IM q12h.
   Available: Monocid 1 gram for reconstitution.
   a. How many mL of diluent will you add?
   b. How many mL will you administer? Shade in the syringe.

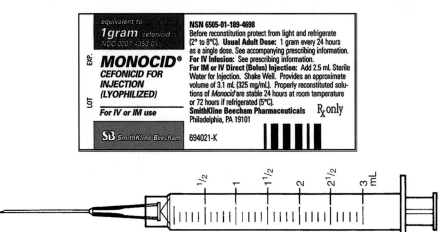

8. Ordered: Penicillin G potassium 100,000 units IM q4h for pneumonia. The directions read: *Sterile solution may be kept in refrigerator for 7 days without significant loss of potency. Add diluent 9.6 mL for 100,000 units/mL concentration of solution; add diluent 4.6 mL for 200,000 units/mL; add diluent 1.6 mL for 500,000 units/mL.*

   a. Which dilution will you use? Why?

   b. How many milliliters will you administer? Shade in the amount on the syringe.

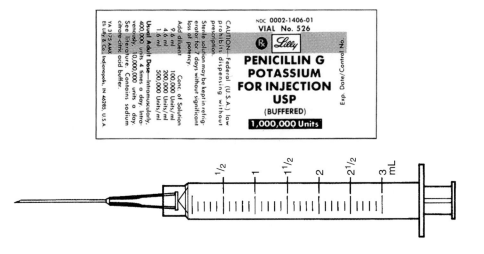

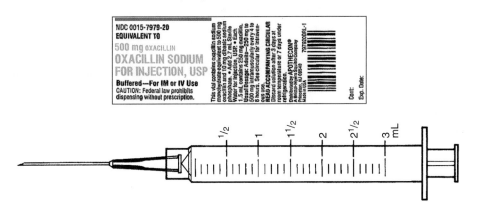

9. Ordered: Oxacillin sodium 250 mg IM q4h for a urinary tract infection (UTI).

   a. How many milliliters of diluent will you add?

   b. How many milliliters of oxacillin sodium will you administer?

   Shade in the amount on the syringe.

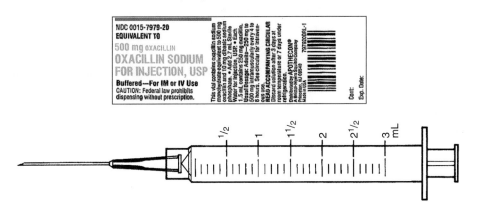

10. Ordered: Keflin 400,000 units IM q12h.

   Available: a vial with 600,000 units/mL. How many milliliters will you administer? Shade in the amount on the syringe.

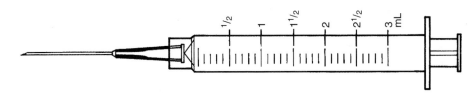

℮volve **Refer to the Basic Calculations section of Drug Calculations Companion, version 4 on Evolve for additional practice problems.**

Basic Intravenous Therapy Calculations

Objectives

- Calculate intravenous (IV) flow rates for drops per min, mL per hr, mg per g per hr, and infusion time.
- Interpret IV labels.
- Identify various electronic IV infusion devices.
- Identify IV sets: primary, primary with a port, IVPB extension tubing, transfusion sets, and venous access devices for intermittent use.
- Calculate the amount of saline or heparin for use in keeping venous access patent.
- Calculate the grams of sodium chloride or dextrose in IV bags.
- Identify osmolarity values for IV solutions.
- Check physician's IV order for type of solution, amount, additives, and rate.
- Set PCA pump using standard protocol.
- Analyze IV orders for safe administration using critical thinking skills.
- Analyze medication errors using critical thinking skills.

Introduction

It is the nurse's responsibility to calculate the milliliters per hour or drops per minute to regulate an intravenous infusion. Knowledge of electronic infusion devices is required as is knowledge of the basic hand-regulated primary sets. The nurse is responsible for calculating the intravenous piggyback (IVPB) infusions that are timed for shorter periods.

IV Infusions

Intravenous (IV) infusions are used more frequently today than intramuscular (IM) injections. Continuous medication therapy can be delivered via an IV route, minimizing multiple injections via the IM route. Intermittent medication therapy can be delivered through a saline/heparin lock (Figure 7-1), which allows the patient free movement until the next scheduled dose. The saline lock is used for intermittent short-duration therapy in acute care, long-term care, and home care. Intermittent therapy can also be delivered as a piggyback with a continuous infusion. A heparin flush can also be used to keep the port patent.

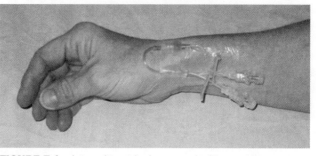

FIGURE 7-1 Intermittent lock covered with a rubber diaphragm. (From Perry AG, Potter PA: Clinical nursing skills and techniques, ed 7, St Louis, 2010, Mosby.)

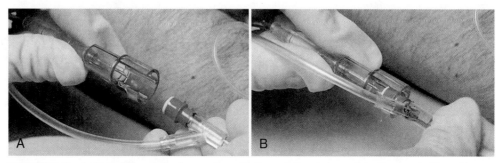

FIGURE 7-2 **A,** Needleless infusion system. **B,** Connection into an injection port. (From Perry AG, Potter PA: Clinical nursing skills and techniques, ed 7, St Louis, 2010, Mosby.)

Medications (additives) can be added to the IV by the manufacturer, pharmacist, or nurse. The physician orders the medication, strength, and amount, as well as the type and amount of diluent. It is important that the person responsible for the IV understand the actions of the medication, flow rate, adverse reactions, and antidotes. IV fluids flow directly into the vein, resulting in immediate action, and cannot be retrieved. Therefore, it is imperative that the correct calculations, medications, and flow rate be administered.

An intermittent IV lock is known by many different terms. Some terms used are saline lock, hep lock, PRN cap, intermittent IV (INT), and intermittent peripheral infusion device (IPD). All have needleless resealable valves (Figure 7-2).

Types of IV Lines

There are many types of IV tubing used for temporary and long-term access to veins and arteries.

Peripheral   A peripheral line is usually used for fluid replacement and temporary intermittent medication administration. The IV line is inserted in the hand, arm, or possibly leg if the hand or arm cannot be accessed. Foot and scalp sites are used for infants.

Peripheral inserted central catheter (PICC)   A PICC line (Figure 7-3) is longer than a central catheter line (approximately 22 inches in length). The insertion point is usually the vein in the antecubital region of the arm, where the line is then advanced into the superior vena cava. It is inserted by a PICC-certified RN or physician. Only solutions with a osmolarity of less than 10% should be administered via peripheral lines.

Central line   A central line (Figure 7-4) is inserted by an MD or DO directly into the jugular or subclavian vein and then into the superior vena cava. This type of line is for therapy requiring a longer period of time.

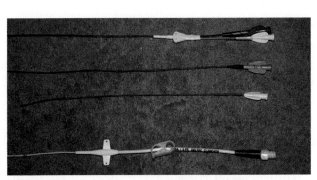

FIGURE 7-3 Peripheral inserted central catheter (PICC lines). The double-lumen catheter is used to draw blood samples.

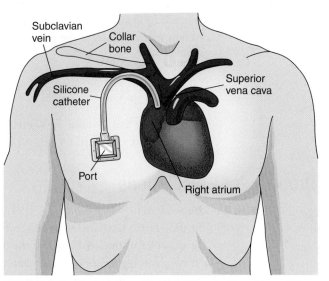

FIGURE 7-4 Central line with a medi-port. (From Perry AG, Potter PA: Clinical nursing skills and techniques, ed 7, St Louis, 2010, Mosby.)

⊖ *CLINICAL ALERT*

Only solutions with an osmolarity of less than 10% should be administered via peripheral lines.

Table 7-1 is a guide that can be used to maintain patency by flushing intermittent access locks. Always refer to hospital protocol for type of solution, volume, and frequency.

Table 7-1 Intermittent Flushing Ranges

Catheter	Flush Solution	Volume (mL)
Peripheral	Normal saline	1-3 mL
Peripherally inserted central catheter (PICC)	Normal saline	3-5 mL
Central venous	Heparinized saline	5-10 mL of saline followed with 3 mL heparin 1:100 units per mL

⊖ *CLINICAL ALERT*

When flushing peripheral IV lines, a 10 mL syringe should be used. A smaller syringe creates greater pressure within the line, which may cause damage to the vein and be harmful to the patient.

IV Calculations

Check IV orders before beginning calculations. There are two steps in IV calculations. The first step is to find out how many *milliliters per hour* (volume) the IV is ordered to infuse. The second step is to calculate the *drops per minute* needed to infuse the ordered volume.

Analyze your problem. If the order says to infuse the IV for 24 hours, calculate the mL per hr by beginning with Step 1. If the order says to infuse the IV at 75 mL per hr, begin with Step 2.

Step 1 mL/hr

RULE When the total volume is given, calculate the mL/hr.

$$\frac{\text{Total volume (TV)}}{\text{Total time (TT) in hours}} = \text{mL per hr}$$

Ordered: 2000 mL D5W (dextrose 5% in water) to be infused for 24 hours. The problem is to find out how many mL per hr the patient must receive for the 2000 mL to be infused in 24 hours.

Formula

$$\frac{\text{Total volume (TV)}}{\text{Total time (TT) in hours}} = \text{mL per hr}$$

Calculation

$$\frac{\text{TV}}{\text{TT}} = \frac{2000}{24} = 83 \text{ mL per hr}$$

We now know that to infuse 2000 mL of fluid in 24 hours, the patient must receive 83 mL per hr. Infusion devices are calibrated for mL per hr.

Drop Factor Calculations

Step 2 Drops per min

The drop factor is needed to calculate drops per min. The drop factor is the number of drops in 1 mL. The diameter of the needle where the drop enters the drip chamber varies from one manufacturer to another. The bigger the needle, the fatter the drop (Figure 7-5, *A*); it takes only 10 macrodrops to make a milliliter. The smallest unit is the microdrop (60 drops per mL) (Figure 7-5, *B*). This is used for people who can tolerate only small amounts of fluid, such as pediatric and geriatric patients and patients who require fluid restrictions. Drop factors of 10, 15, 20, and 60 (microdrip) are the most common. The drop factor is determined by the manufacturer and is found on the IV tubing package.

RULE When the mL per hr is given, calculate the drops per min.

$$\frac{\text{Drop factor or gtt/mL (from IV package)}}{\text{Time in minutes}} \times \text{Total hourly volume (V/hr)} = \text{drops per min}$$

Example Ordered: D5W to infuse at 83 mL per hr. The drop factor (Df) is 10.

$$\frac{\text{Df}}{\text{Time (min)}} \times \text{V/hr} = \frac{10 \text{ (Df)}}{60 \text{ (min)}} \times 83 \text{ (V/hr)}$$

$$\frac{10}{60} \times \frac{83}{1} = \frac{1}{6} \times \frac{83}{1} = \frac{83}{6} = 13.8 \text{ or } 14 \text{ drops per min}$$

Drops cannot be timed in tenths, only in whole numbers. If the decimal is greater than or equal to 0.5, round to the next higher number.

Example Ordered: Antibiotic to infuse at 100 mL in 30 min. The drop factor is 15.

$$\frac{\text{Df}}{\text{Time (min)}} \times \text{V/hr} = \frac{15 \text{ (Df)}}{30 \text{ (min)}} = 100 \text{ (V per hr)}$$

$$\frac{15}{30} \times \frac{100}{1} = \frac{1}{2} \times \frac{100}{1} = \frac{100}{2} = 50 \text{ drops per min}$$

Summary Two-step IV flow rate calculations

Step 1
$$\frac{\text{TV}}{\text{TT in hr}} = \text{mL per hr}$$

Step 2
$$\frac{\text{Df}}{\text{Time in min}} \times \text{V per hr} = \text{drops per min}$$

remember Reduce the fraction Df per min *before* multiplying by the volume.

Example Which would you rather calculate?

$$\frac{12}{60} \times 60 \quad \text{or} \quad \frac{1}{5} \times 60$$

The reduced fraction is easier to calculate.

remember When the IV tubing is microdrip, 60 drops per mL, the drops per min will be the same as the mL per hr.

Example 1000 mL to infuse in 8 hours with a microdrip set.

Step 1

$$\frac{TV}{TT \text{ in hr}} = \frac{1000}{8} = 125 \text{ mL per hr}$$

Step 2

$$\frac{Df}{Time \text{ in min}} \times V \text{ per hr} = \frac{60}{60} \times 125 = 125 \text{ drops per min}$$

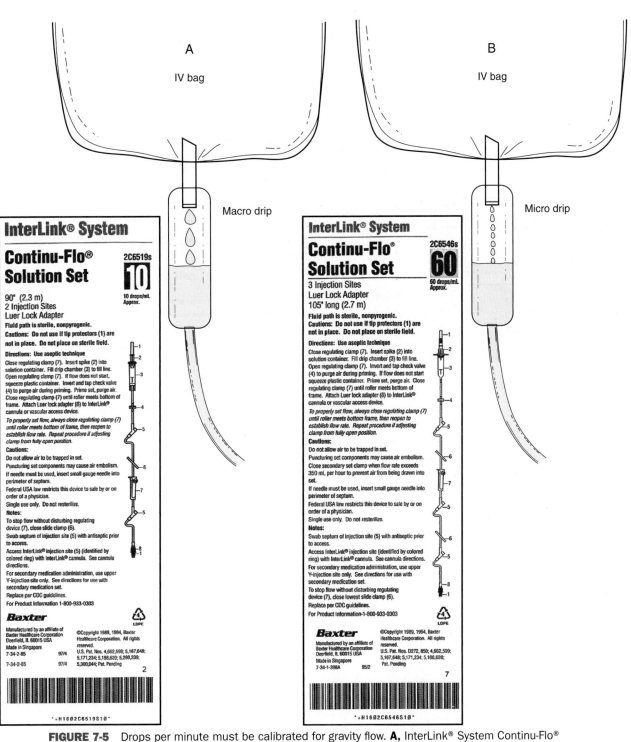

FIGURE 7-5 Drops per minute must be calibrated for gravity flow. **A,** InterLink® System Continu-Flo® Solution Set with drop factor of 10 (10 drops = 1 mL). **B,** InterLink® System Continu-Flo® Solution Set with drop factor of 60 (60 drops = 1 mL).

Drops per Minute by Manufacturer

A simple approach to calculate drops per min after you have determined the mL per hr is to memorize the reduced fraction numbers. Manufacturers have established rates for their products (Figure 7-6). Below is an example.

Product Drip Rates	Minutes	Df	=	Reduced Number
60 drops per mL	60	60	=	1
20 drops per mL	60	20	=	3
15 drops per mL	60	15	=	4
10 drops per mL	60	10	=	6

You may have to memorize only one number because most facilities purchase equipment from a single company.

FIGURE 7-6 Various drop rates from different manufacturers.

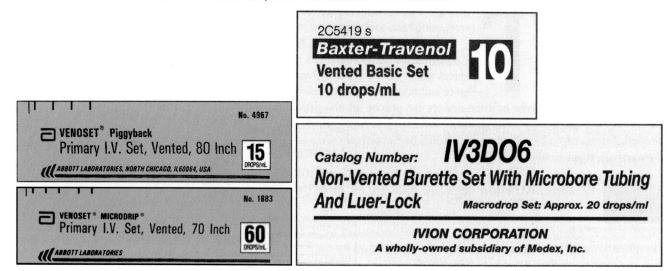

Example If you know you are using a set that delivers 20 drops per mL, divide 3 into the mL per hr.

$$\frac{125}{3} = 41.6 = 42 \text{ drops per min}$$

As you already know, the formula for calculating drops per min is:

$$\frac{Df}{\text{Time in min}} \times V \text{ per hr} \quad \text{or} \quad \frac{20}{60} \times 125 = \frac{1}{3} \times 125 = 41.6 = 42 \text{ drops per min}$$

Now you know two different methods for calculating drops per min.

⊘ CLINICAL ALERT

Check the IV every hour, even if an infusion device is used. Recheck drops per minute rate frequently because the IV rate can vary with position. Time taping the IV has become important as electrical blackouts and brown outs can adversely affect the device.

Flo Meter Tape

The order is to infuse 1000 mL in 10 hr (Figure 7-7). The infusion label shows a starting time of 0700 hr and an ending time of 1700 hr. The IV is scheduled to infuse for 10 hr. Use the 10 hr rate per hr on the tape and initital each hour at 100 mL per hour. The ending time will be 1700 hr.

infusion label

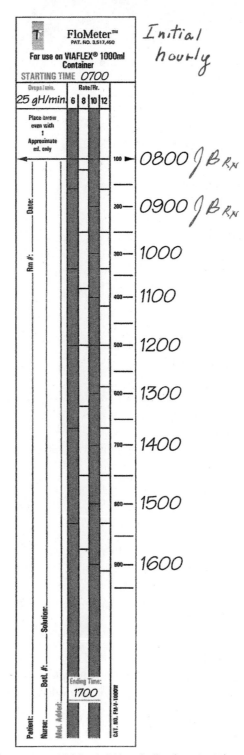

FIGURE 7-7 A FloMeter™ Tape on a 1000 mL IV bag indicating start time and hourly rate at 100 mL per hour and initialed hourly.

| **IV Calculations**

Use either the Step 1 or the Step 2 formula to calculate mL per hr or drop per min to answer the following questions.

Step 1 $\dfrac{TV}{TT \text{ in hr}} = mL \text{ per hr}$

Step 2 $\dfrac{Df}{Time \text{ in min}} \times V \text{ per hr} = \text{drops per min}$ or $\dfrac{mL \text{ per hr}}{\text{reduced drop rate}}$

1. Ordered: 1500 mL to be infused for 12 hr. If the drop factor is 15, how many drops per min is this?

2. Ordered: 50 mL to be infused for 1 hr. How many drops per min will be administered with microdrip?

3. Ordered: 100 mL to be infused for 30 min. How many drops per min is this if the drop factor is 10?

4. Ordered: 1000 mL to be infused for 8 hr. How many drops per min will be administered if the drop factor is 10?

5. Ordered: 200 mL to be infused for 1 hr. If the drop factor is 15, how many drops per min will be administered?

6. Ordered: 1000 mL to be infused at 150 mL per hr. The drop factor is 20. How many drops per min will be infused?

7. Ordered: 75 mL to be infused for 45 min. The drop factor is 10. How many drops per min will be administered?

8. Ordered: 150 mL to be infused for 90 min. The drop factor is microdrip. How many drops per min will be administered?

9. Ordered: 150 mL to be infused for 40 min. The drop factor is 15 drops per mL. How many drops per min is this?

10. Ordered: 1500 mL to be infused for 8 hr. How many mL per hr will be administered?
    a. How many drops per min is this with a drop factor of 10?
    b. How many drops per min is this with a drop factor of 15?

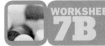

Additional Practice in IV Calculations

Use either the Step 1 or the Step 2 formula to calculate mL per hr or drops per min to answer the following questions.

1. Ordered: 2000 mL for 24 hr. The drop factor is 15. How many drops per min will be administered?

2. You have 500 mL 0.45% NS infusing for 4 hr. The drop factor is 15. How many drops per min will be infused?

3. A solution of 3000 mL D5W with 1.5 g carbenicillin is being infused for 24 hr. The drop factor is 15 drops per minute.
   How many drops per min will be infused?

4. You have 1500 mL normal saline (NS). The drop factor is 15. The solution is to be given for an 8-hr period.
   a. How many mL per hr will be infused?
   b. How many drops per min will be infused?

5. Ordered: 1000 mL to be infused for 12 hr on microdrip. At how many drops per min will you regulate the infusion?

6. Ordered: 100 mL gentamicin to be infused for 30 min. The drop factor is 20.
   a. With which step will you begin?
   b. How many drops per min will be infused?

7. You have 2000 mL D5W being infused for 24 hr. How many mL per hr will be infused?

8. Ordered: 250 mL D5W is to be infused for 10 hr on a microdrip. How many drops per min will be administered?

9. Ordered: 1500 mL of Ringer's lactate solution to be infused for 12 hr.
   a. How many mL per hr will be infused?
   b. The drop factor is 15. How many drops per min will be infused?

10. Write your two-step formula again.
    Step 1   **Step 2**

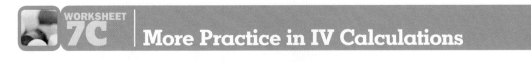

More Practice in IV Calculations

Use either the Step 1 or the Step 2 formula to calculate mL per hr or drops per min to answer the following questions.

1. Ordered: 100 mL to be infused for 30 min. The drop factor is 15. At how many drops per min will you set the IV rate?

2. Ordered: 50 mL to be infused for 30 min. At how many drops per min will you set the IV rate if the drop factor is 10?

3. Ordered: 1000 mL to be infused for 6 hr. How many drops per min will be administered if the drop factor is 15?

4. Ordered: 100 mL to be infused for 60 min. At how many drops per min will you set the IV rate if a microdrip is used? Is this the same as mL per hr?

5. Ordered: D5W continuous infusion at 85 mL per hr. The drop factor is 20. At how many drops per min will you set the IV rate?

6. Ordered: 100 mL per hr. At how many drops per min will you set the IV rate if the drop factor is 10?

7. Ordered: 1500 mL 0.45% NS for 24 hr. The drop factor is 10. At how many drops per min will you set the IV rate?

8. Ordered: 500 mL for 8 hr by microdrip. How many drops per min is this?

9. Ordered: 1000 mL Ringer's lactate solution at 75 mL per hr. The drop factor is 15. How many drops per min will be administered?

10. Ordered: 2000 mL to be infused for 12 hr. The drop factor is 20.
   a. At how many mL per hr will you set the IV rate?
   b. How many drops per min will this be?

Abbreviations for Common IV Solutions

NS	Normal saline; 0.9% sodium chloride (Figure 7-8)
$\frac{1}{2}$ NS	Normal saline; 0.45% saline or $\frac{1}{2}$ strength sodium chloride (Figure 7-9)
D5W or 5% D/W	Dextrose 5% in water (Figure 7-10)
D5RL	Dextrose 5% in Ringer's lactate solution (Figure 7-11)
RL, LR, or RLS	Ringer's lactate solution (Figure 7-12)
D5NS	Dextrose 5% in 0.9% normal saline (Figure 7-13)
D5 and $\frac{1}{2}$ NS (0.45% NS)	Dextrose 5% in $\frac{1}{2}$ normal saline or 0.45% sodium chloride (Figure 7-14)

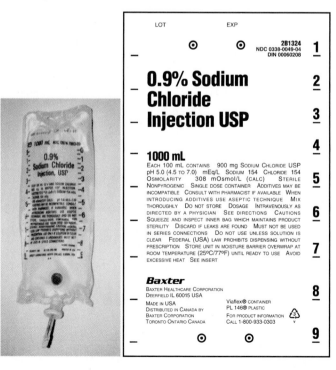

FIGURE 7-8 Normal saline 0.9% (osmolarity range 280-308).

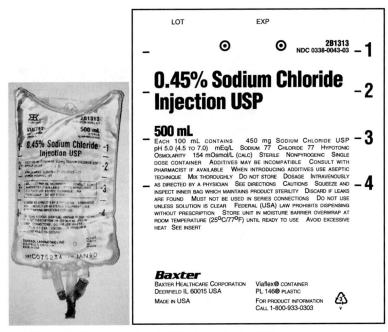

FIGURE 7-9   Normal saline 0.45% (osmolarity 154).

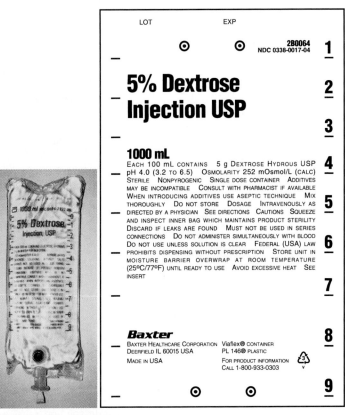

FIGURE 7-10   5% dextrose.

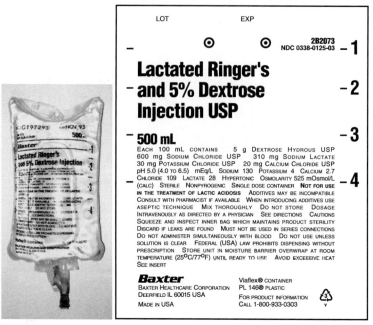

FIGURE 7-11 Ringer's lactate solution and 5% dextrose.

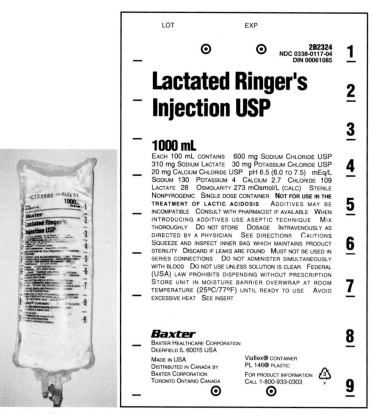

FIGURE 7-12 Ringer's lactate solution.

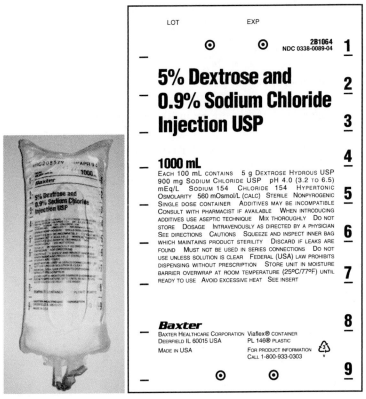

FIGURE 7-13 5% dextrose in normal saline.

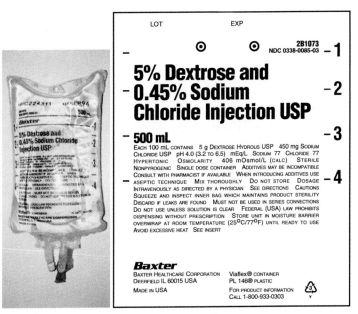

FIGURE 7-14 5% Dextrose in normal saline.

Percentage of Solute in IV Bags

The percentage numbers of the IV bags indicate the amount of dextrose, sodium chloride, or other constituents in the infusion. The type of IV solution ordered is determined by the diagnosis. Patients with diabetes mellitus, kidney diseases, hemotologic disorders, or cardiac problems will need different types of solutions. The nurse must be aware of the diagnosis as it relates to the type of IV solution used. To determine the number of milliliters of dextrose or sodium chloride the percentage (%) represents, use the following formula. The dissolved substance or solute (dextrose, sodium chloride) is represented by a weight measurement (g). However, one mL of water weighs 1 g. Therefore, the solute is weighed in grams per 100 mL of solution. The percentage = g solute per 100 mL solution.

remember Percentage is based on 100.

Example How many g of dextrose are in 1000 mL of D5W?

KNOW   WANT TO KNOW

5 g (solute) : 100 mL :: x g (solute) : 1000 mL

$$\text{or}\quad \frac{5}{100} \times \frac{x}{1000} = \frac{1\emptyset\emptyset x}{5 \times 1\emptyset\emptyset\emptyset} = \frac{1}{50} = 50 \text{ g or mL}$$

$$100x = 5 \times 1000 = 5000$$
$$1\emptyset\emptyset x = 500\emptyset$$
$$x = 50 \text{ g (solute)}$$
$$\text{or mL of dextrose in 1000 mL}$$

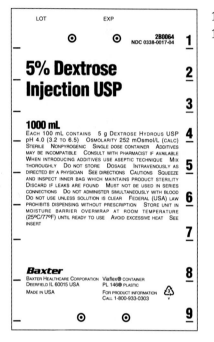

PROOF
100 × 50 = 5000
5 × 1000 = 5000

Intravenous solutions are categorized according to tonicity or osmolarity. Osmolarity is the concentration of active dissolved particles in solution. All IV labels will show the mOsmo/L. Table 7-2 shows the differences between *hypotonic, isotonic,* and *hypertonic* solutions according to the mOsmo/L on the labels.

Table 7-2 Tonicity of Solutions

Hypotonic (less than 250 mOsm/L)	Isotonic (250-375 mOsm/L)	Hypertonic (greater than 375 mOsm/L)
Fluid shifts out of intravascular compartment, hydrating cells	Osmolarity equal to that of serum	Fluid is drawn into the intravascular compartment from the cells
Examples: 0.45% saline (154 mOsm/L)	Examples: 0.9% saline (308 mOsm/L) 0.5% dextrose in water (252 mOsm/L) lactated Ringer solution (273 mOsm/L)	Examples: 5% dextrose and 0.9% NaCl (560 mOsm/L) 5% dextrose and lactated Ringer solution (525 mOsm/L)

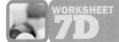

WORKSHEET 7D | IV Solute Calculations

Calculate the g of NaCl dextrose and the osmolarity, HYPO, ISO, HYPER in the following intravenous fluids.

1.

LOT   EXP

2B1064
NDC 0338-0089-04   **1**

5% Dextrose and
2
0.9% Sodium Chloride
Injection USP
3

1000 mL
4
EACH 100 mL CONTAINS   5 g DEXTROSE HYDROUS USP
900 mg SODIUM CHLORIDE USP   pH 4.0 (3.2 TO 6.5)
mEq/L   SODIUM 154   CHLORIDE 154   HYPERTONIC
5
OSMOLARITY 560 mOsmol/L (CALC) STERILE NONPYROGENIC
SINGLE DOSE CONTAINER   ADDITIVES MAY BE INCOMPATIBLE
CONSULT WITH PHARMACIST IF AVAILABLE   WHEN INTRODUCING
ADDITIVES USE ASEPTIC TECHNIQUE   MIX THOROUGHLY   DO NOT
STORE   DOSAGE   INTRAVENOUSLY AS DIRECTED BY A PHYSICIAN
6
SEE DIRECTIONS   CAUTIONS   SQUEEZE AND INSPECT INNER BAG
WHICH MAINTAINS PRODUCT STERILITY   DISCARD IF LEAKS ARE
FOUND   MUST NOT BE USED IN SERIES CONNECTIONS   DO NOT
USE UNLESS SOLUTION IS CLEAR   FEDERAL (USA) LAW PROHIBITS
DISPENSING WITHOUT PRESCRIPTION   STORE UNIT IN MOISTURE
7
BARRIER OVERWRAP AT ROOM TEMPERATURE (25°C/77°F) UNTIL
READY TO USE   AVOID EXCESSIVE HEAT   SEE INSERT

Baxter
8
BAXTER HEALTHCARE CORPORATION   Viaflex® CONTAINER
DEERFIELD IL 60015 USA   PL 146® PLASTIC
MADE IN USA   FOR PRODUCT INFORMATION
CALL 1-800-933-0303
9

g _____ NaCl
g _____ dextrose
osmolarity: _____

2.

LOT   EXP

2B1073
NDC 0338-0085-03 **1**

5% Dextrose and
0.45% Sodium
2
Chloride Injection USP

3
500 mL
EACH 100 mL CONTAINS   5 g DEXTROSE HYDROUS USP   450 mg SODIUM
CHLORIDE USP   pH 4.0 (3.2 TO 6.5)   mEq/L   SODIUM 77   CHLORIDE 77
HYPERTONIC   OSMOLARITY   406 mOsmol/L (CALC)   STERILE
NONPYROGENIC   SINGLE DOSE CONTAINER   ADDITIVES MAY BE INCOMPATIBLE
CONSULT WITH PHARMACIST IF AVAILABLE   WHEN INTRODUCING ADDITIVES USE
4
ASEPTIC TECHNIQUE   MIX THOROUGHLY   DO NOT STORE   DOSAGE
INTRAVENOUSLY AS DIRECTED BY A PHYSICIAN   SEE DIRECTIONS   CAUTIONS
SQUEEZE AND INSPECT INNER BAG WHICH MAINTAINS PRODUCT STERILITY
DISCARD IF LEAKS ARE FOUND   MUST NOT BE USED IN SERIES CONNECTIONS
DO NOT USE UNLESS SOLUTION IS CLEAR   FEDERAL (USA) LAW PROHIBITS
DISPENSING WITHOUT PRESCRIPTION   STORE UNIT IN MOISTURE BARRIER
OVERWRAP AT ROOM TEMPERATURE (25°C/77°F) UNTIL READY TO USE
AVOID EXCESSIVE HEAT   SEE INSERT

Baxter
BAXTER HEALTHCARE CORPORATION   Viaflex® container
DEERFIELD IL 60015 USA   PL 146® PLASTIC
MADE IN USA   FOR PRODUCT INFORMATION
CALL 1-800-933-0303

g _____ dextrose
g _____ NaCl
osmolarity: _____

3.

LOT   EXP

2B1163
NDC 0338-0095-03 **1**

10% Dextrose and
0.9% Sodium Chloride   **2**
Injection USP

3
500 mL
EACH 100 mL CONTAINS   10 g DEXTROSE HYDROUS USP   900 mg SODIUM
CHLORIDE USP   pH 4.0 (3.2 TO 6.5)   mEq/L   SODIUM 154
CHLORIDE 154   OSMOLARITY 813 mOsmol/L (CALC) HYPERTONIC   MAY
CAUSE VEIN DAMAGE   STERILE   NONPYROGENIC   SINGLE DOSE CONTAINER
ADDITIVES MAY BE INCOMPATIBLE   CONSULT WITH PHARMACIST IF AVAILABLE
WHEN INTRODUCING ADDITIVES USE ASEPTIC TECHNIQUE   MIX THOROUGHLY
4
DO NOT STORE   DOSAGE   INTRAVENOUSLY AS DIRECTED BY A PHYSICIAN   SEE
DIRECTIONS   CAUTIONS   SQUEEZE AND INSPECT INNER BAG WHICH MAINTAINS
PRODUCT STERILITY   DISCARD IF LEAKS ARE FOUND   MUST NOT BE USED IN
SERIES CONNECTIONS   DO NOT USE UNLESS SOLUTION IS CLEAR   FEDERAL
(USA) LAW PROHIBITS DISPENSING WITHOUT PRESCRIPTION   STORE UNIT IN
MOISTURE BARRIER OVERWRAP AT ROOM TEMPERATURE (25°C/77°F) UNTIL
READY TO USE   AVOID EXCESSIVE HEAT   SEE INSERT

Baxter
BAXTER HEALTHCARE CORPORATION   Viaflex® container
DEERFIELD IL 60015 USA   PL 146® PLASTIC
MADE IN USA   FOR PRODUCT INFORMATION
CALL 1-800-933-0303

g _____ dextrose
g _____ NaCl
osmolarity: _____

Calculate the g of NaCl in the following intravenous fluids. State the osmolarity.

4. FIGURE 7-8

Normal saline 0.9% (osmolarity range 280-308).

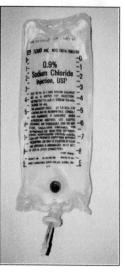

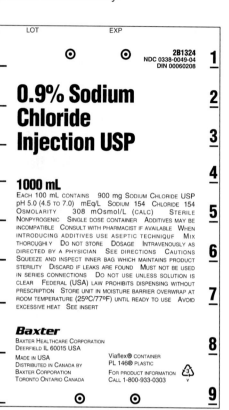

g _____ NaCl

osmolarity: _____

5. FIGURE 7-9

Normal saline 0.45% (osmolarity 154).

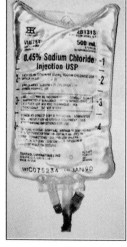

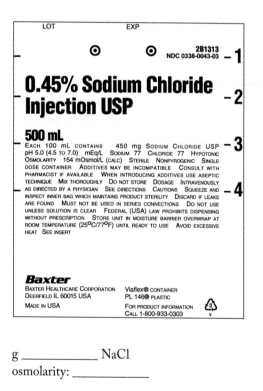

g _____ NaCl

osmolarity: _____

Calculate the g of dextrose and osmolarity in the following intravenous fluids.

6. FIGURE 7-10

5% dextrose.

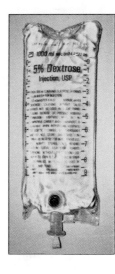

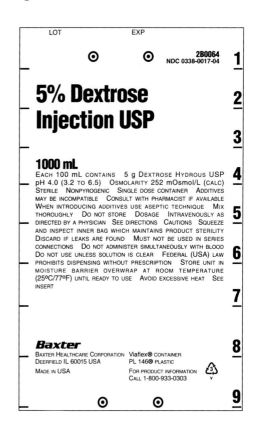

g _____ dextrose

osmolarity: _____

7. FIGURE 7-11

Ringer's lactate solution and 5% dextrose.

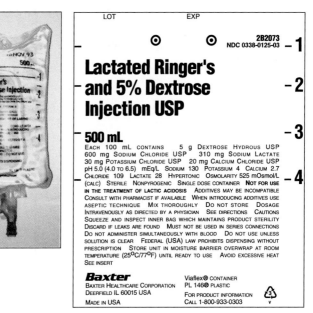

g _____ dextrose

osmolarity: _____

Calculate the g of NaCl and the osmolarity in the following intravenous fluid.

8. FIGURE 7-12

Ringer's lactate solution.

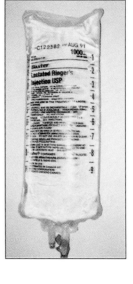 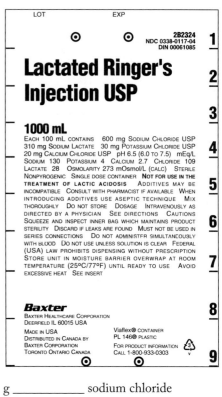

LOT   EXP

2B2324
NDC 0338-0117-04
DIN 00061085

1

Lactated Ringer's Injection USP

2

3

1000 mL

4

EACH 100 mL CONTAINS   600 mg SODIUM CHLORIDE USP
310 mg SODIUM LACTATE   30 mg POTASSIUM CHLORIDE USP
20 mg CALCIUM CHLORIDE USP   pH 6.5 (6.0 TO 7.5)   mEq/L
SODIUM 130   POTASSIUM 4   CALCIUM 2.7   CHLORIDE 109
LACTATE 28   OSMOLARITY 273 mOsmol/L (CALC)   STERILE
NONPYROGENIC   SINGLE DOSE CONTAINER   **NOT FOR USE IN THE
TREATMENT OF LACTIC ACIDOSIS**   ADDITIVES MAY BE
INCOMPATIBLE   CONSULT WITH PHARMACIST IF AVAILABLE   WHEN
INTRODUCING ADDITIVES USE ASEPTIC TECHNIQUE   MIX
THOROUGHLY   DO NOT STORE   DOSAGE   INTRAVENOUSLY AS
DIRECTED BY A PHYSICIAN   SEE DIRECTIONS   CAUTIONS
SQUEEZE AND INSPECT INNER BAG WHICH MAINTAINS PRODUCT
STERILITY   DISCARD IF LEAKS ARE FOUND   MUST NOT BE USED IN
SERIES CONNECTIONS   DO NOT ADMINISTER SIMULTANEOUSLY
WITH BLOOD   DO NOT USE UNLESS SOLUTION IS CLEAR   FEDERAL
(USA) LAW PROHIBITS DISPENSING WITHOUT PRESCRIPTION
STORE UNIT IN MOISTURE BARRIER OVERWRAP AT ROOM
TEMPERATURE (25ºC/77ºF) UNTIL READY TO USE   AVOID
EXCESSIVE HEAT   SEE INSERT

5

6

7

Baxter

BAXTER HEALTHCARE CORPORATION
DEERFIELD IL 60015 USA

MADE IN USA
DISTRIBUTED IN CANADA BY
BAXTER CORPORATION
TORONTO ONTARIO CANADA

VIAFLEX® CONTAINER
PL 146® PLASTIC

FOR PRODUCT INFORMATION
CALL 1-800-933-0303

8

9

g _____ sodium chloride

osmolarity: _____

Calculate the g of NaCl and dextrose and osmolarity in the following intravenous fluids.

9. FIGURE 7-13

5% dextrose in normal saline.

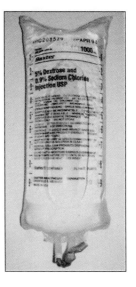

LOT   EXP

2B1064
NDC 0338-0089-04

1

5% Dextrose and 0.9% Sodium Chloride Injection USP

2

3

1000 mL

4

EACH 100 mL CONTAINS   5 g DEXTROSE HYDROUS USP
900 mg SODIUM CHLORIDE USP   pH 4.0 (3.2 TO 6.5)
mEq/L   SODIUM 154   CHLORIDE 154   HYPERTONIC
OSMOLARITY 560 mOsmol/L (CALC)   STERILE NONPYROGENIC
SINGLE DOSE CONTAINER   ADDITIVES MAY BE INCOMPATIBLE
CONSULT WITH PHARMACIST IF AVAILABLE   WHEN INTRODUCING
ADDITIVES USE ASEPTIC TECHNIQUE   MIX THOROUGHLY   DO NOT
STORE   DOSAGE   INTRAVENOUSLY AS DIRECTED BY A PHYSICIAN
SEE DIRECTIONS   CAUTIONS   SQUEEZE AND INSPECT INNER BAG
WHICH MAINTAINS PRODUCT STERILITY   DISCARD IF LEAKS ARE
FOUND   MUST NOT BE USED IN SERIES CONNECTIONS   DO NOT
USE UNLESS SOLUTION IS CLEAR   FEDERAL (USA) LAW PROHIBITS
DISPENSING WITHOUT PRESCRIPTION   STORE UNIT IN MOISTURE
BARRIER OVERWRAP AT ROOM TEMPERATURE (25ºC/77ºF) UNTIL
READY TO USE   AVOID EXCESSIVE HEAT   SEE INSERT

5

6

7

Baxter

BAXTER HEALTHCARE CORPORATION   VIAFLEX® CONTAINER
DEERFIELD IL 60015 USA   PL 146® PLASTIC
MADE IN USA

FOR PRODUCT INFORMATION
CALL 1-800-933-0303

8

9

g _____ dextrose

g _____ NaCl

osmolarity: _____

10. FIGURE 7-14

Calculate the dextrose, NaCl and osmolarity.

5% dextrose in $\frac{1}{2}$ normal saline.

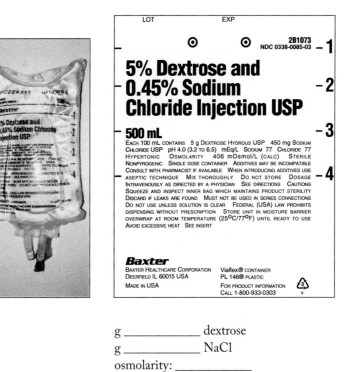

g _____ dextrose

g _____ NaCl

osmolarity: _____

Answers on page 390

WORKSHEET 7E | IV Calculations

Directions: Calculate mL per hr, hours to infuse, and completion time on problems 2, 4, 6 and 8.

1. Ordered: 1500 mL D5W to infuse in 4 hr. How many mL per hr should be delivered?

2. Ordered: 1000 mL of lactated Ringer solution to infuse at 125 mL per hour. The IV was started at 0900. When will the infusion be completed?

3. Ordered: 5 g Rocephin IV to infuse in 6 hr.
   Available: 5 g Rocephin in 1000 mL of D5W.
   How many mL per hour should infuse?

4. Ordered: 1000 mL normal saline with 500 mg erythromycin to infuse in 8 hr. The infusion was started at 0715 hours. When will the infusion be complete?

5. The patient is receiving an IV of D5W at 125 mL per hr. How many grams of dextrose per hour is the patient receiving?

6. Ordered: 500 mg aminophylline in 250 mL normal saline IVPB to infuse at 30 mL per hr. The IV started at 1330 hours. When will the infusion be complete?

7. Ordered: Magnesium sulfate per 2 g over 4 hr.
   Available: 500 mL D5W with 2 g of magnesium sulfate.
   How many mL per hr should be infused?

8. Ordered: Aminophylline 1 g in 500 mL D5W to infuse at 40 mL per hr.
   Available: 1 g of aminophylline in 500 mL of D5W. The IV was started at 2100 hours.
   When will the infusion be complete?

9. Ordered: 2 g Keflin in 200 mL normal saline IVPB to infuse in 3 hr. How many mL per hour will the infusion device be set for?

10. Ordered: Rocephin 1 gm in 500 mL of normal saline to infuse in 4 hr. At what rate will you set the IV pump?

IV medications must be charted on a flow sheet (Figure 7-15).

HOSPITAL

NURSING CARE RECORD
Medical/Surgical

DATA FLOW RECORD   Date ___1-12-12___

TIME	0600	1600															
PULSE	84	80															
RESPIRATION	20	22															
BLOOD PRESSURE	150/92	152/90															
COUGH/ DEEP BREATH	✓	✓															
INITIALS	JG	CB															

The IV flow sheet may record the vital signs prior to initiating IV therapy and again on every shift. The IV site and location is recorded along with the time and date it was started.
The catheter type and needle size are recorded next to the type and rate of the IV solution.
Additional IV solutions are recorded in the date/time inserted column. When the IV is discontinued, the reason is recorded under the comments column.

IV THERAPY

SITE	DATE/TIME INSERTED	SITE LOCATION	CATH TYPE/ SIZE	IV SOLUTION	RATE	DEVICE	TUBING CHANGE	APPEARANCE 7-3	3-11	11-7	SITE D/C'd	COMMENTS
R	1-12-12 0600	LPF	22 angio	1000 D5W	75°			1				
R	1-12-12 1900	LPF	22 angio	1000 D5W	75°		△		1			
R	1-12-12 2200	LPF	22 angio						2		✓	*Slight redness noted at site pt denies pain or tenderness.*

HEALTH DEVIATION NEEDS

DCP ASSESSED: In Progress ☐   Revise Plan ☐
DCP Conference ☐ _____

REFERRAL MADE: SS ☐   HHC ☐   Dietary ☐   Pharmacy ☐
Other _____

PATIENT/FAMILY TEACHING:
Pt/Other _____
_____
_____
_____

_____   PT/FAMILY TEACHING RESPONSE CODES
_____   1 = Received Literature
_____   2 = Communicates Understanding
_____   3 = Requires Reinforcement
_____   4 = Previous Experience
_____   5 = Return Demonstration
_____   6 = Objective Achieved
_____   7 = Referral Initiated
_____   8 = Refused
_____   9 = Preprinted Teaching Protocol

IV CODES
Site Location
				Catheter	Appearance
L = Left	AC = Antecubital	UAF = Upper Anterior		S.G. = Swan Ganz	1 = Asymptomatic
R = Right	UA = Upper Arm			H.D. = Hemodialysis	2 = Red
S = Scalp	UPF = Upper Posterior Forearm	LAF = Lower Anterior Forearm		Hick = Hickman	3 = Swollen
Ft = Foot				G = Groshong	4 = Ecchymotic
F = Femoral				Port = Port-A-Cath or other implanted port	5 = Warm
H = Hand	LPF = Lower Posterior Forearm				6 = Cool
W = Wrist			IJ = Internal Jugular		7 = Draining
		SC = Subclavian		I = Introducer	8 = Leaking
				PP = Pace Port	Lumen
					d = distal
					m = middle
					p = proximal

EMOTIONAL SUPPORT CODES
1 = Active Listening
2 = Reassurance/Comfort
3 = Relaxation
   A = Breathing
   B = Visualization/Imagery
4 = Coping Skills Review

△ = Change

PROCEDURES

TIME	DEPT.	MODE	TRANSPORTER	RETURN

INITIAL	SIGNATURE/TITLE	INITIAL	SIGNATURE/TITLE
hz	*J Jahle, RN*		

FIGURE 7-15 Example of an IV therapy medication administration record (MAR).

IV Delivery Sets

Figure 7-16, *A,* shows a primary set. This is the basic set that delivers IV fluids for a short duration. It does not have a port for additions. This is a needleless connector.

Figure 7-16, *B,* shows a primary set with a port for adding piggyback medications. This set has a manual dial for the mL per hr rate.

Safety Systems for IV Ports

Needleless IV systems (Figure 7-17) are designed to protect caregivers from accidental punctures by contaminated needles. The BD SafetyGlide™ needle (Figure 7-18) used to inject medication into IV ports is another measure to avoid accidental punctures.

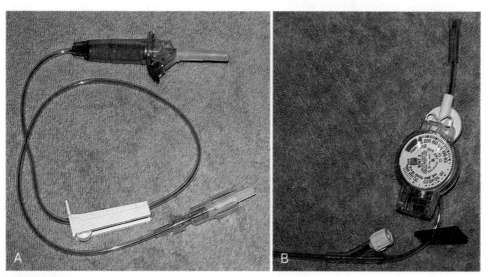

FIGURE 7-16   A, Primary set with a roller clamp to regulate the IV set. **B,** Primary set with a port for adding piggyback medications.

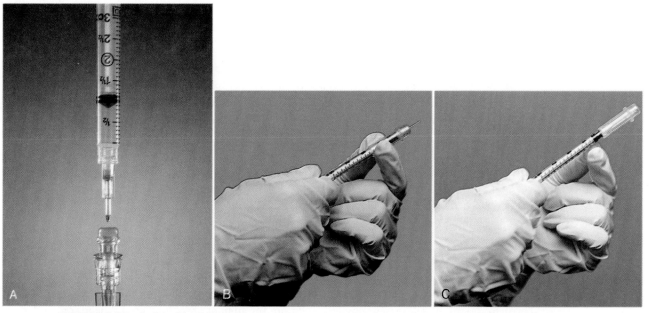

FIGURE 7-17   A, InterLink® IV Access System, an example of a needleless system. **B,** Needle with plastic guard to prevent needle sticks. **B,** Position of guard before injection. **C,** After injection the guard locks in place, covering the needle. (*A,* From Becton, Dickinson, and Company, Franklin Lakes, NJ. *B* and *C,* From Perry AG, Potter PA: Clinical nursing skills and techniques, ed 7, St Louis, 2010, Mosby.)

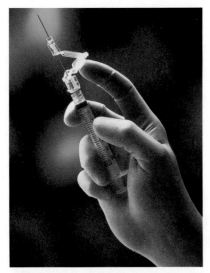

FIGURE 7-18 BD SafetyGlide™ needle. (From Becton, Dickinson, and Company, Franklin Lakes, NJ.)

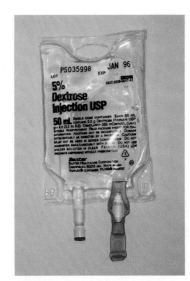

FIGURE 7-19 50 mL of solution for IV piggyback infusion.

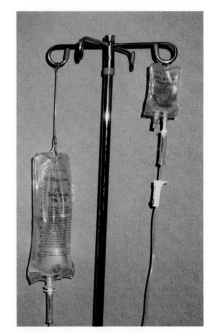

FIGURE 7-20 Gravity flow IV piggyback. The IV piggyback is elevated above the existing IV, allowing it to infuse by gravity.

⊜ *CLINICAL ALERT*

All ports must be cleaned with antiseptic prior to puncture.

Gravity Piggyback Infusions

The acronym for intravenous piggyback is IVPB (Figure 7-19). When special medications are ordered intermittently, the primary IV can be bypassed by introducing the medication through a special entry or portal. Piggyback (PB) medications are infused intermittently via the existing IV line. A secondary IV tube with a needle attachment is inserted into the portal or entry site. The PB infusion amount is usually 50 to 250 mL of medicated solution.

Elevating the IVPB 12 inches above the existing IV allows the PB to infuse by gravity (Figure 7-20). When all of the medication has been infused, the existing IV will resume to the rate set for the PB infusion. The nurse must remember to regulate the primary IV to the previous rate. If an infusion device is used, the IV can be programmed to resume to the primary infusion rate at the completion of the PB.

Piggyback medications are premixed by the pharmacy, drug manufacturer, or nurse. The manufacturer's insert provides recommended times for IVPBs to infuse if the physician does not state the rate in the order.

remember Gravity-flow sets are delivered in drops per minute.

⊜ *CLINICAL ALERT*

The nurse must ensure that the additive medication is compatible with the IV solution.

Piggyback Premixed IVs

Piggyback IV additions are premixed by the pharmacy or the manufacturer. The medication is diluted in 50 to 250 mL of an iso-osmotic sterile solution. The amount of solution used depends on the type of medication, the presence of fluid restrictions, and the weight of the patient.

IVPB admixtures (Figure 7-21) are usually prepared in bulk by the pharmacist for more efficient use of time. If more than one day's supply is prepared, the IVPB can be frozen without altering its stability.

Premixed frozen IVPBs should be thawed in the refrigerator or at room temperature. Never thaw in a microwave oven or in hot or warm water.

All IVPB admixtures must be visually inspected before starting. Check the order, label, medication, strength, and quantity. Make sure that the admixture is clear and free from particles and the expiration date has not passed.

Nurse-Activated Piggyback Systems

The Abbott ADD-Vantage and the Baxter Mini-Bag Plus (Figure 7-22) are used in home care as well as in hospitals and long-term care centers. The IVPB mini-bag has a vial of medication attached to a special port. The pharmacy dispenses the IVPB with the unreconstituted drug vial attached to the mini-bag. At the time of delivery, the nurse breaks the seal between the vial and the mini-bag. This allows the medication to flow into the mini-bag. The medication vial remains attached to the mini-bag, which is a safety feature created to decrease potential medication errors. Figure 7-23 shows the steps for assembling and using the ADD-Vantage system.

Electronic Infusion Devices

Electronic infusion devices are used in hospitals, extended care facilities, home care, and ambulatory care settings. They deliver a set amount of intravenous fluids per hour. Some examples of electronic infusion devices are shown in Figure 7-24. They are individually programmed to deliver a set amount of IV solution per hour.

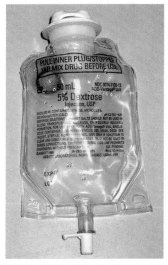

FIGURE 7-21 50 mL of dextrose. Medication can be added for infusion as an IV piggyback.

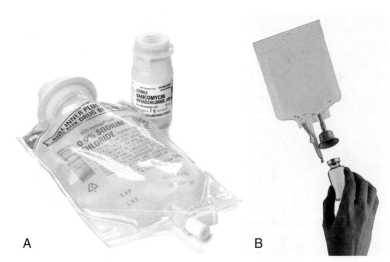

A   B

FIGURE 7-22 **A,** Hospira ADD-Vantage® with a drug vial of vancomycin. **B,** The Mini-Bag™ Plus Container is a "ready-to-mix drug delivery system for reconstituting and administering IV drug dosages. The system consists of a Mini-Bag™ container with a built-in vial adaptor that fits powered drug vials with standard 20-mm closures. The system can be assembled without immediately mixing the drug and diluent. The drug admixture may be prepared just before administration by breaking the seal between the vial and the IV solution container. The medication vial remains attached to the Mini-Bag™ Plus Container, which reduces the potential for medication errors. The Mini-Bag™ Plus Container may be used in home care as well as in hospitals and long-term care centers. (A, From Hospira, Inc., Lake Forest, IL. B, From Baxter Healthcare Corporation, Deerfield, IL.)

ADD-Vantage® System

As Easy as **1, 2, 3**

1 Assemble
— Use Aseptic Technique

Swing the pull ring over the top of the vial and pull down far enough to start the opening. Then pull straight up to remove the cap. Avoid touching the rubber stopper and vial threads.

Hold diluent container and gently grasp the tab on the pull ring. Pull up to break the tie membrane. Pull back to remove the cover. Avoid touching the inside of the vial port.

Screw the vial into the vial port until it will go no further. Recheck the vial to assure that it is tight. Label appropriately.

2 Activate
— Pull Plug/Stopper to Mix Drug with Diluent

Hold the vial as shown. Push the drug vial down into container and grasp the inner cap of the vial through the walls of the container.

Pull the inner plug from the drug vial; allow drug to fall into diluent container for fast mixing. Do not force stopper by pushing on one side of inner cap at a time.

Verify that the plug and rubber stopper have been removed from the vial. The floating stopper is an indication that the system has been activated.

3 Mix and Administer
— Within Specified Time

Mix container contents thoroughly to assure complete dissolution. Look through bottom of vial to verify complete mixing. Check for leaks by squeezing container firmly. If leaks are found, discard unit.

Pull up hanger on the vial.

Remove the white administration port cover and spike (pierce) the container with the piercing pin. Administer within the specified time.

For more information on Advancing Wellness with ADD-Vantage® family of devices, contact your Hospira representative at **1-877-9467(1-877-9Hospira)** or visit www.Hospira.com

®Hospira, Inc. - 275 North Field Drive, Lake Forest, IL 60045

6-131-1-Nov. 04

THE ADD-Vantage® SYSTEM

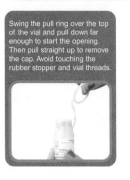
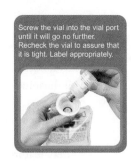
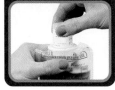
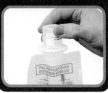
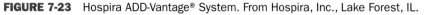

FIGURE 7-23 Hospira ADD-Vantage® System. From Hospira, Inc., Lake Forest, IL.

CADD-Prizm (see Figure 7-24, *A*) is a battery-operated pump that provides IV medications to confined or ambulatory patients. There are four delivery modes:

- Patient-controlled analgesia (PCA)
- Continuous infusion
- Intermittent infusion
- Total parenteral nutrition

⊜ *CLINICAL ALERT*

All ports must be cleaned with antiseptic prior to puncture.

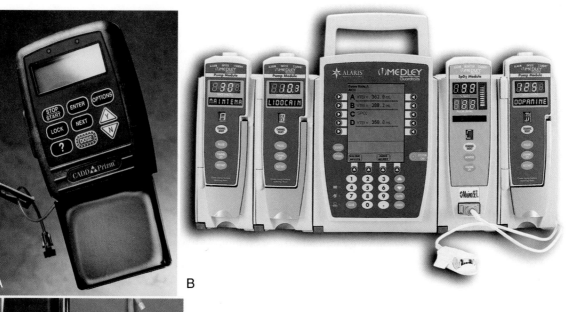

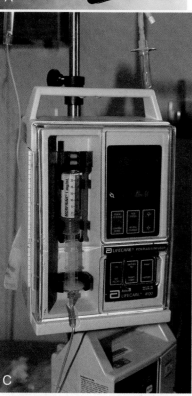

FIGURE 7-24 Electronic infusion devices. **A,** CADD-Prizm VIP ambulatory battery-operated infusion device used for IV parenteral nutrition. **B,** Medley™ Medication Safety System. **C,** A PCA electronic infusion device. (*A,* From SIMS Deltec, Inc., St Paul, MN. *B,* From ALARIS Medical Systems, Inc., San Diego, CA. *C,* From Elkin MK, Perry AG, Potter PA: Nursing interventions and clinical skills, ed 4, St Louis, 2007, Mosby.)

PCA Protocol

The patient-controlled analgesia (PCA) device allows a prespecified amount of narcotic to be available to the patient upon demand. This provides a more constant blood level of analgesia and better pain control (Fig 7-24, *C*). The patient can control the pain level by pushing the control button. Pain medication, usually an opioid such as morphine, is usually the medication of choice. The nurse programs the amount and frequency of the ordered morphine as well as the safety lockout time. The usual programmed amount is minimal effective analgesic concentration (MEAC), which can be *1 mg with a 6-minute lockout; 1.5 mg with a 9-minute lockout* or a *2 mg with a 12-minute lockout*. The device also stores information about how frequenctly the patient pushed the button during the lockout phase. This information allows the nurse to adjust the morphine level or lockout time to achieve the MEAC after consulting with the physician. Evaluation of the patient's pain and respiratory status must be monitored every half hour.

Total Parenteral Nutrition Device

The total parenteral nutrition (TPN) delivery mode allows the infusion of nutritional elements slowly at the beginning of the administration. This keeps the glucose level from rising too rapidly. The system slowly tapers up and then tapers down toward the end of the infusion.

Pressure-Flow Infusion Device

The ambulatory infusion device system was developed for ambulatory use. It can be put in a pocket, inside a shirt, or in any other convenient place where it can be concealed. The flow rate is pre-set. Figure 7-25 shows an example of an ambulatory infusion device.

Piggyback Infusions

Examples
- Ordered: Cefazolin 1 g IV in 50 mL for 30 min. At how many mL per hr should the infusion pump be set?

KNOW   WANT TO KNOW
50 mL : 30 min : : x mL : 60 min   **OR** $\frac{50}{30} = \frac{x}{60} = \frac{300}{3} = 100$ mL per hr

$3\emptyset\ x = 300\emptyset$

$x = 100$ mL per hr

PROOF
$3\emptyset \times 10\emptyset = 30$
$5\emptyset \times 6\emptyset = 30$

Set the infusion pump for 100 mL per hr.

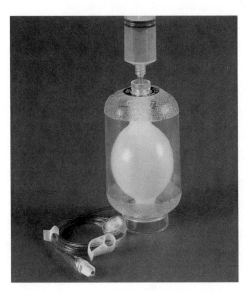

FIGURE 7-25 MedFlo® Post operative pain management system ambulatory infusion device. (From Smith & Nephew Endoscopy, Andover, MA.)

- Ordered: Ampicillin 500 mg IV in 100 mL NS for 45 min. At how many mL per hr should the infusion pump be set?

KNOW   WANT TO KNOW

100 mL : 45 min :: x mL : 60 min   Convert minutes into a decimal

45 x = 100 × 60 = 6000   **OR**   45 min ÷ 60 = 0.75

45 x = 6000

     x = 133.3 = 133 mL per hr   100 mL ÷ 0.75 = 133 mL per hr

> **PROOF**
> 45 × 133.3 = 5998.5
> 60 × 100 = 6000

Set the infusion pump at 133 mL per hr.

CLINICAL ALERT

Electronic infusion devices are set to infuse mL per hr. When administering a small amount of medication for less than 1 hour, the device must be set at mL per hr even though the medication will infuse in less than 1 hour.

Answers on page 391

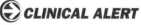

WORKSHEET 7F | Infusion Device and Solute g/mL and gtt/min Calculations

Use the two-step formula to answer the following questions.

1. **Ordered:** 100 mL with 1 g cephalothin to be infused for 30 min by microdrip (microdrip = 60 drops per min).
   a. How many drops per min will be infused on a gravity flow if the drop factor is used?
   b. At how many mL per hr will you set the infusion device?

2. **Ordered:** Aqueous penicillin 600,000 units in 100 mL IVPB to be infused for 1 hr. At how many mL per hr will you set the infusion device?

3. **Ordered:** 250 mL NS to be infused at 150 mL per hr. The drop factor is 15 drops per mL. How long will it take to infuse?

4. **Ordered:** Ampicillin 1 g in 50 mL IVPB ADD-Vantage® System to be infused for 20 min.
   a. At how many mL per hr would you set the infusion device?
   b. How many drops per min will be administered on a gravity flow if the drop factor is 15?

5. **Ordered:** Keflin 2 g in 100 mL IVPB to be infused for 1 hr. The drop factor is 15. How many drops per min is this? At how many mL per hr will you set the infusion device?

6. **Ordered:** Gentamicin 80 mg in 50 mL IVPB to be infused for 30 min.
   a. At how many mL per hr will you set an infusion device?
   b. How many drops per min will infuse for a gravity flow if the drop factor is 60?

7. **Ordered:** 200 mL Foscavir to infuse for 90 min. The drop factor is microdrip.
   a. How many drops per min will infuse?
   b. At how many mL per hr will you set the infusion pump?

8. **Ordered:** 1000 mL 0.9% saline to infuse for 12 hr. The drop factor is 15 drops per mL.
   a. How many drops per min will infuse?
   b. At how many mL per hr will you set the infusion pump?
   c. How many milliliters of sodium chloride will the patient receive?

9. **Ordered:** 2000 mL D5W to be infused for 8 hr. The drop factor is 15 drops per mL.
   a. How many mL per hr will infuse?
   b. How many drops per min will infuse?
   c. How many milliliters of dextrose will the patient receive in 8 hours?

10. **Ordered:** Kantrex 300 mg in 150 mL IVPB. Label reads to infuse for 40 to 60 min. The drop factor is microdrip.
    a. What is the fastest rate for the IVPB to infuse? At what rate will you set the infusion device?
    b. What is the slowest rate for the IVPB to infuse? At what rate will you set the device?

Answers on page 393

 WORKSHEET 7G | **Multiple-Choice Practice**

Circle the letter of the correct answer in the following problems. Remember: To convert tenths of an hour into minutes, multiply by 60. Example: 0.65 hr × 60 = 39 min

1. **Ordered:** 2500 mL to be infused for 24 hr. Available: An IV tubing with 15 drops per mL. At what rate will you set the IV device?
   a. 52 drops per min   b. 35 drops per min   c. 26 drops per min   d. 104 drops per min

2. Administer 50 mL of an IV antibiotic for 15 min. The IV set is calibrated at 15 drops per mL. At how many drops per min will you set the rate?
   a. 100 drops per min   b. 60 drops per min   c. 25 drops per min   d. 50 drops per min

3. **Ordered:** 50 mL piggyback to be infused for 30 min. The drop factor is 20. At how many drops per min will you set the rate?
   a. 17 drops per min   b. 100 drops per min   c. 20 drops per min   d. 33 drops per min

4. **Ordered:** 300 mL of 0.9% NS for 6 hr. The IV set is microdrip. At how many drops per min will you set the rate?
   a. 60 drops per min   b. 50 drops per min   c. 30 drops per min   d. 45 drops per min

5. **Ordered:** Dobutrex 150 mg in 150 mL Ringer's lactate (RL). The infusion device is set at 12 mL per hr. How long will it take to infuse?
   a. 6 hr, 15 min   b. 12 hr, 50 min   c. 8 hr, 15 min   d. 12 hr, 30 min

6. The IV is infusing at 30 drops per min. The drop factor is 20 drops per mL. The IV bag label reads 500 mL of 0.45% NS. How many hours will it take to infuse?
   a. 5 hr, 50 min   b. 3 hr, 36 min   c. 4 hr, 40 min   d. 5 hr, 30 min

7. Calculate the infusion time for an IV of 1000 mL of D5W infusing at 25 drops per min with a drop factor of 10 drops per mL.
   a. 6 hr, 40 min   b. 6 hr, 10 min   c. 5 hr, 57 min   d. 4 hr, 17 min

8. A pint of blood (500 mL) is hung at 1100 hours. The flow rate is 42 drops per min. The drop factor on the administration set is 10 drops per mL. When will the infusion be complete?
   a. 1733 hours   b. 1920 hours   c. 1300 hours   d. 1654 hours

9. Tridil is infusing at 30 mL per hr. The IV label reads: *500 mL D5W with Tridil 5 mcg per 3 mL.* How many hours will it take to infuse?

    a. 15 hr, 10 min   **b.** 18 hr, 45 min   **c.** 16 hr, 40 min   **d.** 12 hr, 48 min

10. **Ordered:** Amicar 5 g in 250 mL for 2 hr. At how many mL per hr should the infusion device be set?

    a. 150 mL per hr   **b.** 100 mL per hr   **c.** 175 mL per hr   **d.** 125 mL per hr

Critical Thinking Exercises

Analyze the following scenarios

1. It is the change of shift. The patient with congestive heart failure (CHF) is being infused with an IV of 1000 mL D5W. The patient complains of being very short of breath. After checking the IV rate, you find that it is infusing at 175 mL per hr. Taking into consideration the patient's diagnosis, you check the IV order and it reads 500 mL D5W in 24 hr.

    Ordered:

    Given:

    Error(s):

    Potential adverse drug event:

    Preventive measures:

    Discussion
    • What would be your first action?
    • What are the serious effects that might jeopordize the patient's safety?
    • At what rate should the IV be infusing?
    • How can this type of error be reconciled to reduce potential risks?

2. Mr. K. has been transferred from the PACU to the surgical floor at 1400 hr after having a pneumonectomy. An IV with 1 gram of Rocephin in 500 mL of D5W is infusing at 42 mL per hr. The PACU nurse indicated on the chart that she had given Mr. K. 4 mg of morphine IV push about 10 minutes ago. Orders are to continue the Rocephin and start a PCA with 1 mg of morphine with a 6-minute lockout. At 1800 hr the nurse noticed that Mr. K. has pushed the lockout button three times, which indicated that the dose of 1 mg every 6 minutes was not adequate. The physician then gave a verbal order to increase the dosage to 1.5 mg. The nurse increased the morphine to 1.5 mg. At 2200 hr the evening nurse reported that Mr. K.'s respirations were 10 per min.

    Discussion

    What will be your first action?

    What is the potential risk to the patient?

    Was the physician's order incomplete?

    How frequently should a patient on a PCA be checked?

    What is the protocol for a lockout time for 1.5 mg of morphine?

    To promote safety using a PCA, how would you reconcile this error?

3. Your 75-year old patient, Mrs. J. has an IV of Ampicillin 1 g in 500 mL D5W to be infused in 6 hours. The IV was started at 0730 hr. At 0830 hr when you checked the IV, you notice that Mrs. J.'s face is flushed. You ask if she feels OK and she answers yes. The nurse asks Mrs. J. if she has any allergies and she said that a long time ago when she was little she had a rash when she was given what she thought was penicillin but never thought anything more about it because it was so long ago. The nurse checked Mrs. J.'s chart and found that Penicillin was listed as an allergy. At 1030 hr Mrs. J. was frightened and said she has a hard time breathing and feels as if her throat is closing. At this time the nurse stopped the IV and notified the physican, and then gave the patient Epinephrine, as was the protocol for allergy emergencies. The nurse noticed that the IV had 150 mL left to be infused.

Discussion:

Do you think the nurse acted prudently?

What was the correct rate for IV? At what rate was it infusing?

What was the potential risk to the patient?

How can a situation like this be reconciled for patient safety?

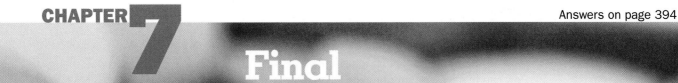

CHAPTER 7

Final

Answers on page 394

1. **Ordered:** 3000 mL for 24 hr. The drop factor is 15. How many drops per min will infuse via a gravity device?

2. **Ordered:** 75 mL to be infused for 45 min. The drop factor is 10. At how many mL per hr will you set the infusion device? How many drops per min will infuse via a gravity device if the drop factor is 10?

3. **Ordered:** 1000 mL to be infused for 12 hr IV. At how many mL per hr will you set the infusion device? How many drops per min will be administered via a gravity device if the drop factor is 20?

4. **Ordered:** 1200 mL to be infused for 8 hr. The drop factor is microdrip. How many drops per min will infuse using a gravity device?

5. **Ordered:** Infuse 2000 mL D5W for 24 hr. The drop factor is 10. At how many mL per hr will you set the infusion device? How many drops per min will be administered using a gravity device?

6. **Ordered:** 1500 mL NS to infuse for 12 hr. The drop factor is 15. How many mL per hr will be administered? How many drops per min will infuse?

7. **Ordered:** 3000 mL D5W to infuse for 24 hr with 0.5 g of penicillin in each 1000 mL. The drop factor is 20, by microdrip. How many mL per hr will infuse? How many drops per min will be administered?

8. **Ordered:** 200 mL cefazolin to infuse for 45 min via the infusion device. At how many mL per hr will you set the infusion device?

9. **Ordered:** 1000 mL to run for 12 hr on microdrip. At how many drops per min will you regulate the flow?

10. **Ordered:** 250 mL to infuse for 90 min. How many mL per hr will infuse if the electronic infusion device is used? How many drops per min will infuse using a drop factor of 15?

ⓔvolve **Refer to the Intravenous Calculations section of Drug Calculations Companion, version 4 on Evolve for additional practice problems.**

Advanced Intravenous Calculations

8

Objectives
- Calculate milligrams per kilogram and micrograms per kilogram per minute and per hour.
- Calculate hourly drug dose and hourly flow rate for IV solutions.
- Estimate and calculate infusion rates and drug doses using ratio and proportion.
- Calculate time and dose intervals for direct IV push (bolus) medications administered by a syringe.
- Evaluate existing infusions for correct flow rate and/or drug dose, and obtain order to change if incorrect.
- Analyze IV medication errors using critical thinking.

Introduction
This chapter builds on the mastery of the basic IV calculations learned in Chapter 6. Taking the time to work through each set of problems will facilitate the acquisition of the logic needed to solve complex IV solution calculations. When each step has been mastered, you will be able to identify and use basic safe calculation shortcuts.

Advanced IV Calculations

Advanced IV calculations are used to determine the amount of IV drug and flow rate per minute and/or per hour for HIGH-ALERT potent medications based on the patient's weight, condition, and response to treatment. If an infusion device is not available, microdrip tubing should be used with a volume-control device (Figure 8-1 on page 182). High alert medications must be delivered on an IV pump.

The choice of administration and equipment depends not only on the orders and the patient's condition but also on hospital policy, accrediting body policy, the current literature and pharmacy recommendations, and the equipment available.

The nurse must be able to evaluate orders and existing solutions for safe and correct dose/flow rates, preferred routes, and compatibilities with existing solutions. Table 8-1 provides the ISMP's list of High-Alert medications.

Titrated Infusions

Dose/flow rate adjustments may be made, particularly with powerful solutions of medications, based on the patient's condition, weight, and physiologic response to the medication. For example, an order may call for an IV to be **titrated** (adjusted) to maintain a certain blood pressure range. The most potent IV medications are administered and adjusted in micrograms per kilogram per minute or milligrams per kilogram per minute. For purposes of reducing errors and simplifying mathematics in flow rate calculations, many of these infusions now have a standardized **total drug/total volume ratio** of 1:1, 1:2, and 1:4 (e.g., 250 mg/250 mL [1:1]; 250 mg/500 mL [1:2], 250 mg/1000 mL [1:4]). If the patient requires fluid restriction, the physician may order a stronger concentration of drug to solution (4:1 or 2:1 drug in solution, such as 1 g:250 mL [4:1] or 500 mg:250 mL [2:1]).

⊙ CLINICAL ALERT

If you consult flow rate and compatibility charts, examine the source and the date published. If the publisher is a reputable source, such as the laboratory that furnishes the IV solutions in use, and if the chart is current, then take further care to examine the layout and content of the tables to ensure that the information needed is selected.

IV solutions that contain powerful medications are usually prepared by the pharmacy and administered by a volumetric infusion pump. There are several sophisticated devices on the market (Figure 8-1). The data to be entered can range from the traditional mL/hr to drug doses ordered per minute in mg/min or mcg/min, along with the patient's weight, if necessary (mg/kg/min) (Figure 8-2).

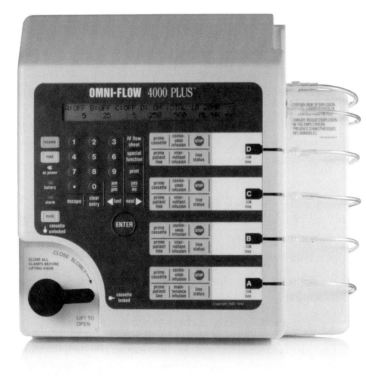

FIGURE 8-1 Omni-Flow® 4000 Plus Medication Management System 4-Channel IV Pump. (From Hospira, Inc., Lake Forest, IL.)

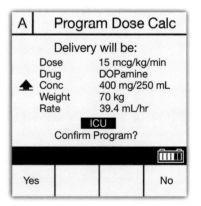

FIGURE 8-2 Plum A+® Drug Confirmation Screen. (Note that this machine shows a delivery rate in tenths of a mL/hr.) (From Hospira, Inc., Lake Forest, IL.)

Table 8-1 ISMP's List of *High-Alert* Medications

Institute for Safe Medication Practices

ISMP's List of *High-Alert Medications*

High-alert medications are drugs that bear a heightened risk of causing significant patient harm when they are used in error. Although mistakes may or may not be more common with these drugs, the consequences of an error are clearly more devastating to patients. We hope you will use this list to determine which medications require special safeguards to reduce the risk of errors. This may include strategies like improving access to information about these drugs; limiting access to high-alert medications; using auxiliary labels and automated alerts; standardizing the ordering, storage, preparation, and administration of these products; and employing redundancies such as automated or independent double-checks when necessary. (Note: manual independent double-checks are not always the optimal error-reduction strategy and may not be practical for all of the medications on the list).

Classes/Categories of Medications
adrenergic agonists, IV (e.g., epinephrine, phenylephrine, norepinephrine)
adrenergic antagonists, IV (e.g., propranolol, metoprolol, labetalol)
anesthetic agents, general, inhaled and IV (e.g., propofol, ketamine)
antiarrhythmics, IV (e.g., lidocaine, amiodarone)
antithrombotic agents (anticoagulants), including warfarin, low-molecular-weight heparin, IV unfractionated heparin, Factor Xa inhibitors (fondaparinux), direct thrombin inhibitors (e.g., argatroban, lepirudin, bivalirudin), thrombolytics (e.g., alteplase, reteplase, tenecteplase), and glycoprotein IIb/IIIa inhibitors (e.g., eptifibatide)
cardioplegic solutions
chemotherapeutic agents, parenteral and oral
dextrose, hypertonic, 20% or greater
dialysis solutions, peritoneal and hemodialysis
epidural or intrathecal medications
hypoglycemics, oral
inotropic medications, IV (e.g., digoxin, milrinone)
liposomal forms of drugs (e.g., liposomal amphotericin B)
moderate sedation agents, IV (e.g., midazolam)
moderate sedation agents, oral, for children (e.g., chloral hydrate)
narcotics/opiates, IV, transdermal, and oral (including liquid concentrates, immediate and sustained-release formulations)
neuromuscular blocking agents (e.g., succinylcholine, rocuronium, vecuronium)
radiocontrast agents, IV
total parenteral nutrition solutions

Specific Medications
epoprostenol (Flolan), IV
insulin, subcutaneous and IV
magnesium sulfate injection
methotrexate, oral, non-oncologic use
opium tincture
oxytocin, IV
nitroprusside sodium for injection
potassium chloride for injection concentrate
potassium phosphates injection
promethazine, IV
sodium chloride for injection, hypertonic (greater than 0.9% concentration)
sterile water for injection, inhalation, and irrigation (excluding pour bottles) in containers of 100 mL or more

Background
Based on error reports submitted to the USP-ISMP Medication Errors Reporting Program, reports of harmful errors in the literature, and input from practitioners and safety experts, ISMP created and periodically updates a list of potential high-alert medications. During February-April 2007, 770 practitioners responded to an ISMP survey designed to identify which medications were most frequently considered high-alert drugs by individuals and organizations. Further, to assure relevance and completeness, the clinical staff at ISMP, members of our advisory board, and safety experts throughout the US were asked to review the potential list. This list of drugs and drug categories reflects the collective thinking of all who provided input.

© ISMP 2008

⊖ CLINICAL ALERT

It has been recommended that all high-alert drug calculations be double checked independently by a second licensed person.

Institute for Safe
Medication Practices
www.ismp.org

New High Technology Infusion Devices Called "Smart Pumps"

A variety of infusion pump devices have been developed to reduce medication errors. Grave adverse drug events with powerful IV pump-infused drugs have occurred due to programming errors such as entering mL for mg, mg for mcg, or pounds for kg.* The smart pumps are preprogrammed with specific guidelines on kg weight-based dose limits, and usual doses for drugs used in specialized clinical areas such as adult and infant ICU areas, obstetrics, and so on. Hospital pharmacies often manage the multiple sources of preprogrammed software information including drug libraries and specific patient care area safe dose ranges.

The nurse selects the drug from the software on the pump, enters the drug concentration, the order, and the patient's weight in kg to obtain the flow rate and is "alerted" if the data entered exceed safe dose limits for the target population. Some smart pumps also alert the nurse if the same drug is being infused on another line. All alerts are logged so that problems can be audited by the agency's safety committees.

---

*Kg-based weights for drugs are the standard recommendation.

⊛ CLINICAL ALERT

Interpretation of drug concentrations on labels; awareness of differences among mcg, mg, mL, and units, and the difference between lb and kg; familiarity with safe dose ranges for the target population, pump equipment operation, and potential equipment flaws all are essential to safe administration. The nurse has a chance to confirm all the data before initiating the flow of the drug.

⊛ CLINICAL ALERT

Although these pumps can reduce errors, the nurse cannot be overly reliant on pump alerts. The alerts depend upon the accuracy and scope of preprogrammed information as well as the function of the pump.

Solving Titrated Infusion Problems

Steps for Solving Titrated Infusion Problems

1. Calculate the safe dose range (SDR) per kilogram per minute (mcg/kg/min or mg/kg/min) from the literature.
2. Compare the SDR in the literature with the physician's order, using the same terms (micrograms or milligrams) and evaluate for the SDR as shown below.
3. If the order is safe, calculate the hourly drug and flow rate using the formula below.

Hourly Drug and Flow Rate Formula for Titrated Infusions

	HAVE				WANT TO HAVE		
TD	:	TV	::	HD	:	HV	
Total drug	:	Total volume	::	Hourly drug	:	Hourly volume	

in
Lowest reduced ratio

One of these will be x.
One of these will be known.

remember IV orders may necessitate converting mcg or mg/min to mg/hr.

▶ **Example**   Ordered: 3 mcg/kg/min of Intropin (dopamine HCl) for a new patient with heart failure. Available: 400 mg dissolved in 500 mL D5W. The literature recommends an initial dose of 2 to 5 mcg/kg/min, (not to exceed a total of 50 mcg/kg/min). The dose is to be titrated to the patient's systolic blood pressure at the level ordered by the physician. This patient weighs 242 lb. What flow rate should be set?

Step 1   **a. Convert** pounds to kilograms using a calculator (2.2 lb = 1 kg).
  242 lb ÷ 2.2 = 110 kg
  b. Calculate the SDR if needed.
  (SDR and order are in the same terms. Calculation is not needed.)

Step 2   **Compare** the SDR recommended in the literature with the order:
  Ordered: 3 mcg/kg/min for new patient
  SDR: 2-5 mcg/kg/min for initial dosing
  Decision: Safe to give. Order is within the SDR.

⊖ *CLINICAL ALERT*

Titrated infusions seldom require a high flow rate. It is essential that the flow rates be correct. Speeding up or slowing down an IV without a physician's order, to compensate for incorrect flow rate, is hazardous. Be aware that abrupt changes in the flow rates of IV fluids and therefore in medication levels can cause serious side effects.

Step 3   **a. Calculate** the ordered hourly drug dose in milligrams (same terms as drug [400 mg] on hand) using a calculator (recalling that 1000 mcg = 1 mg).
  3 mcg × 110 kg × 60 min ÷ 1000 = 19.8 mg/hr, rounded to 20 mg/hr.
  b. Calculate the hourly flow rate (HV) after reducing the total drug/total volume ratio to lowest terms.

$$
\begin{array}{cc}
\textbf{HAVE} & \textbf{WANT TO HAVE} \\
TD : TV & :: HD : HV \\
400 \text{ mg} : 500 \text{ mL} & :: 20 \text{ mg} : x \text{ mL} \\
4 : 5 & :: 20 : x \\
& x = 25 \text{ mL/hr}
\end{array}
$$

Set the flow rate on the IV infusion device to 25 mL/hr.

Alternative   If the hourly volume is known but the hourly drug dose is not, just place the unknown (x) under the
Step 3   hourly drug dose and fill in the hourly volume ordered in this equation. Check the answer with the literature for the SDR (e.g., the order was for 25 mL/hr or is infusing at 25 mL/hr when you arrive; how much drug is the patient receiving per hour and per minute so that the SDR can be checked?).

  Use the same formula. Read the total drug, total volume, and hourly volume on the IV devices in the patient's room:

$$
\begin{array}{cc}
\textbf{HAVE} & \textbf{WANT TO HAVE} \\
TD : TV & :: HD : HV \\
400 \text{ mg} : 500 \text{ mL} & :: x \text{ mg} : 25 \text{ mL} \\
(\text{reduce ratio}) \ 4 : 5 & :: x : 25 \\
5x = 100 & x = 20 \text{ mg/hr of drug being infused} \\
\end{array}
$$
20 mg/hr ÷ 110 kg ÷ 60 min × 1000 mcg = 3 mcg/kg/min

The SDR states 2 to 5 mcg/kg/min. Now you know that the order was followed properly, and that the flow rate is correct and within the SDR. The next few worksheets provide the necessary basic skills practice to understand and perform these calculations rapidly.

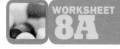

WORKSHEET 8A

Advanced IV Calculation Practice

1. Change the drug per minute to drug per hour in micrograms, then in milligrams, for each given weight. The use of a calculator is permissible, or a ratio of given drug × kg : 1 min :: x drug : 60 min (1000 mcg = 1 mg).

	Drug/kg/min	Weight	mcg/hr	mg/hr
Example	**a.** 5 mcg/kg/min	Wt: 5 kg	$5 \times 5 \times 60 = 1500$	1.500. = 1.5
	b. 8 mcg/kg/min	Wt: 20 kg	_____	_____
	c. 3 mcg/kg/min	Wt: 121 lb	_____	_____
	d. 4 mcg/kg/min	Wt: 50 kg	_____	_____
	e. 20 mcg/kg/min	Wt: 60 kg	_____	_____

2. Reduce the total drug/total volume ratio to lowest terms (e.g., 1000 : 250 = 4 : 1)

	TD : TV	Lowest Ratio
Example	**a.** 250 mg : 1000 mL	1 : 4
	b. 500 mg : 500 mL	_____
	c. 100 mg : 1000 mL	_____
	d. 250 mg : 500 mL	_____
	e. 500 mg : 1000 mL	_____

3. Estimate the value of x (hourly volume) after reducing the ratio of total drug to total volume. The ratio of hourly drug to hourly volume will be the same as total drug to total volume.

	TD : TV :: HD HV	ANSWER
Example	**a.** 250 mg : 1000 mL :: 10 mg : x mL	1 : 4 :: 10 : 40 mL/hr
	b. 500 mg : 500 mL :: 30 mg : x mL	_____ mL/hr
	c. 100 mg : 1000 mL :: 5 mg : x mL	_____ mL/hr
	d. 250 mg : 500 mL :: 3 mg : x mL	_____ mL/hr
	e. 500 mg : 250 mL :: 10 mg : x mL	_____ mL/hr
		_____

4. If you came on duty and evaluated these IV solutions and rates in a patient-care setting, you would estimate the hourly drug after first reducing the total drug/total volume ratio and then examining the rate set on the infusion device.

   Estimate the hourly drug (x).

	TD : TV :: HD : HV	ANSWER
Example	**a.** 250 mg : 250 mL :: x mg : 20 mL	1 : 1 :: 20 : 20 20 mg/hr
	b. 1000 mg : 500 mL :: x mg : 6 mL	_____ __ mg/hr
	c. 250 mg : 500 mL :: x mg : 18 mL	_____ __ mg/hr
	d. 400 mg : 1000 mL :: x mg : 10 mL	_____ __ mg/hr
	e. 500 mg : 250 mL :: x mg : 18 mL	_____ __ mg/hr

5. Change micrograms to milligrams by moving the decimal three places to the left. Reduce the total drug/total volume ratio to the lowest terms. Finally, estimate the hourly volume. (The hourly drug must always be calculated in the same terms as the total drug.)

TD : TV :: HD : HV

ANSWER

Example
a. 250 mg : 1000 mL ::　(4000 mcg) $\underline{4}$ mg : x mL　　$\underline{1 : 4 :: 4 : 16}$ mL/hr
b. 500 mg :　500 mL ::　(9000 mcg) ___ mg : x mL　　_____ mL/hr
c. 1000 mg :　500 mL :: (20,000 mcg) ___ mg : x mL　　_____ mL/hr
d. 250 mg :　500 mL :: (15,000 mcg) ___ mg : x mL　　_____ mL/hr
e. 400 mg :　250 mL ::　(8000 mcg) ___ mg : x mL　　_____ mL/hr

Answers on page 395

WORKSHEET 8B | IV Drug/Flow Rates

Tip: Being able to convert drug, weight, time, and volume parameters within the metric system with ease facilitates advanced IV calculations.

1. Fill in the table by using a calculator and/or by moving decimals.

mg/hr	mcg/hr	mg/min	mcg/min
a. 0.050	50	0.050 = 60 = 0.0008	0.8
b.		0.4	
c. 30			
d.			20
e. 7.5			

2. Fill in the table using a calculator.

kg	mg/hr	mg/kg/min	mcg/kg/min
a. 85	25	25 ÷ 85 ÷ 60 = 0.005	5
b. 70		10	
c. 62			0.1
d. 55	75		
e. 48			50

3. Fill in the table for these IV drug/flow rate calculations using the TD : TV :: HD : HV formula.

IV Contents	TD : TV Reduced Ratio	HD (mg/hr)	HV (mL/hr)	mg/mL
a. 500 mg/1000 mL	1 : 2	5	1 : 2 :: 5 : 10	500 = 1000 = 0.5
b. 250 mg/500 mL			30	
c. 400 mg/250 mL		24		
d. 500 mg/500 mL			75	
e. 500 mg/250 mL		16		

CLINICAL ALERT

Remember that the difference between a microgram (mcg) and a milligram (mg) is "× 1000." The difference between drug per minute and hourly drug is "× 60."

The difference between mcg/kg/min and mcg/min is equal to "× the weight in kilograms." Manipulating these differences is critical for safe medication administration.

Answers on page 395

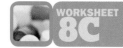

Medication Doses Infusing in Existing Solutions

It is often necessary to verify the amount of drug being delivered in an existing solution. The amount of drug in the IV solution is frequently a milligram dose, whereas the amount of drug the patient is receiving is a microgram dose or a microgram/kilogram dose.

Note the example in Problem 1 and do the following in the remaining problems:
- Set up your TD : TV :: HD : HV ratio and determine mg/hr. Prove your answer.
- Move decimals to change milligrams to micrograms (×1000).
- Use a calculator to change hourly drug (HD) to drug/minute (divide by 60).
- Use a calculator to determine kilograms, and divide micrograms by kilogram weight to obtain mcg/kg/min. Enter all calculator data twice for verification.

Example

1. An IV of Drug Y 100 mg in 1000 mL is infusing at 20 mL/hr. The physician asks, "How many *mg/hr* is the patient receiving? How many *mcg/min*? How many *mcg/kg/min*?" The patient weighs 143 lb today.

   a. TD : TV reduced ratio: 100 : 1000 = 1 : 10
   b. TD : TV :: HD : HV   1 mg : 10 mL :: 2 mg : 20 mL
   c. mg/hr: 2
   d. mcg/hr: 2 × 1000 = 2000
   e. mcg/min: 2000 ÷ 60 = 33.3
   f. mcg/kg/min: 33.3 = 65 kg = 0.5

PROOF	1 × 20 = 20
	10 × 2 = 20

2. An IV of Drug Y 250 mg in 500 mL is infusing at 15 mL/hr. The patient weighs 110 lb today.
   a. TD : TV :: HD : HV reduced ratio:
   b. mcg/hr:
   c. mcg/min:
   d. mcg/kg/min:

PROOF

3. An IV of Drug Y 400 mg in 1000 mL is infusing at 5 mL/hr. The patient weighs 121 lb today.
   a. TD : TV :: HD : HV reduced ratio:
   b. mcg/hr:
   c. mcg/min:
   d. mcg/kg/min:

PROOF

4. An IV of Drug Y 1000 mg in 250 mL is infusing at 10 mL/hr. The patient weighs 132 lb today.
   a. TD : TV :: HD : HV reduced ratio:
   b. mcg/hr:
   c. mcg/min:
   d. mcg/kg/min:

PROOF

5. An IV of Drug Y 500 mg in 250 mL is infusing at 8 mL/hr. The patient weighs 175 lb today. (Calculate kilograms to nearest tenth.)
   a. TD : TV :: HD : HV reduced ratio:
   b. mcg/hr:

   PROOF

   c. mcg/min:
   d. mcg/kg/min:

Answers on page 395

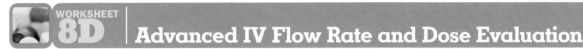

WORKSHEET 8D | **Advanced IV Flow Rate and Dose Evaluation**

Perform the requested calculations. Use a calculator for long division or multiplication. Evaluate flow rates.

▶ Example 1. Nitroprusside sodium infusion is ordered at 0.3 mcg per kg per minute IV and is being infused on a patient with hypertension in a pharmacy prepared solution of 50 mg in 500 mL of D5W. Pharmacy directions instruct to set a flow rate of 12.6 mL an hr for this patient and administer on an IV pump. The patient's weight is 70 kg.
   a. Hourly drug order in mcg: a. 0.3 × 70 × 60 = 1269 mcg per hr
   b. Hourly drug order in mg: b. 1.26 mg per hr (decimal moved 3 places to left)
   c. TD : TV reduced ratio: c. 1:10 (50:500)
   d. Hourly flow rate ordered to   d. 12.6 mL per hr (1 mg:10 mL::1.26 mg:12.6 mL per hr)
      nearest tenth of a mL:
   e. Is the pharmacy direction   e. Yes
      correct?

2. Azithromycin 500 mg IV is ordered for a patient with pelvic inflammatory disease. Directions state that each 500 mg vial must be reconstituted first with 4.8 mL SW to give 100 mg per mL. Further dilute each 500 mg to 250 mL with D5W or other compatible solutions. For 2 mg per mL dilution, give over 1 hr. The nurse you are replacing on shift states that IV rate should be 500 mL per hour.
   a. Mg per mL final dilution:
   b. Is flow rate correct?
   c. If not, what should it be?

3. Cefepime HCl 1 g is ordered IV q12h for a patient with severe pneumonia. Supplied is an ADD Vantage vial. 1 g vial to be diluted to 50 mL with NS in an ADD Vantage infusion container. Dose concentrations between 1 mg per mL and 40 mg per mL are acceptable. Current IV drug reference text for intermittent infusions states, "Infuse over 30 minutes."
   a. Mg per mL concentration after dilution:
   b. Is the concentration safe to administer?
   c. Flow rate to administer over 30 minutes:

4. Pantroprazole sodium 40 mg IV infusion once daily for 10 days is ordered for a patient with severe gastroesophageal reflux disease (GERD). A 40 mg dose is reconstituted first with 10 mL NS and further diluted to total volume of 100 mL with D5W and infused over at least 15 minutes, per label instructions. The IV is programmed when you come on duty for 6.7 mL per minute on a pump.
   a. Mg per mL after first dilution:
   b. Mg per mL after final dilution:
   c. Is the IV program approximately correct?
   d. IV flow rate per hr: (to the nearest tenth of a mL)

CHAPTER 8 Advanced Intravenous Calculations   **189**

5. Cytoxan 5 mg per kg IV two times a week is ordered for an adult patient with malignant disease. The patient's weight is 50 kg. The pharmacy has sent a diluted solution of 250 mg in 250 mL NS. Directions in current pharmacy reference say to infuse over at least 60 minutes. This order is to infuse over 90 minutes. When you arrive on duty, the IV is infusing at 100 mL per hr.

    a. Drug order in mg:

    b. TD : TV reduced ratio:

    c. Hr equivalent of 90 min:

    d. Flow rate in mL per hr:

    e. Is current infusion rate correct?

    f. Nurse action:

⊘ CLINICAL ALERT

Patient Safety Issue: Each nurse needs to refer to manufacturer instructions, current drug references, and personal calculations to protect the patient from prescriber, pharmacy, and prior caretaker IV drug, dosage, and/or flow rate errors and ADE or sentinel events.

    High-risk drugs and powerful drugs are administered on an IV pump. Beware of prescribing, programming, and mechanical errors.

Answers on page 396

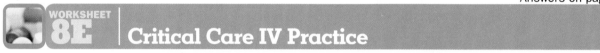

WORKSHEET 8E | Critical Care IV Practice

Evaluate the following orders and infusions for safety. Use a calculator to determine kilogram weights to the nearest tenth. Change micrograms to milligrams, when applicable, by moving decimals. Use a calculator to determine the SDR when needed. Double check and label all calculations. Prove the hourly flow rate calculation. If requested, decide whether the order/infusion is:

1. Safe/Correct

2. Unsafe/Incorrect. Consult with physician.

Example 1. Ordered: Dopamine HCl (Intropin) 4 mcg/kg/min IV for a 110-lb patient. The literature states that the usual dose is 2 to 5 mcg/kg/min. Available: Dopamine 200 mg in 250 mL D5W.

a. Patient's weight in kg:	$110 \div 2.2 = 50$	
b. SDR/min:	$100 - 250$ mcg/min	
c. Is the order safe?	Yes. 4 mcg $\times$ 50 = 200 mcg/min.	
	200 mcg/min is within the SDR	
d. Hourly drug order in mcg:	12,000 (200 mcg $\times$ 60 min)	
e. Hourly drug order in mg*:	12 (decimal moved 3 places to left)	
f. TD : TV reduced ratio:	4 : 5 (200 mg : 250 mL)	
g. Hourly flow rate to be set on infusion device:	12 mL/hr (4 : 5 :: 12 : x)	
	$4x = 60$	**PROOF** $4 \times 15 = 60$
	$x = 15$ mL/hr	$5 \times 12 = 60$

2. Ordered: Dobutamine HCl (Dobutrex) 5 mcg/kg/min IV for a 132-lb patient. Available: Dobutamine 250 mg in 250 mL D5W. The flow rate is currently infusing at 36 mL/hr.
   a. Patient's weight in kg:
   b. Hourly drug order in mcg:
   c. Hourly drug order in mg*:
   d. TD : TV reduced ratio:
   e. Hourly flow rate to be set on infusion device:
   f. Is current infusion correct?
   g. Evaluation and decision:

   PROOF

3. Ordered: Lidocaine 4 mg/min. Available: 1 g of lidocaine in 500 mL of D5W.
   a. TD : TV reduced ratio (mg : mL):
   b. Hourly drug ordered:
   c. Hourly flow rate to be set on infusion device:

   PROOF

4. Ordered: Isuprel (isoproterenol hydrochloride) 5 mcg/min. Available: Isoproterenol hydrochloride 1 mg in 250 mL D5W.
   a. TD : TV reduced ratio:
   b. Hourly drug ordered in mcg and in mg:
   c. TD : TV :: HD : HV ratio:
   d. Hourly flow rate to be set on infusion device:

   PROOF

*Because the available drug (250 mg) is in mg, the hourly drug order must also be entered in mg.

5. Ordered: Initial infusion of norepinephrine at 50 mL/hr. Available: Norepinephrine 1 mg in 250 mL normal saline (NS). The SDR is 8 to 12 mcg/min initially.
   a. TD : TV :: HD :: HV ratio:
   b. Hourly drug being infused in mg:
   c. Hourly drug order in mcg/hr:
   d. Hourly drug order in mcg/min:
   e. SDR for this patient:
   f. Evaluation and decision:

   PROOF

CLINICAL ALERT

Document IVs carefully according to hospital policies. Consult the prescriber if the flow rate needs adjustment.

WORKSHEET 8F | IV Calculations for Obstetrics

Calculate and evaluate the following orders. Remember that the terms must be the same in your TD : TV :: HD : HV ratio and proportion.

Example **1.** Ordered: Magnesium sulfate 2 g/hr IV. Available: Magnesium sulfate 40 g/250 mL Ringer's lactate solution on an infusion device infusing at 13 mL/hr.
   a. TD : TV :: HD : HV   40 g : 250 mL :: 2 g : x mL
   b. mL/hr ordered (HV):   4x = 50, x = 12.5 mL/hr
   c. mL/hr infusing: 13 mL/hr

   d. Evaluation and decision: Rate is correct.

   > **PROOF** 4 × 12.5 = 50
   >   25 × 2 = 50

2. Ordered: Pitocin (oxytocin) 20 milliunits/min. Available: 1000 mL D5NS with 10 units of Pitocin (1000 milliunits = 1 unit). The IV is infusing at 100 mL/hr. (Hint: Change units to milliunits to obtain the total drug equivalent for the equation.)
   a. TD : TV reduced ratio:
   b. TD (milliunits) : TV :: HD (milliunits) : HV ordered:
   c. Evaluation and decision:

   > **PROOF**

3. Ordered: Terbutaline 10 mcg/min for 30 min. Available: Terbutaline 5 mg in 500 mL/D5W.
   a. TD : TV reduced ratio:
   b. Hourly drug ordered in mcg:
   c. Hourly drug ordered in mg:
   d. TD : TV :: HD : HV ratio:
   e. Hourly flow rate to be set on infusion device:

   > **PROOF**

4. Ordered: Magnesium sulfate 25 mL/hr. Call the doctor when 2 g have been infused. Available: 500 mL D5W with 20 g of magnesium sulfate on infusion device.
   a. TD (g) : TV reduced ratio in infusion:
   b. TD : TV :: HD : HV (existing infusion):
   c. g/hr ordered at 25 mL/hr:
   d. Length of time 2 g to be infused:

   > **PROOF**

5. Ordered: Pitocin (oxytocin) 2 milliunits/min. Available: 10 units Pitocin in 1000 mL of D5NS.
   a. milliunits/mL of Pitocin in IV container:
   b. TD : TV reduced ratio:
   c. Hourly drug ordered:
   d. TD : TV :: HD : HV ratio:
   e. Flow rate on infusion device to be set:

   > **PROOF**

WORKSHEET 8G | **More IV Practice Problems**

Calculate and evaluate the following infusion problems.

1. Ordered: Esmolol hydrochloride at 39 mL/hr. Available: 5 g in 500 mL 5% D Ringer's lactated solution. The patient weighs 143 lb. The SDR is 50 to 200 mcg/kg/min.
   a. Patient's weight in kg:
   b. SDR for this patient in mcg/min:
   c. SDR in mg/hr:
   d. TD : TV :: HD : HV ratio ordered:
   e. Hourly drug delivered in mg:
   f. mg/min ordered:
   g. mcg/min ordered:
   h. mcg/kg/min ordered:
   i. Evaluation and decision:

2. Ordered: Nitroglycerin IV at 10 mcg/min. Available: Nitroglycerin IV 50 mg in 500 mL D5W. The infusion is flowing at 6 mL/hr.
   a. TD : TV :: HD : HV ratio ordered:
   b. Hourly drug ordered in mg:
   c. TD : TV :: HD : HV infusing
   d. mcg/min being delivered:
   e. Is flow rate correct?
   f. Evaluation and decision:

3. Ordered: Pronestyl (procainamide hydrochloride) at 50 mL/hr. Available: 1 g in 500 mL D5W. The SDR for maintenance is 1 to 6 mg/min.
   a. TD : TV :: HD : HV ratio:
   b. Hourly drug delivered in mg:
   c. mg/min ordered:
   d. Evaluation and decision:

4. Ordered: Nipride (sodium nitroprusside) at 0.3 mcg/kg/min. Available: 50 mg sodium nitroprusside in 250 mL NS. The infusion is flowing at 15 mL/hr. The patient weighs 220 lb.
   a. Weight in kg:
   b. Hourly drug ordered in mg:
   c. TD : TV :: HD : HV ratio ordered:
   d. TD : TV :: HD : HV ratio infusing:
   e. Hourly drug infusing in mg:
   f. Evaluation and decision:

5. Ordered: Cardizem (diltiazem hydrochloride) at 15 mg/hr. Available: Diltiazem hydrochloride 125 mg in 25 mL diluent to be added to 100 mL D5W. Infusion is flowing at 15 mL/hr.
   a. TD : TV :: HD : HV ratio:
   b. Evaluation and decision:

Direct IV (Bolus) Administration with a Syringe

Direct IV administration (IV push) is used to administer small amounts of diluted or undiluted medication over a brief period (seconds or minutes), preferably into a vascular access device.

Medications such as morphine, Dilantin, or furosemide may be prepared in a syringe and then delivered directly via an intermittent IV med-lock or the proximal port of an existing continuous IV.

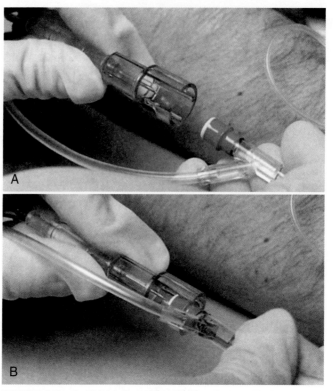

FIGURE 8-3 **A,** Shielded needle infusion system. **B,** Connection into an injection port. (From Perry AG, Potter PA: Clinical nursing skills and techniques, ed 7, St Louis, 2010, Mosby.)

⊖ CLINICAL ALERT

Many of the medications that are administered in this manner must be diluted. A wide barrel (diameter) syringe such as a 10-mL syringe is preferred in order to reduce pressure during administration. Check agency policies for flushes and other direct IV push medications.

It is crucial that the literature be consulted for safe-dose limits, rates of flow, dilutions, compatible solutions, and routes, and that the patient's response be closely monitored during the administration and afterwards.

To reduce needlestick injuries, the trend is to use infusion systems with safety features (Figure 8-3).

There are two ways to time IV push medications for direct administration of medication through a syringe. Regardless of the method you select, the first step is always to calculate and prepare the correct volume.

Timing IV Push Medications—Method 1 (mL per Minute)

This method calculates the amount in milliliters to be slowly and gradually pushed over each minute.

Formula   TV   :   TM   :: x mL   : 1 min
Total volume : Total minutes :: x volume (mL) : 1 min

▶ **Example**   Ordered: Digoxin 0.5 mg IV over 5 min. Dilute to 4 mL sterile water for injection.

TV : TM :: x mL : 1 min

4 mL : 5 min :: mL : 1 min

$$\frac{\cancel{5}}{\cancel{5}}x = \frac{4}{5}$$

$x = 0.8$ mL to be pushed slowly each minute

PROOF	$4 \times 1 = 4$
	$5 \times 0.8 = 4$

1600 : 00   4 mL in syringe
            1601   3.2 mL remaining
            1602   2.4 mL remaining
            1603   1.6 mL remaining
            1604   0.8 mL remaining
            1605   0 remaining

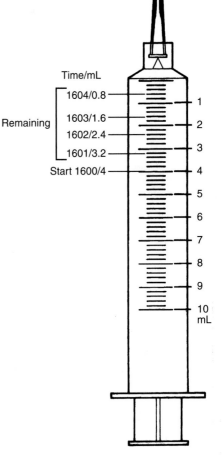

Time/mL

Remaining
1604/0.8 ———— 1
1603/1.6 ———— 2
1602/2.4 ———— 3
1601/3.2 ————
Start 1600/4 ———— 4
5
6
7
8
9
10
mL

The schedule above reflects a start time of 1600 hours. It is helpful to write your start time and a schedule of "markers" (increments of time and volume) when you need to push over several minutes. Write this before beginning to inject and have it in front of you to avoid errors caused by distraction.

Safety syringes and needleless syringes are being used to reduce needlestick injuries (Figure 8-4).

Timing IV Push Medications—Method 2 (Seconds per Calibration)

Many IV push medications have dilutions that permit 1 mL/min so that the timing is easy to maintain. Occasionally, when the timing is to be very slow and is not 1 mL/min, counting seconds per calibration permits more precise timing of the injection.

RULE   Divide the number of seconds of total time of administration by the number of calibrated increments in a syringe prepared with medication (lines on the syringe within each milliliter). This will yield the seconds per increment to be pushed.

Formula $\dfrac{\text{Total seconds}}{\text{Total increments}}$ = Seconds to deliver each increment

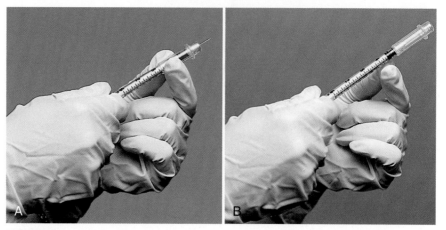

FIGURE 8-4 Needle with plastic guard to prevent needle sticks. **A,** Position of guard before injection. **B,** After injection, the guard locks in place, covering the needle. (From Perry AG, Potter PA: Clinical nursing skills and techniques, ed 7, St Louis, 2010, Mosby.)

Example Give 0.5 mg digoxin IV over 5 min. Directions say to dilute to 4 mL of sterile water for injection. There are 20 calibrations in 4 mL on this syringe.

$$\frac{300 \text{ seconds}}{20 \text{ calibrations } (0.2 \text{ mL ea})} = 1 \text{ calibration } (0.2 \text{ mL}) \text{ every 15 seconds}$$

Use the second hand on your watch and/or count each cycle (1 to 15) as you administer the medication, 1 calibration (0.2 mL) every 15 seconds.

Tip: start count when the second hand is on 12.

4 mL occupies
20 calibrated lines
5 minutes = 300 seconds

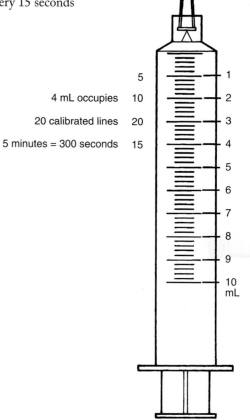

WORKSHEET 8H | IV Push Calculations

Solve the following problems using the syringes shown to calculate the seconds per calibration, if applicable, and mL/min to be administered.

1. Ordered: 10% calcium chloride (10 mL) over 5 min.
   a. For how many seconds will you administer each calibration?
   b. How many mL/min will be injected?

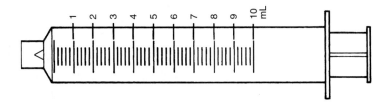

2. Ordered: Digoxin 0.5 mg IV over 10 min. (The literature specifies a minimum of 5 min for administration.) Available: Digoxin 250 mcg/mL.
   a. Total mL you will inject:
   b. Total seconds for injection:
   c. Seconds per calibration:
   d. mL/min to be injected:

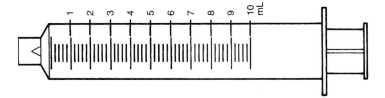

3. Ordered: Phenytoin sodium IV loading dose of 900 mg at 50 mg/min on an infusion device (Figure 8-5). Available: Phenytoin 100 mg/mL.
   a. Total mL to be injected:
   b. Total time for injection:
   c. mL/min to be administered:

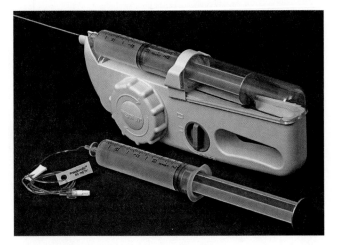

FIGURE 8-5 Freedom 60 infusion pump. This portable reusable manual infusion uses standard 60 mL syringes and can be filled from 1 to 60 mL. It offers flow rates with rate-controlled tubing from 0.5 to 1200 mL per hr. It does not permit free flow. From Repro-Med Systems, Inc., Chester, NY.

4. Ordered: Furosemide 20 mg IV undiluted over 2 min. Available: Furosemide 10 mg/mL.
   a. Total mL to be injected:
   b. Total time in seconds:
   c. Seconds per calibration:
   d. mL/min to be administered:

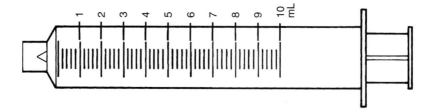

5. Ordered: Morphine Sulfate 4 mg IV injection. The literature states that a single dose should be administered over 4 to 5 min and that the dose may be diluted in 4 to 5 mL with sterile water or normal saline for injection. The nurse dilutes it to 5 (mL) with NS.
   a. Total mL to be injected:
   b. Total time in minutes.
   c. mL/min to be administered:

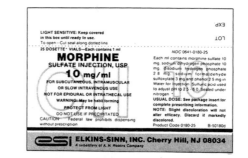

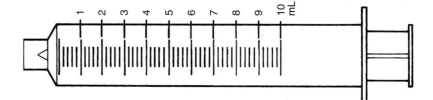

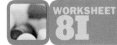

Multiple-Choice Practice

Use a calculator. Estimate your answers for each applicable step in the mathematics. Establish the reduced total drug/total volume ratio for the infusions, move decimals to convert between micrograms and milligrams, and use logical shortcuts such as multiplying by 60 to change minutes to hours where applicable.

1. Ordered: Isoproterenol HCl IV at 5 mcg/min. How many mg/hr would be infused?
   a. 0.5 mg
   b. 50 mg
   c. 0.3 mg
   d. 300 mg

2. Available: Aminophylline 250 mg in 1000 mL of D5W. How many milligrams are in each milliliter of the IV solution (mg/mL)?
   a. 0.25 mg
   b. 0.5 mg
   c. 1 mg
   d. 4 mg

3. Available: 1 g of lidocaine in 500 mL of D5W. What is the total drug ratio in mg to the total volume of IV solution?
   a. 2:1
   b. 4:1
   c. 1:2
   d. 1:4

4. Available: Norepinephrine 1 mg in 250 mL of NS. The SDR is 8 to 12 mcg/min initially. What is the minimum flow rate recommendation in mL/hr? *Hint: Change the SDR to milligrams after you obtain the SDR in mcg/hr so that you can compare milligrams to milligrams.*
   a. 48 mL/hr
   b. 60 mL/hr
   c. 120 mL/hr
   d. 480 mL/hr

5. Ordered: Furosemide 30 mg IV push over 2 min. Available: Furosemide 10 mg/mL. How many mL/min are to be administered?
   a. 0.5 mL/min
   b. 0.7 mL/min
   c. 1 mL/min
   d. 1.5 mL/min

6. Ordered: Lanoxin IV push 0.5 mg over 5 min. Available: Lanoxin 250 mcg/mL. How many mL/min will be injected?
   a. 0.25 mL/min
   b. 0.4 mL/min
   c. 1 mL/min
   d. 1.5 mL/min

7. Procainamide hydrochloride is infusing at 40 mL/hr (per the prescriber order) for maintenance in an adult with an arrhythmia. Available: 1 g in 500 mL D5W. The SDR for maintenance is 1 to 6 mg/min. What decision will the nurse make?
   a. The order is within SDR. Proceed with the IV.
   b. The order is above the SDR. Hold the infusion and clarify with the physician.
   c. The order is below SDR. Start the infusion and consult with the physician.
   d. The order is unclear. Consult with a knowledgable colleague.

8. Ordered: Procainamide hydrochloride at 60 mg/hr on an infusion device. Available: 1 g in 1000 mL D5W. What flow rate in mL/hr will the nurse set?
   a. 30 mL/hr
   b. 60 mL/hr
   c. 100 mL/hr
   d. 120 mL/hr

9. Ordered: Magnesium sulfate 30 mL/hr. Call the physician when 3 g have been infused. Available: 500 mL D5W with 20 g of magnesium sulfate on an infusion device. In how much time will you expect to call the physician at this flow rate? *Hint: Determine how much drug per hour is infusing.*
   a. 30 min
   b. 1 hr 50 min
   c. 2 hr 30 min
   d. 3 hr

10. Ordered: Dobutamine HCl 2.5 mcg/kg/min for a 70-kg patient. Available: Dobutamine HCl IV concentration 500 mcg/mL. What flow rate will you set in mL/hr?
    a. 10 mL/hr
    b. 11 mL/hr
    c. 20 mL/hr
    d. 21 mL/hr

Critical Thinking Exercises

Analyze the following scenarios.

1. During a bedside emergency for ventricular fibrillation, a physician called for Potassium Chloride (KCl) 30 mEq to be added to an IV line of D5W, and for Bretylium tosylate to be given by direct push into a second, separate IV line. As the orders were called out, one nurse prepared the medications and handed them to the nurse who was assisting, who then administered the medications. At one point, the nurse was handed two syringes of medication. She was told that one was bretylium tosylate and that the other syringe contained KCl 30 mEq. The KCl was administered undiluted to the patient by direct push, and the bretylium was placed in D5W.

   Error(s):

   Causes of error(s):

   Potential injuries:

   Nursing actions:

   Preventive measures:

2. A patient in the ICU weighing 60 kg was to receive an IV infusion of Dobutrex ordered to start at 3 mcg/kg/min. The nurse programmed the IV pump to infuse at 3 mg/kg/min.

Error(s):

Causes of error(s):

Potential injuries:

Nursing interventions:

Recommendations for the patient safety committee to prevent this type of error:

3. A patient was admitted with seizures. Phenobarbital 120 mg IV push stat was ordered. The nurse diluted the medication in 3 mL of sterile water for injection. It was administered over 1 minute. Check the label directions.

NDC 0002-7213-01
VIAL No. 358

Lilly

STERILE
PHENOBARBITAL
SODIUM, USP
120 mg
WARNING—May be habit forming.

Store at 59° to 86° F
YD 1101 AMX
Eli Lilly & Co. Indpls, IN 46285 U.S.A.
Expiration Date/Control No.

See accompanying literature for uses and method of administration. To prepare a solution for intramuscular injection, add 1 mL of Sterile Water for injection to the powder in the vial and dissolve.

CAUTION—If used intravenously, dissolve in 3 mL of Sterile Water for Injection. The rate of injection should not exceed 1 mL per minute. Under no circumstances should any solution be injected which is not absolutely clear.

Lyophilized

Error:

Cause(s) of error:

Potential adverse drug event(s) (ADE):
(Refer to side effects of Phenobarbital IV in current IV drug reference)

Nursing interventions and antidotes needed:
(Refer to current IV drug reference)

Recommendations for the patient safety committee to prevent this type of error:

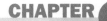
Final

Solve the following problems using a calculator, moving decimals, reducing ratios, and labeling your answers. Prove your work.

Make a decision:

A. Safe to give   **B.** Unsafe; consult with physician

1. Ordered: Dobutamine HCl 5 mcg/kg/min. Available: Dobutamine HCl 2000 mcg/mL in an infusion device. Patient's weight is 50 kg.
   a. mcg/hr needed:
   b. Flow rate to be set on IV infusion device: _____ hr

2. Ordered: Potassium chloride 10 mEq to be administered to a 44-lb child with hypokalemia. Administer over 4 hr. Dilute in 100 mL of D5W. The literature states that the rate should not exceed 3 mEq/kg/24 hr for a child.
   a. Patient's weight in kg:
   b. SDR for this child per 24 hr:
   c. Total drug ordered:
   d. Decision (Safe/Unsafe):
   e. Amount of drug in mL to be added to IV (refer to label for mEq/mL):
   f. Hourly flow rate on infusion device in mL:

POTASSIUM CHLORIDE
For Injection Concentrate, USP

N 63323-965-20   Preservative Free   96520

Concentrate Must Be
Diluted Before Use

40 mEq   (2 mEq/mL)

20 mL Single Dose Vial

MUST BE DILUTED PRIOR TO IV ADMINISTRATION Sterile, Nonpyrogenic. Each mL contains: Potassium chloride 2 mEq (149 mg). Water for injection q.s. HCl and/or KOH may have been added for pH adjustment. 4000 mOsmol/L (calc.) Usual Dosage: See Insert. Store at controlled room temperature 15°-30°C (59°-86°F). Rx only

401701

LOT
EXP

3. Ordered: Dopamine HCl at 2 mcg/kg/min. Infusing when you enter the room: Dopamine HCl at 15 mL/hr. Available: Dopamine HCl 400 mg/500 mL. Patient's weight is 80 kg.
   a. mg/hr needed:
   b. Actual mg/hr infusing:
   c. Flow rate ordered:
   d. Actual flow rate in mL/hr:
   e. Decision (correct or needs order for change):

4. Ordered: Dopamine IV at 4 mcg/kg/min for a patient in septic shock who weighs 110 lb today. The SDR is 2 to 10 mcg/kg/min. The IV solution contains 200 mg in 250 mL of solution. The IV is flowing at 15 mL/hr when you enter the room.
   a. Patient's weight in kg:
   b. SDR for this patient:
   c. Ordered drug rate/min:
   d. Decision (Safe/Unsafe):
   e. TD : TV ratio:
   f. mg/hr of drug ordered:

g. Hourly flow rate needed:

h. Decision (correct or needs order for change):

LOT   EXP

200 mg   2B0832
NDC 0338-1005-02

Dopamine   <u>50</u>

(800 mcg/mL)
Dopamine Hydrochloride
and 5% Dextrose Injection USP   <u>100</u>

250 mL

Each 100 mL contains 80 mg Dopamine   <u>150</u>
Hydrochloride USP 5 g Dextrose Hydrous USP
5 mEq/L Sodium Bisulfite added as a stabilizer pH
adjusted with hydrochloric acid pH 3.5 (2.5 to
4.5) Osmolarity 261 mOsmol/L (calc) Sterile
Nonpyrogenic Single dose container Drug
additives should not be made to this solution
Dosage Intravenously as directed by a physician
See directions Cautions Must not be used in
series connections Do not administer   **200**
simultaneously with blood Do not use unless
solution is clear and is not darker than slightly
yellow Federal (USA) law prohibits dispensing
without prescription

Baxter

Baxter Healthcare Corporation Viaflex® Plus container
Deerfield IL 60015 USA   PL 2207 plastic

Made in USA   For product information
                     Call 1-800-933-0303   v

5. Ordered: Dilaudid (hydromorphone HCl) 3 mg direct IV for a patient with severe pain.
Directions state it may be given undiluted slowly or diluted up to 5 mL with SW or NS to facilitate titration. It may be administered over 2 to 5 minutes slowly. The nurse dilutes it to 3 mL
and plans to administer it over 3 minutes.*

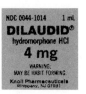

NDC 0044-1014   1 mL
DILAUDID®
hydromorphone HCl
4 mg
WARNING:
MAY BE HABIT FORMING.
Knoll Pharmaceuticals
Whippany, NJ 07031

a. Total amount of Dilaudid to be prepared (in mL, round to nearest tenth):

b. Total amount of diluted volume to be administered in mL:

c. Total number of minutes for injection:

d. Amount in mL/min to be administered:

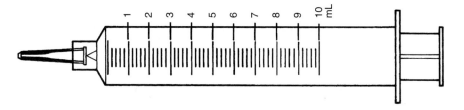

🜲 CLINICAL ALERT

*When small amounts of medication are ordered, dilution makes it easier to con-
trol the rate of injection. This nurse wants to administer 1 mL per minute for ease
of administration. There were other options. Always read the directions for dilution
and rate of administration. If the patient begins to have side effects, the medication will be withdrawn. It is safer and always preferable to inject into an existing IV
port or line so that side effects can be countered quickly when necessary.

⊝volve **Refer to the Advanced Calculation section of Drug Calculations Companion, version 4 on
Evolve for additional practice problems.**

Parenteral Nutrition

Objectives
- Calculate grams of protein, dextrose, and lipids per order.
- Calculate the percentage of protein, dextrose, and lipids per infusion.
- Discuss the reasons that different concentrations of additives are used in peripheral and central lines.
- Calculate the percentage of additives per infusion.
- Calculate the kilocalories for protein, dextrose, and lipids per infusion.
- Calculate the total kilocalories per infusion.
- Compare the ordered amount of parenteral nutrition with the infusion label.
- Analyze medication errors using critical thinking.

Introduction The IV requirements for patients who are unable to ingest food are calculated on a daily basis. Concentrations of nutrients are calculated to show the differing strengths and percentages of additives for peripheral and central lines. The percentage of additives is calculated to ensure that the electrolyte and mineral requirements are being met. Standard orders for peripheral and central lines are compared. Medication administration records are discussed. The importance of parenteral orders and verification of the labels on the bag are stressed.

Total Parenteral Nutrition

Nutritional support of the sick patient in the hospital as well as in the home has become increasingly important. More people are being treated with total parenteral nutrition (TPN) in the home and it is the nurse's responsibility to teach the patient and the family to care for the catheter insertion site, the infusion pump, and possible side effects of the infusion. Survival of the patient with a gastrointestinal problem is made possible by advances in the field of parenteral nutrition.

⊖ CLINICAL ALERT
Medication incompatibility can occur when IV medications are delivered with TPN administration. A TPN IV pharmacist should be consulted to determine compatibility.

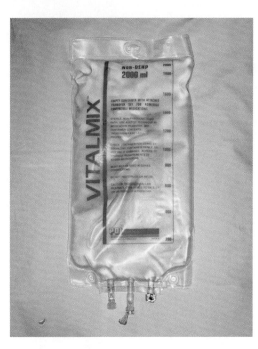

FIGURE 9-1 TPN bag. The content label will be put on the bag by the pharmacist.

TPN permits the venous administration of dextrose, amino acids, lipids, electrolytes, and vitamins to sustain life when the gastrointestinal system must be bypassed or during serious illness or injury (e.g., burns). A TPN bag is shown in Figure 9-1.

A routine maintenance IV solution of 1000 mL with 5% dextrose delivered over an 8-hour period provides approximately 200 calories derived from dextrose. If a patient is restricted from ingesting anything by mouth (npo) and receives 3 liters of D5W a day, the 600 total calories received would not be enough to promote or maintain health for a sustained period. In contrast, TPN may deliver as much as 1 cal/mL, depending on the concentration of nutrients.

TPN is administered via a central vein such as the subclavian or internal jugular. This is known as *central parenteral nutrition (CPN)*. Peripheral administration, known as *peripheral parenteral nutrition (PPN)*, is given via peripheral veins. The choice depends on the patient, the vein condition, and how long the patient will need the therapy. The larger central veins are selected for longer term therapy and higher concentrations of nutrients. The contents of TPN are customized according to the patient's condition and need, the venous route, relevant laboratory values, and the patient's weight. Orders for the contents may be changed daily. Special formulas are created for renal, hepatic, diabetic, burn and cardiac patients. TPN formulas are specific and are determined by energy, protein, fluid, and caloric requirements.

PPN is used for nutritional therapy of 2 weeks or less. A PPN solution must be kept at the following concentration levels to prevent vein irritation: amino acids, 5.5%; dextrose, 10%; lipids, 10%. CPN permits high levels of concentration because it is infused into large veins. CPN solutions are hypertonic and have high osmolarity. CPN is used when nutrition therapy is needed for longer than 2 weeks. CPN concentrations usually are as follows: amino acids, 8.5% to 15%; dextrose, 20% to 70%; lipids, 20%. Dextrose administered with amino acids spares the protein for tissue repair. Parenteral nutrition must always be administered by an infusion pump, **never** by gravity. There are many types of electronic delivery devices. Figure 9-2 shows two such devices.

A three-in-one solution, or total nutrition admixture, combines lipids, amino acids, and dextrose. The solution is white because of the lipids, which make precipitation difficult to observe. The three-in-one solution is used for both hospital and home therapy. When lipids are administered with dextrose and amino acids, the osmolarity of the solution will improve the tolerance for peripheral venous administration. The lipids can also be administered separately (Figure 9-3). Lipids help control hyperglycemia, which is a complication of parenteral nutrition. After 12 hours lipids may become unstable; therefore, monitor carefully. Lipids are isotonic and can therefore be administered either peripherally or centrally. If a fat embolus could be a problem, monitor the patient closely. Amino acids, vitamins, and other life supporting additives are easily denigrated when exposed to sunlight. Home therapy TPN is usually run for 12 hours to give the patient some infusion free time.

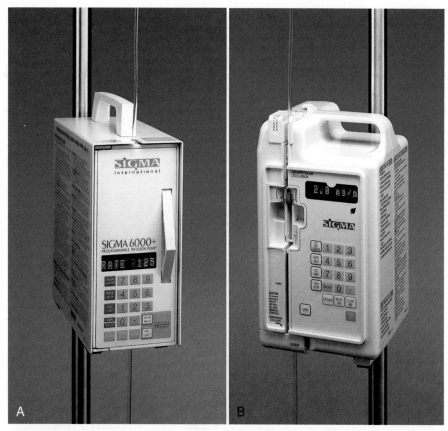

FIGURE 9-2 **A,** Sigma international 6000 programmable infusion device. **B,** Sigma 8000 automatic dose-related calculation device. (From Sigma International, Inc., Medina, NY.)

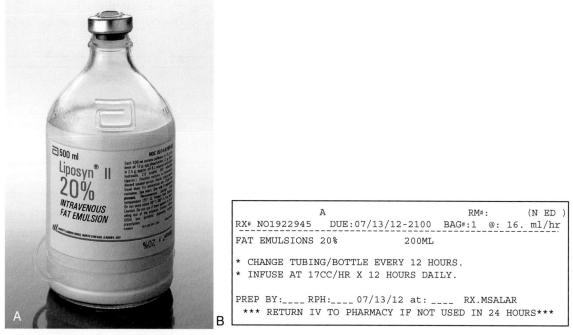

```
                    A                    RM#:         (N ED )
RX# NO1922945   DUE:07/13/12-2100   BAG#:1  @: 16. ml/hr
---------------------------------------------------------
FAT EMULSIONS 20%              200ML

* CHANGE TUBING/BOTTLE EVERY 12 HOURS.
* INFUSE AT 17CC/HR X 12 HOURS DAILY.

PREP BY:____ RPH:____ 07/13/12 at: ____  RX.MSALAR
 *** RETURN IV TO PHARMACY IF NOT USED IN 24 HOURS***
```

FIGURE 9-3 **A,** Liposyn II (fat emulsion) 20% for parenteral nutrition. Notice the opaque contents contrasted with the parenteral infusion without lipids (fat emulsion). **B,** Fat emulsion (lipid) order. (**A,** From Abbott Laboratories, Abbott Park, IL.)

HOME HEALTH		DATE
PATIENT	ADDRESS	

TPN FORMULA:

AMINO ACIDS: ☐ 5.5% ☐ 8.5% ☑ 10% ☐ WITH STANDARD ELECTROLYTES	mL *425*
DEXTROSE: ☐ 10% ☐ 20% ☐ 40% ☐ 50% ☑ 70% (check one)	mL *357*
LIPIDS: ☐ 10% ☑ 20% FOR ALL-IN-ONE FORMULA	mL *125*

FINAL VOLUME qsad STERILE WATER FOR INJECTION *400 mL*	*1248* mL

Calcium Gluconate	0.465 mEq/mL	*5* mEq
Magnesium Sulfate	4 mEq/mL	*5* mEq
Potassium Acetate	2 mEq/mL	mEq
Potassium Chloride	2 mEq/mL	mEq
Potassium Phosphate	3 mM/mL	*15* mM
Sodium Acetate	2 mEq/mL	mEq
Sodium Chloride	4 mEq/mL	*35* mEq
Sodium Phosphate	3 mM/mL	mM
TRACE ELEMENTS CONCENTRATE	☐ 4 ☐ 5 ☐ 6	mL

Patient Additives:

☐ MVC 9 + 3 10 mL Daily

☐ HUMULIN-R *10* units DAILY

☐ FOLIC ACID _____ mg
_____ times weekly

☐ VITAMIN K _____ mg
_____ times weekly

☐ OTHER: *MVI 10 mL/daily*

☐ OTHER: _____

Directions:

INFUSE: ☐ DAILY

☐ _____ TIMES WEEKLY

OTHER DIRECTIONS:

_____

_____

_____

Rate: ☐ CYCLIC INFUSION:	"	☐ CONTINUOUS INFUSION:	"	☑ STANDARD RATE:
OVER _____ HOURS	"	AT _____ mL PER HOUR	"	AT *104* mL PER HOUR
(TAPER UP AND DOWN)	"		"	FOR *12* HOURS

LAB ORDERS:

☐ STANDARD LAB ORDERS
SMAC-20, CO2, Mg+2 TWICE WEEKLY
CBC WITH AUTO DIFF WEEKLY
UNTIL STABLE, THEN:
SMAC-20, CO2, Mg+2 WEEKLY
CBC WITH AUTO DIFF MONTHLY

☐ OTHER: _____

_____

_____

VALIDATION:

_____
DOCTOR'S SIGNATURE

Print Name: _____

Office Address: _____

_____

Phone: _____

WHITE: Home Health   CANARY: Physician

FIGURE 9-4 Sample physician's order form for TPN example calculation on page 209.

Validation of TPN Label With the Physician's Order

Validate the contents listed on the TPN bag label (see Figure 9-5), with the physician's order (Figure 9-6).

The 341 mL of qsad (quantity sufficient additive) sterile water includes the volume for the additives of calcium gluconate, magnesium sulfate, potassium phosphate, sodium chloride, and multivitamins. In this order, the pharmacist included all of the additives (except for the 10 units of insulin, which the nurse will add immediately before administration).

TPN Bag label

```
      HOME  INFUSION  PHARMACY
████████████████████████████████
 RX#37856      █████████
██████████████

AMINO*ACIDS 10%=425ML DEXTROSE*70%=357ML
STER*WATER=341ML LIPIDS*20%=125ML
MVI=10ML/DAY *ADDITIVES PER LITER*
SOD*CHLOR=35mEq POT*PHOS=15mM CALCIUM=5mEq
MAGNESIUM=5mEq


QTY#      TPN 40-51GM PROTEIN+LIPIDS
INFUSE NIGHTLY 8PM TO 8AM THRU IV PICC LINE
VIA SIGMA PUMP. *****ADD 10 UNITS
HUMULIN-R TO EACH BAG JUST PRIOR TO
INFUSION***** **NOTE:CONTAINS TPN
SOLN+LIPIDS:RATE ADJUSTED** SETTINGS:
RATE=104ML/HR VOLUME=1248ML
        *** REFRIGERATE ***

EXPIRATION DATE:01/06/15
```

FIGURE 9-5 TPN bag label. It is the nurse's responsibility to check the label on the TPN bag with the physician's order. Quantities of nutrients and additives are calculated based on 1 liter. The total volume (TV) is calculated by adding the amount over 1 liter as a decimal (e.g., 1248 mL = 1.248 L).

⊖ *CLINICAL ALERT*

The nurse's responsibility is to check the physician's order to determine if the pharmacy has filled the order according to the directions in Figure 9-4. Compare the order with the label (Figure 9-5).

Example   Refer to Figure 9-4, a sample physician's order form.

⊖ *CLINICAL ALERT*

It is not recommended to administer other medications via the Y-port or piggy back before consulting with the pharmacist for compatibility. There can be many metabolic complications due to the type of additives in the TPN solution.

Calculate grams, percentage of concentration, and kilocalories per bag of TPN.

Total Grams Per Bag

Formula: % × mL = g/L

Step 1
Amino acids (AA) 10% in 425 mL
$0.10 × 425 = 42.5$ g/L

Formula: g/L × TV*/L = g/bag

Step 2
42.5 g/L × 1.248 TV/L = 53 g/bag
There are 53 g of AA in 1248 mL of TPN.

Shortcut method: % × mL = g/L × TV/L = g/bag
AA 10% in 425 mL
$0.10 × 425 = 42.5$ g/L × 1.248 TV/L = 53 g

---

*TV, total volume.

To calculate the answer for g/L, multiply by the TV to determine the total g/bag. There are 55.5 g of AA in 1248 mL of TPN.

Shortcut method: % × mL = g/L × TV/L = g/bag

Dextrose 70% in 357 mL
$0.70 \times 357 = 250$ g/L $\times 1.248$ TV/L $= 312$ g/bag

To calculate the answer for g/L, multiply by the TV to determine the total g/bag. There are 312 g of dextrose in 1248 mL of TPN.

Shortcut method: % × mL = g/L × TV/L = g/bag

Lipids 20% in 125 mL

Step 1   Step 2
$0.20 \times 125 = 25$ g/L $\times$ TV/L $1.248 = 31.2$ g/bag
There are 31.2 g of lipids in 1248 mL.

Percentage of Concentration Per Bag

Formula: $\frac{g/bag}{TV} = \%/bag$

AA $\frac{53}{1248} = 0.044 = 4.2\%$ of bag is AA (PRO)

Dextrose $\frac{312}{1248} = 0.250 = 25\%$ dextrose (CHO)

Lipids $\frac{30.2}{1248} = 0.0250 = 25\%$ lipids (FAT)

Percentage of Additives

Formula:	Step 1	**mEq/L × TV/L = mEq/bag**
	Step 2	**mEq/bag ÷ TV = % in bag**
Shortcut method:		mEq/L × TV/L ÷ TV = % in bag
Calcium gluconate		5 mEq × 1.248 TV = 6.24 mEq/bag
		6.24 ÷ 1248 = 0.005 = 0.5% in bag
Magnesium sulfate		5 mEq × 1.248 = 6.24 ÷ 1248 = 0.5% in bag
Potassium phosphate		15 mEq × 1.248 = 18.72 ÷ 1248 = 1.5% in bag
Sodium chloride		35 mEq × 1.248 = 43.68 ÷ 1248 = 3.5% in bag

A milliequivalent (mEq) is a measurement of weight that represents 1000th of a gram.

mL/hr to Set the Pump

$$\frac{TV}{\text{Total Time (hr)}} = \text{mL/hr} \quad \frac{1248}{12} = 104 \text{ mL/hr}$$

Kilocalories (kcal) Per Bag

Formula: kcal/g × g/bag = kcal/bag

1 g CHO = 4 kcal	312 g × 4 kcal = 1248 kcal of CHO
1 g PRO = 4 kcal	53 g × 4 kcal = 212 kcal of PRO
1 g FAT = 9 kcal	31.2 g × 9 kcal = 281 kcal of FAT
	Total kcal = 1741/bag of TPN

⊜ CLINICAL ALERT

Begin TPN at a slow rate of 25 to 50 mL/hr and gradually increase by 25 mL/hr every 6 hours to the ordered rate, according to hospital protocol. Maintain a steady rate of infusion (within 10% of the ordered dose) to reduce the chance of a sudden onset of hyperglycemia.

Nursing Considerations for TPN

- Patients receiving TPN must be monitored for hyperglycemia and serum potassium levels as well as for all electrolytes.
- The TPN and lipid administration set should be changed every 24 hours. When administering lipids only, change tubing every 12 hours.
- The fat emulsions filter should be a 1.2-micron size.
- The TPN and lipid solutions should be refrigerated at 39° F or 4° C until time of administration.
- TPN solutions should be filtered with a 0.22-micron filter.

RULE Always compare the order with the label to ensure correct percentage of nutritional elements.

➔ CLINICAL ALERT

It is not recommended to administer other medications via the Y port line or piggy back before consulting with the pharmacist for compatibility. There can be many metabolic complications due to the type of additives in the TPN solution.

➔ CLINICAL ALERT

The admixture of fat emulsions with the dextrose and amino acids may produce bacterial growth. Discard the solution after 24 hours.

Answers on page 401

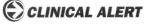

WORKSHEET 9A | Central Parenteral Nutrition Calculations

Use Figure 9-6 to answer the following questions.

1. What are the total grams per bag of:
   a. Amino acids (AA)
   b. Dextrose
   c. Lipids

2. What are the percentages of concentration per bag of:
   a. AA
   b. Dextrose
   c. Lipids

3. What are the percentages of concentration per bag of:
   a. Calcium gluconate
   b. Magnesium sulfate
   c. Potassium acetate
   d. Sodium chloride

4. How many kilocalories are there per bag of:
   a. CHO
   b. PRO
   c. FAT
   d. What is the total number of kilocalories per bag?

5. For how many mL/hr will you set the infusion device?

A sample MAR for parenteral nutrition is shown in Figure 9-8.

TPN FORMULA:

HOME HEALTH

DATE

PATIENT

ADDRESS

	mL
AMINO ACIDS: ☑ 5.5% ☐ 8.5% ☐ 10% ☐ WITH STANDARD ELECTROLYTES	*400*
DEXTROSE: ☑ 10% ☐ 20% ☐ 40% ☐ 50% ☐ 70% (check one)	*350*
LIPIDS: ☑ 10% ☐ 20% FOR ALL-IN-ONE FORMULA	*200*

FINAL VOLUME qsad STERILE WATER FOR INJECTION *400 mL*	*1350* mL

Calcium Gluconate	0.465 mEq/mL	*5*	mEq
Magnesium Sulfate	4 mEq/mL	*10*	mEq
Potassium Acetate	2 mEq/mL		mEq
Potassium Chloride	2 mEq/mL	*20*	mEq
Potassium Phosphate	3 mM/mL		mM
Sodium Acetate	2 mEq/mL		mEq
Sodium Chloride	4 mEq/mL	*30*	mEq
Sodium Phosphate	3 mM/mL		mM
TRACE ELEMENTS CONCENTRATE	☐ 4 ☐ 5 ☐ 6		mL

Patient Additives:

☐ MVC 9 + 3 10 mL Daily

☐ HUMULIN-R _____ units DAILY

☐ FOLIC ACID _____ mg
_____ times weekly

☐ VITAMIN K _____ mg
_____ times weekly

☐ OTHER: _____

☐ OTHER: _____

Directions:

INFUSE: ☐ DAILY

☐ _____ TIMES WEEKLY

OTHER DIRECTIONS:

_____

_____

_____

_____

Rate: ☐ CYCLIC INFUSION: "   ☐ CONTINUOUS INFUSION: "   ☑ STANDARD RATE:
OVER _____ HOURS "   AT _____ mL PER HOUR "   AT _____ mL PER HOUR
(TAPER UP AND DOWN) "   "   FOR *12* HOURS

LAB ORDERS:

☐ STANDARD LAB ORDERS
SMAC-20, CO2, Mg+2 TWICE WEEKLY
CBC WITH AUTO DIFF WEEKLY
UNTIL STABLE, THEN:
SMAC-20, CO2, Mg+2 WEEKLY
CBC WITH AUTO DIFF MONTHLY

☐ OTHER: _____

_____

_____

WHITE: Home Health

VALIDATION:

_____
DOCTOR'S SIGNATURE

Print Name: _____

Office Address: _____

_____

Phone: _____

CANARY: Physician

FIGURE 9-6 Sample physician's order for Worksheet 9A.

Acct: Admitted: Att Phys: Diagnosis: Allergies:	MR#: Age: HT: WT:		M A R	MEDICATION AMINISTRATION RECORD
			Page: 3 From: 10/10/12 0730 Thru: 10/11/12 0730	

Start Date/Time	Stop Date/Time	RN/ LPN	Medication	0731-1530	1531-2330	2331-0730
10/05/12 1800	11/04/12 1759		**PICC Line Flush**　　　　　　　(1 Inject) **FLush**　　　　Q12H **IV**　　　　　　　　　　　　#022 **Flush PICC Q 12 HRS with NS 10 ML** **when PICC line used for TPN**		1800	0600
10/09/12 1800	11/08/12 1759		**Amino Acid 8.5% 600 ML**　　(600 ML) **Dextrose 50% 600 ML**　　　(600 ML) **Sodium Chloride CO 58 MEQ**　(14.5 ML) **Potassium Acetate 12 MEQ**　　(6 ML) **Magnesium Sulfate 6 MEQ**　　(1.5 ML)		1800	
			Calcium Gluconate 6 MEQ　(12.84 ML) **Infuvite Multivitamin 10 ML**　(10 ML) **Trace Elements 1 ML**　　　　(1 ML) **Sodium Phosphate 26 MEQ**　(6.5 ML) **Insulin Humulin Regu 21 units**　(0.21 ML)			
			50 ML/HR　　Q24H　　　　#047 **IV** **Central**			
			Store in Refrigerator			

The preprinted MAR from the pharmacy shows the contents of the TPN, the time it is to be started and the times and amount of NS to be used to flush the Central and PICC Lines. The nurse will initial next to the pre-printed time as well as initial and sign the bottom of the MAR. The MAR is for 24 hours only.

Order Date	RN INIT.	Date/Time To Be Given	One Time Orders and Pre-Operatives Medication-Dose-Route	Actual Time Given	Site Codes		Dose Omission Code
					Arm　　　　　　LA	RA	A = pt absent
					Deltoid　　　　LD	RD	H = hold
					Ventrogluteal　LVG	RVG	M = med absent
					Gluteal　　　　LG	RG	N = NPO
					Abdomen　　　LUQ	RUQ	O = other
					Abdomen　　　LLQ	RLQ	R = refused
							U = unable to tolerate

INIT	Signature	INIT	Signature

60321 (8/98)A　　　　　　　　　　　　　　　CHART

FIGURE 9-7 Sample medication administration record (MAR).

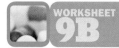

WORKSHEET

9B | Peripheral Parenteral Nutrition Calculations

Use Figure 9-8 to answer the following questions.

1. What are the total grams per bag of:
    a. Amino acids (AA)
    b. Dextrose
    c. Lipids

2. What are the percentages of concentration per bag of:
    a. AA
    b. Dextrose
    c. Lipids

3. What are the percentages of concentration per bag of:
    a. Calcium gluconate
    b. Magnesium sulfate
    c. Potassium phosphate
    d. Sodium chloride

4. How many kilocalories are there per bag of:
    a. PRO
    b. CHO
    c. FAT
    d. What is the total number of kilocalories per bag?

5. For how many mL/hr will you set the infusion device?

HOME HEALTH

DATE

PATIENT

ADDRESS

TPN FORMULA:

AMICO ACIDS: ☐ 5.5% ☑ 8.5% ☐ 10%	mL
☐ WITH STANDARD ELECTROLYTES	*500*

DEXTROSE: ☐ 10% ☐ 20% ☐ 40% ☑ 50% ☐ 70%	mL
(check one)	*500*

LIPIDS: ☑ 10% ☐ 20%	mL
FOR ALL-IN-ONE FORMULA	*250*

FINAL VOLUME qsad STERILE WATER FOR INJECTION	*1500* mL

Calcium Gluconate	0.465 mEq/mL	*5* mEq
Magnesium Sulfate	4 mEq/mL	*15* mEq
Potassium Acetate	2 mEq/mL	*8.3* mEq
Potassium Chloride	2 mEq/mL	mEq
Potassium Phosphate	3 mM/mL	*35* mM
Sodium Acetate	2 mEq/mL	mEq
Sodium Chloride	4 mEq/mL	*35* mEq
Sodium Phosphate	3 mM/mL	mM
TRACE ELEMENTS CONCENTRATE	☐ 4 ☐ 5 ☐ 6	mL

Patient Additives:

☐ MVC 9 + 3 10 ml Daily

☐ HUMULIN-R __*10*__ units DAILY

☐ FOLIC ACID _____ mg _____ times weekly

☐ VITAMIN K _____ mg _____ times weekly

☑ OTHER: *MVI 12 1.5mL/daily*

☐ OTHER: _____

Directions:

INFUSE: ☑ DAILY

☐ _____ TIMES WEEKLY

OTHER DIRECTIONS:

Rate: ☐ CYCLIC INFUSION: OVER *12* HOURS (TAPER UP AND DOWN) ☐ CONTINUOUS INFUSION: AT _____ mL PER HOUR ☑ STANDARD RATE: AT _____ mL PER HOUR FOR *12* HOURS

LAB ORDERS:

☑ STANDARD LAB ORDERS
SMAC-20, CO2, Mg+2 TWICE WEEKLY
CBC WITH AUTO DIFF WEEKLY
UNTIL STABLE, THEN:
SMAC-20, CO2, Mg+2 WEEKLY
CBC WITH AUTO DIFF MONTHLY

☐ OTHER: _____

VALIDATION:

DOCTOR'S SIGNATURE

Print Name: _____

Office Address: _____

Phone: _____

WHITE: Home Health   CANARY: Physician

FIGURE 9-8 Sample physician's order form for Worksheet 9B.

Central Parenteral Nutrition Calculations

Refer to Figure 9-9 to answer the following questions. Use the formulas on pages 209 and 210.

1. Total grams per bag:
   a. How many total grams of amino acids (AA) are there per bag?
   b. How many total grams of dextrose are there per bag?

2. Percentage of concentrations per bag:
   a. What is the percentage of amino acids per bag?
   b. What is the percentage of dextrose per bag?

3. Percentage of additives per bag:
   a. Sodium chloride
   b. Potassium phosphate
   c. Potassium chloride
   d. Magnesium sulfate
   e. Calcium gluconate

4. Kilocalories per bag:
   a. AA
   b. CHO
   c. Total kcal

5. How many hours will it take for the contents of the parenteral nutrition bag to be infused?

Amino Acid 10%	(900 ML)
Dextrose 70%	(430 ML)
Sterile Water For Injection	(70 ML)
Sodium Chloride Conc 140 MEQ	(35 ML)
Potassium Phosphate 41 MEQ	(9.318 ML)
Potassium Chloride 43 MEQ	(21.5 ML)
Magnesium Sulfate 7 MEQ	(1.75 ML)
Calcium Gluconate 7 MEQ	(14.98 ML)
Insulin Humulin Regular 20 units	(0.2 ML)
Infuvite Multivitamin A 10 ML	(10 ML)

Total: 1492.748

** Continued **

DO NOT START AFTER 24 HOURS

Rate: 55 ml/hr   Freq: Q24H
Modified Central TPN
Hang Date/Time: 1800 11/19/12
Expir:
Init: DF
Refrigerate
Prep. By: /_____

DO NOT START AFTER 24 HOURS

FIGURE 9-9 Sample CPN label for Worksheet 9C. Notice that the three-in-one formula with lipids is not used. The time to hang the CPN is 1800 hours.

WORKSHEET 9D | Peripheral Parenteral Nutrition Calculations

Refer to Figure 9-10 to answer the following questions. Use the formulas on pages xxx and xxx.

1. Total grams per bag:
   a. Amino acids
   b. Dextrose

2. Percentage of concentrations per bag:
   a. Amino acids
   b. Dextrose

3. Percentage of additives per bag:
   a. Sodium chloride
   b. Potassium phosphate
   c. Potassium acetate
   d. Calcium gluconate
   e. Magnesium sulfate

4. Kilocalories per bag:
   a. AA
   b. CHO
   c. Total kcal

5. How many hours will it take for the contents to be infused?

Amino Acid 8% (Hepatic)	(600 ML)
Dextrose 20%	(600 ML)
Sodium Chloride Conc 42 MEQ	(10.5 ML)
Potassium Phosphate 26 MEQ	(5.909 ML)
Potassium Acetate 10 MEQ	(5 ML)
Calcium Gluconate 6 MEQ	(12.84 ML)
Magnesium Sulfate 6 MEQ	(1.5 ML)
Infuvite Multivitamin A 10 ML	(10 ML)
Insulin Humulin Regular 24 units	(0.24 ML)

Total: 1245.989

** Continued **

DO NOT START AFTER 24 HOURS

Rate: 50 ml/hr   Freq: Q24H
Peripheral
Hang Date/Time: 1800 11/19/12
Expir:
Init: MM

Prep. By: /_____

DO NOT START AFTER 24 HOURS

FIGURE 9-10 Sample PCN label for Worksheet 9D. Peripheral central line is to be infused at 1800 hours.

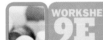

WORKSHEET 9E | Central Parenteral Nutrition Calculations

The central line parenteral (CPN) order is for a patient with a diagnosis of short bowel syndrome. The pharmacist has included the total infused mL and trace elements per bag and not per liter. Answer the following questions using the infused volume of 1399.5 mL rounded to 1400 mL and the final concentrations of Aminosyn II and dextrose 70%. Refer to Figure 9-11.

1. The final concentration of dextrose is 14.3%. How many mL of dextrose 70% are in the total infused volume of 1400 mL?

2. The final concentration of Aminosyn II is 5%. How many mL of Aminosyn II 15% are in the total infused volume of 1400 mL?

3. How many total kcal of dextrose will the patient receive?

4. How many total kcal of protein will the patient receive?

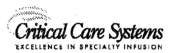

Critical Care Systems

EXCELLENCE IN SPECIALTY INFUSION

Pharmacist in Charge: _____

Caution: Federal law prohibits the transfer of this drug to any person other than the
patient for whom it was prescribed.

Fill Date: 01/13/2010
Original Date: 09/30/2009

RX#:   GIH/JEP

Contents		Final Conc
AMINOSYN II 15%	70 gm/Bag	5 %
DEXTROSE 70%	200 gm/Bag	14.3 %
STERILE WATER FOR INJ	647 ml/Bag	

Additives
CALCIUM GLUCONATE	10 MEQ/Bag
MAGNESIUM SULFATE	16 MEQ/Bag
POTASSIUM ACETATE	25 MEQ/Bag
POTASSIUM CHLORIDE	45 MEQ/Bag
SOD CHLORIDE	53 MEQ/Bag
SODIUM ACETATE INJ	80 MEQ/Bag
CHROMIUM	10 MCG/Bag
COPPER	1000 MCG/Bag
MANGANESE	250 MCG/Bag
SELENIUM	60 MCG/Bag
ZINC	5000 MCG/Bag

Patient to add just prior to infusion
FAMOTIDINE	40 MG	ADD FAMOTIDINE 40MG/4ML TO TPN PRIOR TO INFUSING
MULTIPLE VITAMINS	10 ML	ADD BOTH VIALS TO A BAG OF TPN PRIOR TO INFUSION
DEXFERRUM	20 MG	EVERY OTHER WEEK

Infused Volume: 1399.5 ml
Total Volume: 1468.7 ml
Freq: 1 DAY PER WEEK
Rate: Cycle over 12 hour(s) with a 1 hour(s) taper up
and a 1 hour(s) taper down
Route: INTRAVENOUS
Storage: REFRIGERATED
Qty: 1

FIGURE 9-11 From Accredo Health Group, Inc., Memphis, TN.

Answers on page 404

WORKSHEET 9F

Multiple-Choice Practice

1. Have: CPN solution with 8.5% AA in 375 mL. The total volume (TV) is 1500 mL. How many grams of protein are in the solution?

   a. 50 g/bag   **b.** 77.7 g/bag   **c.** 62 g/bag   **d.** 47.8 g/bag

2. What is the percentage of concentration of grams per bag of the AA in question 1?

   a. 4.6%   **b.** 3%   **c.** 8.2%   **d.** 4.7%

3. Have: CPN solution with 40% dextrose in 400 mL. The TV is 1450. How many grams of dextrose are in the solution?

   a. 232 g/bag   **b.** 130 g/bag   **c.** 160 g/bag   **d.** 260 g/bag

4. What is the percentage of concentration per bag for dextrose in question 3?

   a. 18%   **b.** 16%   **c.** 160%   **d.** 180%

5. Have: A three-in-one TPN solution with 20% lipids in 175 mL. The TV is 1200 mL. How many grams of lipids are in the solution?

   a. 42 g/bag   **b.** 48 g/bag   **c.** 52 g/bag   **d.** 36 g/bag

6. What is the percentage of concentration of grams per bag for lipids in question 5?

   a. 2.7%   **b.** 3.5%   **c.** 5.6%   **d.** 7%

7. Have: Calcium gluconate additive of 6 mEq/L. The TV of the TPN is 1350 mL. What is the percentage of calcium gluconate in the bag?

   a. 0.3%   **b.** 1%   **c.** 0.4%   **d.** 0.6%

8. Have: Magnesium sulfate additive 10 mEq/L. The TV is 1258 mL. What is the percentage of magnesium sulfate in the bag?

   a. 1%   **b.** 10.2%   **c.** 1.8%   **d.** 11%

9. Have: Potassium acetate 12 mEq/L. The TV is 1385 mL. What is the percentage of potassium acetate in the bag?

   a. 2.2%   **b.** 3.6%   **c.** 1.2%   **d.** 2.6%

10. The TV of the parenteral nutrition (PN) solution is 1275 mL. The infusion rate is 110 mL/hr. The infusion is started at 1800 hr. What time will it be completed?

    a. 0659 hr   **b.** 0459 hr   **c.** 0535 hr   **d.** 0345 hr

Critical Thinking Exercises

Analyze the following scenarios.

1. Your patient, Mary Braun, is receiving peripheral parenteral nutrition (PPN). On assessment, she complains that the IV site burns. When the site is checked, the solution is infusing well at the correct rate. The label on the solution is 8.5% amino acids and 70% dextrose.

   Error(s):

   Causes of error(s):

   Nursing interventions:

   Preventive measures:

   Discussion

   What will be your first action?

   Why are the percentages of amino acids and dextrose important to know?

   What is the percentage difference for PPN and CPN infusions?

   How can this situation be reconciled to reduce potential risks?

2. Mrs. S. had been hospitalized for 5 days for ulcerative colitis that was not responding to the treatment. During this time she was receiving a TPN solution with 8.5% amino acid and 40% dextrose with multivitamins 1.5 mL daily. She was then scheduled for a total colectomy. After the surgery, Mrs. S. was returned to the surgical unit. The post operative orders were PCA 1.5 mg morphine every 6 minutes, Ambien 10 mg prn for sleep, and continue daily TPN with Aminosyn II 15%, dextrose 40%, multivitamins 10 mL, and 10 units of Humulin R added to the bag. After 3 days, Mrs. S. complained of nausea, and her skin appeared flushed.

What would be your first reaction to her signs and symptoms?

What medication is she receiving that might cause an adverse reaction?

If this is an adverse reaction, do you think that the benefit of the medication outweighs the reaction?

How can you make Mrs. S. more comfortable to alleviate the signs and symptoms?

3. The 1500 mL TPN infusion of 5% amino acids, 40% dextrose, and 10% lipids is ordered to be infused in 12 hours. The infusion was started at 1430 hr. At 0630 hr, the nurse checked the infusion and found that it still had 300 mL in the bag. She checked the infusion pump, which was set at 100 mL per hour.

Ordered:

Error:

Discussion:

What would be your first action?

Why do you think the infusion time of 12 hours is important?

How was the patient's safety jeopardized?

At what rate should the TPN be infusing?

You are the person who found the error. Will you make out the incident report?

How would an error like this be reconciled in the future?

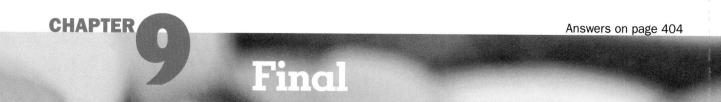

Answers on page 404

CHAPTER 9 Final

Calculate and solve the following problems using a calculator, moving decimals, reducing ratios, and labeling your answers. Prove your work.*

1. A TPN order reads amino acids 8.5% in 550 mL. The total volume of the TPN infusion is 1430 mL.
   a. How many grams of AA will the patient receive through the central line?
   b. How many kilocalories of protein will the patient receive?

2. A TPN order reads dextrose 10% in 475 mL.
   a. How many grams of dextrose will be infused?
   The total volume is 1550 mL in the peripheral line.
   b. How many kilocalories of dextrose will the patient receive?

3. A PPN order reads: Amino acids 5% in 350 mL. The TV is 1280 mL.
   a. How many grams of AA will the patient receive?
   b. How many kilocalories of protein will the patient receive?

*It may be acceptable to withdraw small amounts of large-volume IV solutions equal to the number of milliliters of drug to be added so as to simplify calculations and flow rates. Follow your hospital's policy.

4. The TPN order reads: Dextrose 40% in 400 mL. The TV is 1325 mL.
   a. How many grams of dextrose will the patient receive?
   b. How many kilocalories of carbohydrate will the patient receive?

5. The TPN formula has potassium chloride 4 mEq. The TV is 1250 mL.
   What is the percentage of potassium chloride in the bag?

6. The parenteral nutrition formula has 25 mEq of sodium chloride (NaCl). The TV of the bag is 1425 mL.
   What is the percentage of NaCl in the bag?

7. A TPN solution has 48 g of protein, 255 g of carbohydrate, and 38.6 g of fat.
   How many total kilocalories will the patient receive?

8. A three-in-one TPN solution has lipids 20% in 110 mL. The TV is 1145 mL.
   a. How many grams of lipids will the patient receive?
   b. How many kilocalories of fat will the patient receive?

9. The TPN of 1420 mL is to start at 1800 hr. The rate is 108 mL/hr.
   What time will the infusion be completed?

10. A TPN of 1320 mL is infusing at 120 mL/hr.
    How many hours will it take to infuse?

Insulin Administration

Objectives

- Identify sites for insulin injections.
- Identify the different types of insulin labels.
- Compare the actions of fast-, intermediate-, and long-acting insulins.
- Read calibrations on 30-, 50-, and 100-unit insulin syringes.
- Prepare single- and mixed-dose insulin injections.
- Calculate units of insulin based on CHO grams.
- Interpret the sliding scale using the BMBG method.
- Use electronic intravenous devices to administer insulin dosages.
- Calculate IV insulin for units/hr and mL/hr and duration.
- Analyze medication errors using critical thinking.

Introduction

According to the USP and the ISMP, insulin is the drug most commonly involved in errors. Insulin has been given as an overdose or confused with other unit measured medications such as heparin. The importance of measuring the correct amount of insulin is stressed. Different types of insulin syringes are shown for the practice of selecting the most appropriate syringe for the ordered dose. Mixing two types of insulin is shown in drawings. The bedside monitor blood glucose (BMBG) flow sheet shows how to use the sliding scale to chart hourly insulin needs. IV infusions are calculated for units per hour based on the BMBG level.

Insulin

Insulin is an aqueous solution of the principal hormone of the pancreas. Insulin affects metabolism by allowing glucose to leave the blood and enter the body cells, preventing hyperglycemia.

Diabetes Mellitus

Diabetes mellitus is a deficiency of insulin and is classified according to cause. In type 1, which usually affects people before the age of 30, the pancreatic beta cells do not produce insulin. Insulin injections must be taken every day to control blood glucose levels.

The onset of type 2 diabetes usually occurs after 30 years of age; however, obesity has contributed to a rise in the diagnosis of type 2 diabetes in children and young adults. The pancreas produces *some* insulin but not enough to metabolize the glucose. In some cases, the insulin that is produced is not effective; this is known as *insulin resistance.* Of people with diabetes, 95% have type 2, and 40% of people with type 2 diabetes take insulin injections in conjunction with oral diabetes medications.

The most common complication of insulin therapy is hypoglycemia. This may be caused by injecting too much insulin (a risk in home care), by missing or delaying meals, or by being involved in more physical activity than usual. To treat hypoglycemia, a patient should always carry sugar in some form. The treatment of choice, if the patient can swallow, is glucose tablets (4 to 5 g carbohydrate [CHO] per tablet). Wait 15 minutes to retest the blood glucose. A glucose gel of 15 g is also available for the treatment of hypoglycemia. The glucose gel is to be used if the person cannot swallow but is still conscious. Put gel in the cheek along the gumline and rub vigorously. If the blood glucose level gets very low, unconsciousness may occur. At that point, the patient will need a glucagon injection. Emergency kits are available for home use (Figure 10-1). For patients weighing over 20 kg, use 1 mL. For patients weighing less than 20 kg, use 0.5 mg of glucagon.

Injection Sites

The abdomen is the preferred site for insulin injections. When insulin injections are required on a daily basis, it is important to rotate within that site (Figure 10-2). The abdomen absorbs insulin more rapidly and is safer as an injection site than the upper arm, back, or thigh. If use of the abdomen is medically contraindicated, alternative sites may be used.

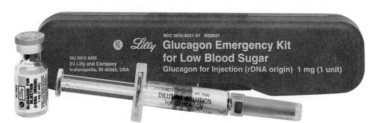

FIGURE 10-1 Glucagon emergency kit for home use. (Copyright Eli Lilly and Company. All rights reserved. Used with permission.)

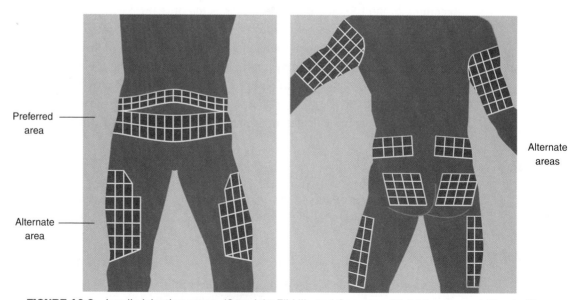

FIGURE 10-2 Insulin injection areas. (Copyright Eli Lilly and Company. All rights reserved. Used with permission.)

Types of Insulin

The source of insulin is either human or animal. This is known as the *species* of the insulin. Human insulin is manufactured to be the same as insulin produced by the body. Human insulin is made in one of two ways:

- By recombinant DNA technology, a chemical process used to produce unlimited amounts of human insulin; or
- By a process that chemically changes animal insulin into human insulin.

Humalog insulin (lispro) is recombinant DNA insulin with a rapid action of 5 to 15 minutes, allowing patients to dose and eat.

Recombinant DNA insulins cause fewer allergies than those from animal sources.

All insulin is supplied in units denoting strength. Insulin is given via special insulin syringes (Figure 10-3) and pens (Figure 10-4). Byetta stimulates glucose-dependent insulin from pancreatic beta cells (GLP-1 and GIP) and decreases glucagon production when glucose levels are elevated (Figure 10-5). Byetta is not insulin.

⊖ CLINICAL ALERT

It is essential that nurses know the signs and symptoms of hypoglycemia (too much insulin) and hyperglycemia (too little insulin) when caring for diabetic patients.

Hypoglycemia Signs and Symptoms	Hyperglycemia Signs and Symptoms
rapid onset	several hour onset
cold clammy skin	warm skin
diaphoretic	flushed dry skin
nervous	lethargic
blood glucose below 70 mg/dL	blood glucose above 300 mg/dL

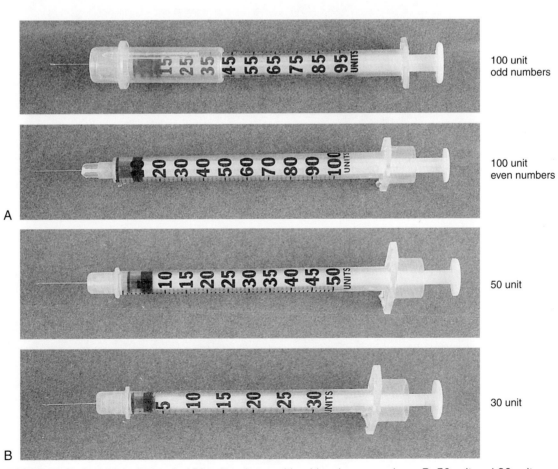

FIGURE 10-3 Insulin syringes. **A,** 100-unit syringes with odd and even numbers. **B,** 50-unit and 30-unit syringes. (From Becton, Dickinson and Company, Franklin Lakes, NJ.)

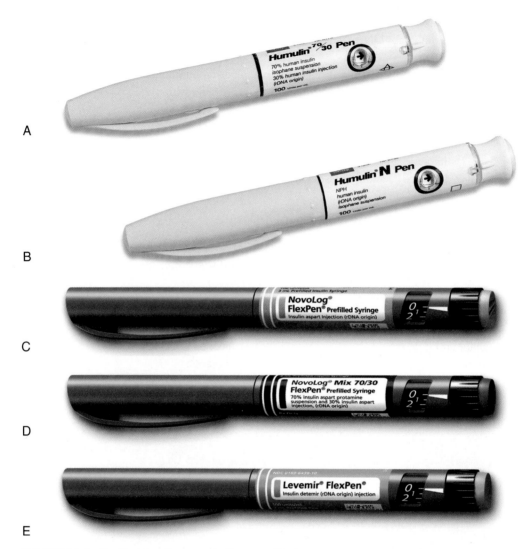

A

B

C

D

E

FIGURE 10-4 Prefilled insulin pens. **A,** Humulin 70/30 short- and intermediate-acting. **B,** Humulin N intermediate-acting. **C,** Novolog® rapid-acting. **D,** Novolog® 70/30 short- and intermediate-acting. **E,** Levemir® long-acting. (A and B, Copyright Eli Lilly and Company. All rights reserved. Used with permission. C-E, From Novo Nordisk Inc., Princeton, NJ.)

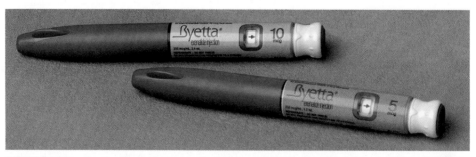

FIGURE 10-5 Byetta Pens. From Amylin Pharmaceuticals, Inc. (San Diego, CA) and Eli Lilly and Company (Indianapolis, IN). Used with permission.

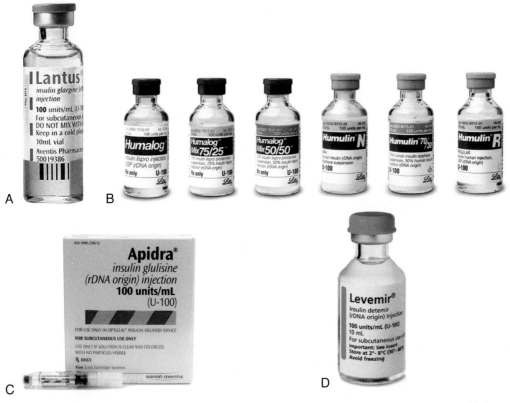

FIGURE 10-6 **A,** Lantus (insulin glargine). The Lantus vial is taller and narrower than the NPH, Regular, and Humalog vials. Lantus is written in purple letters. **B,** Various insulin vials. HUMULIN® and HUMALOG® are registered trademarks of Eli Lilly and Company. **C,** Rapid-acting Apidra. **D,** Long-acting Levemir. (A and C from Sanofi Aventis U.S. Inc., Bridgewater, NJ. B, Copyright Eli Lilly and Company. All rights reserved. Used with permission. D from Novo Nordisk Inc., Princeton, NJ.)

There are different types of cartridges used with insulin pens. Attached needles are usually 24- to 26-gauge with a ⁵⁄₁₆- or ½-inch needle. Insulin is supplied in 10 mL vials labeled U-100, which means there are 100 units/mL (Figure 10-6). Insulin is also supplied in *10 mL vials of U-500, which means there are 500 units/mL. This strength is used for those whose blood glucose levels fluctuate to very high levels. This type of insulin is rarely used and rarely kept on the nursing unit.* Table 10-1 lists the duration of activity of various types of insulins and other injectables. See examples of various U-100 insulins on pages 229 and 230.

⊙ CLINICAL ALERT

Loss of vision is a complication of diabetes. U-30 and U-50 syringes have large numbers and are easier to read than the U-100 (1 mL) syringes. Tactile insulin measuring devices like the Jordan Medical Count-a-Dose enable nonvisual insulin measurement and mixing.

Table 10-1 Insulins and Other Injectables for Diabetes Management

Type	Onset	Peak	Duration	Appearance	When to Take	Mixed with
Insulins						
Rapid-Acting						
Aspart (Novolog)	5-15 min	1-3 hr	3-5 hr	Clear	15 min before a meal	NPH
Lispro (Humalog)	15 min	1-2 hr	3-4 hr	Clear		
Glulisine (Apidra)	15 min	1-2 hr	3-4 hr	Clear		
Short-Acting						
Regular (Novolin R)	30-60 min	2-5 hr	6-8 hr	Clear	30 min before a meal	NPH
Regular (Humulin R)	40-60 min	2-3 hr	4-6 hr	Clear		
Intermediate-Acting						
NPH (Novolin N)	90 min	4-12 hr	up to 24 hr	Cloudy	30 min before a meal	Regular, rapids
NPH (Humulin N)	2-4 hr	4-10 hr	14-18 hr	Cloudy		
Long-Acting						
Glargine (Lantus)	3-5 hr	Peakless	22-26 hr	Clear	At bedtime	**Do not mix**
Detemir (Levemir)	2-4 hr	Peakless	13-20 hr	Clear	At supper or bedtime	**Do not mix**
Short- and Intermediate-Acting	Premixed insulins are taken twice a day The first number is the intermediate-acting insulin					
70/30	1-4 hr	2-4 hr and 6-10 hr	3-4 hr and 10-16 hr	Cloudy	30 min before a meal	Premixed
50/50						
Rapid- and Intermediate-Acting						
75/25	15 min-4 hr	1-2 hr and 6-10 hr	3-4 hr and 10-16 hr	Cloudy	15 min before a meal	Premixed
70/30 Novolog Mix	15 min-4 hr	30-90 min and 6-10 hr	4-5 hr and 10-16 hr	Cloudy	15 min before a meal	Premixed

Other Injectables for Diabetes Management

Brand Name	Generic Name	Dosing	Action	When to Take
Other				
Symlin	Pramlintide acetate	Given subcutaneously. Prefilled pen. Titrate starting at 15 mcg to 60 mcg. (Reduce the rapid- or short-acting insulin by 50%.)	This is a synthetic version of human Amylin, a hormone co-secreted with insulin by the beta cells in the pancreas. Works with insulin to help maintain normal glucose concentrations. It has three actions: (1) helps control blood glucose levels by reducing the postmeal release of glucose from the liver; (2) slows the absorption of carbohydrate by slowing the rate of stomach emptying; (3) reduces appetite.	Is taken with meals or snacks when more than 30 g of carbohydrates are eaten.
Byetta	Exenatide	Given subcutaneously. Pre-filled pen. 5 mcg × 1 month, then 10 mcg	This is a new class of drugs called incretin mimetics. These drugs mimic the action of gut hormones that stimulate the release of insulin in response to increased blood glucose levels. These drugs work by slowing the emptying of the stomach, suppressing the release of glucose from the liver after eating, and stimulating the beta cells of the pancreas to produce more insulin when blood glucose levels rise. They also reduce food intake, thus decreasing body weight.	Within 60 min before breakfast and the evening meal

Types of U-100 Insulins

Short-Acting

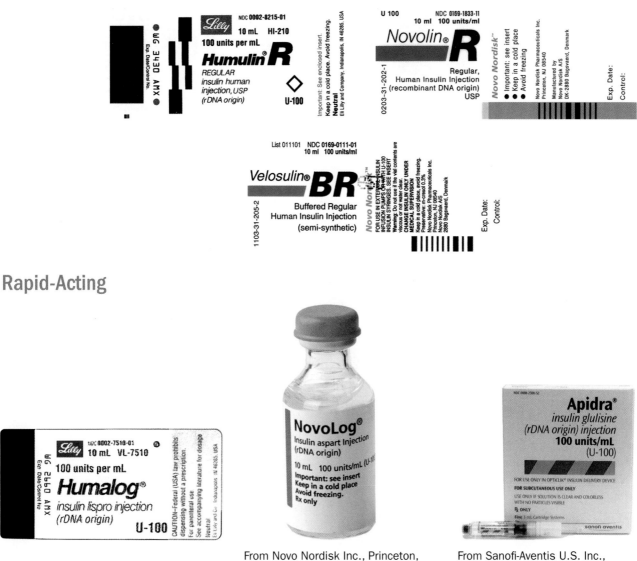

From Novo Nordisk Inc., Princeton, NJ.

From Sanofi-Aventis U.S. Inc., Bridgewater, NJ.

Rapid-Acting

🔆 **CLINICAL ALERT**

Regular insulin should always be clear. Discard if unclear.

Mix insulins only with those of the same name because they may have differing amounts of preservatives. For example, Humulin R should be combined only with Humulin L or N. Humulin is a brand name.

Intermediate-Acting

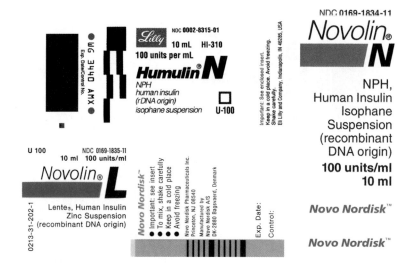

Intermediate- and Rapid-Acting Mixtures

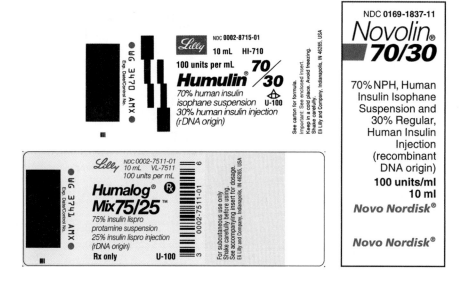

The insulin combination of NPH and Regular is used to give a 24-hour effect.

In 1 mL of Humulin 70/30, there are 70 units of intermediate-acting insulin and 30 units of rapid-acting insulin. In 1 mL of Humulin 50/50, there are 50 units of intermediate-acting insulin and 50 units of rapid-acting insulin.

Note: Mix before administration by rolling *gently* between the palms. Never shake because this creates bubbles.

⊝ CLINICAL ALERT

Insulin is available in various strengths: rapid acting, regular, intermediate-acting, long-acting, and combinations of rapid- and intermediate-acting. READ LABELS CAREFULLY TO AVOID GIVING THE WRONG STRENGTH.

Long-Acting

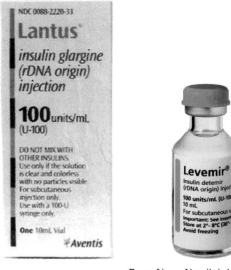

From Novo Nordisk Inc., Princeton, NJ.

⊖ CLINICAL ALERT

Lantus must NOT be mixed in the same syringe with any other insulin or be diluted. It is NOT intended for IV administration. Caution: Lantus is clear like Regular Humalog. Lantus is given anytime for 24-hour coverage without a peak. Consistency in administration is necessary.

Insulin Syringes

Insulin is usually given in a 1 mL or 0.5 mL insulin syringe calibrated to U-100 insulin. The 0.5 mL insulin syringe is used for smaller doses because the calibrations are larger and easier to read. The most commonly used insulin syringes are 50- and 100-unit syringes, as shown in Figure 10-3.

⊖ CLINICAL ALERT

Tuberculin syringes are calibrated in tenths and must never be substituted for insulin syringes, which are calibrated from 1 to 100 units.

Types of U-100 Insulin Syringes

Each calibration in the syringe shown in Figure 10-7 represents 1 unit. This syringe is used for small doses of 50 units or less and is used with U-100 insulin only. Needles are usually 24 to 26 gauge for subcutaneous injections. Clip-on magnifiers for syringes are available to enlarge the calibrations and numbers.

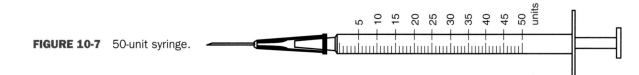

FIGURE 10-7   50-unit syringe.

Each calibration in the syringe shown in Figure 10-8 equals 2 units. This syringe is for use with U-100 insulin only.

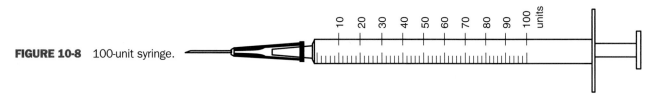

FIGURE 10-8   100-unit syringe.

Each calibration in the syringe shown in Figure 10-9 represents 1 unit. This syringe is used for small doses of 30 units or less as a safety feature for people with diabetes who have vision problems (a Magni-Guide may also be useful for those people [Figure 10-10]) or for children who require small doses of insulin. This syringe is for use with U-100 insulin only.

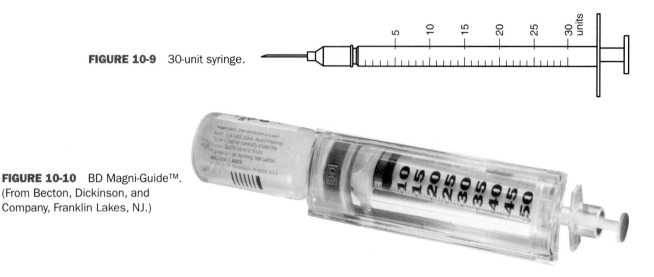

FIGURE 10-9   30-unit syringe.

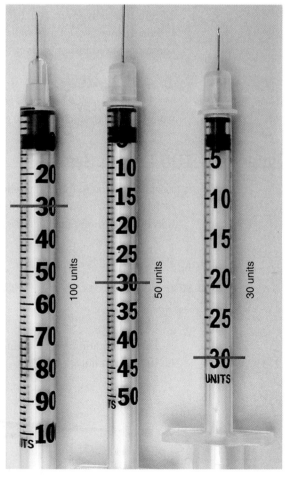

FIGURE 10-10   BD Magni-Guide™. (From Becton, Dickinson, and Company, Franklin Lakes, NJ.)

Insulin Orders

A typical order for insulin must include the following:

A. The *name* of the insulin: Humulin, Novolin, Lantus.

B. The *type* of the insulin: regular, lispro, aspart, N, detemir, or glargine.

C. The *number* of units or amount the patient will receive: 10 units.

D. The *time* to be given: AM, $\frac{1}{2}$ hr before a meal.

E. The *route* is subcutaneous unless IV is specified.

Example   Prepare 30 units of Humulin R insulin subcutaneously $\frac{1}{2}$ hr before a meal. Using a 100 unit syringe, 50 unit syringe, or 30 unit syringe fill the syringe to the 30 units calibration (Figure 10-11). (All insulins come in U-100 so orders no longer specify U-100.)

ⓢ CLINICAL ALERT

Units must be spelled out (not abbreviated by a U) because abbreviating can be a source of medication errors (e.g., mistaking the U for a zero). Insulin dosages require two licensed nurses to double check for accuracy.

FIGURE 10-11   From left to right: 30 units measured on a 100 unit syringe (each calibration is 2 units), a 50 unit syringe (each calibration is 1 unit), and a 30 unit syringe (each calibration is 1 unit). (From Macklin D, Chernecky C, Infortuna H. Math for clinical practice, ed 2, St Louis, 2011, Mosby.)

WORKSHEET 10A | Single-Dose Measures

Read the syringes and write your answers in the spaces provided.

1. Units measured: _____

2. Units measured: _____

3. Units measured: _____

4. Units measured: _____

5. Units measured: _____

6. Units measured: _____

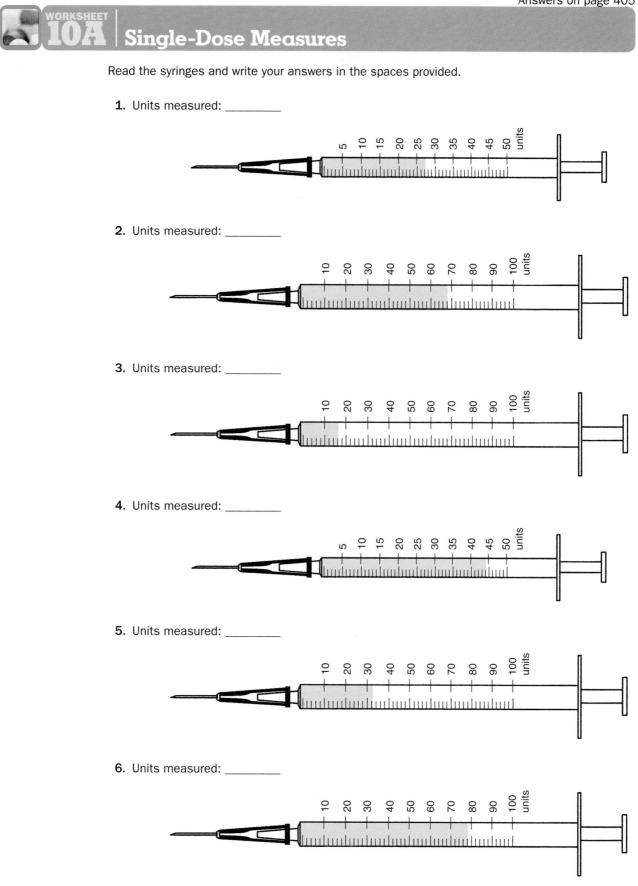

7. Units measured: _____

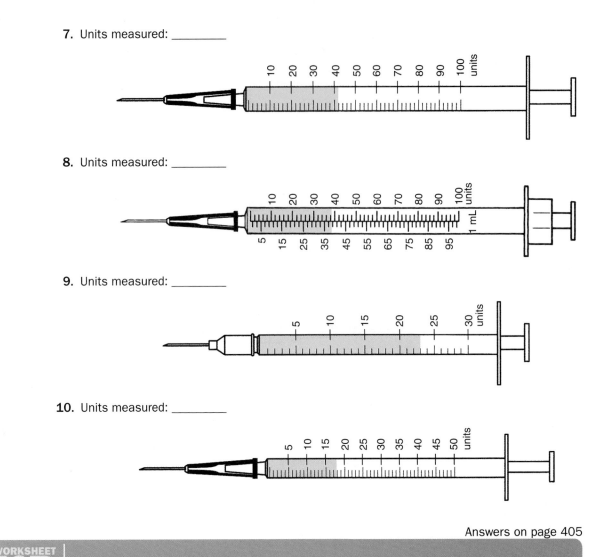

8. Units measured: _____

9. Units measured: _____

10. Units measured: _____

Answers on page 405

| # Additional Practice in Single-Dose Measures

Circle the letter of the syringe with the correct ordered amount.

1. Ordered: 12 units of Novolin Regular subcutaneous 30 min before a meal.

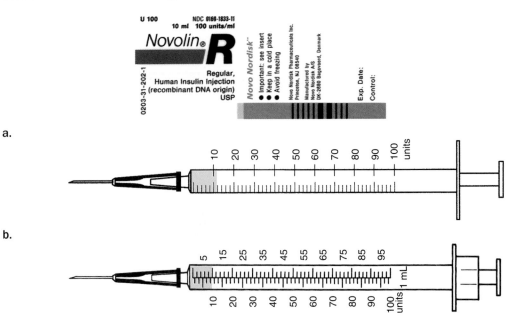

U 100   NDC 0169-1833-11
10 ml   100 units/ml

Novolin® R

0203-31-202-1

Regular,
Human Insulin Injection
(recombinant DNA origin)
USP

Novo Nordisk™

● Important: see insert
● Keep in a cold place
● Avoid freezing

Novo Nordisk Pharmaceuticals Inc.
Princeton, NJ 08540

Manufactured by
Novo Nordisk A/S
DK-2880 Bagsvaerd, Denmark

Exp. Date:

Control:

a.

b.

2. Ordered: 6 units of Humulin Regular subcutaneous $\frac{1}{2}$ hr before a meal.

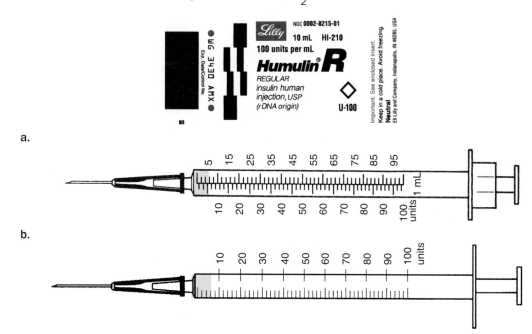

a.

b.

3. Ordered: 13 units of Humulin NPH subcutaneous at 1100 hr.

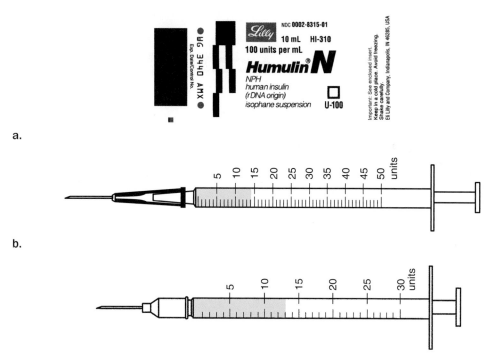

a.

b.

4. Ordered: 12 units of Lantus subcutaneous at 2200 hr.

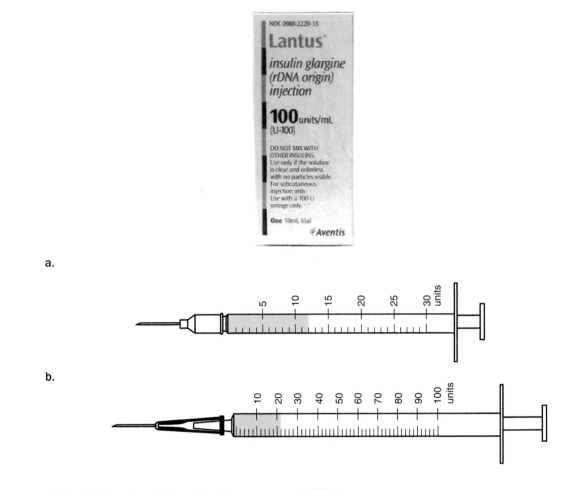

a.

b.

5. Ordered: 40 units of detemir subcutaneous at 0930.

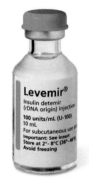

From Novo Nordisk Inc., Princeton, NJ.

a.

b.

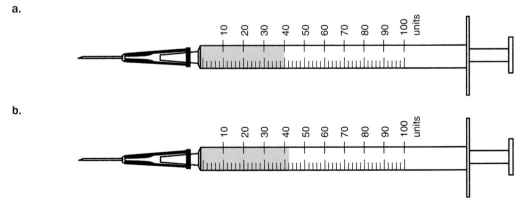

Mixing Insulin

Insulin dosages are drawn up *exactly* as ordered. An incorrect dosage could be devastating to the patient. Frequently, regular or rapid-acting insulin is combined with an intermediate-acting insulin. This gives insulin coverage (glucose control) within 15 to 60 minutes and lasts 10 to 16 hours. This technique of combining the two types of insulin is important for the nurse, patient, and family to master. The regular insulin vial should *not* be contaminated with the longer-acting insulin; therefore, the regular insulin should be drawn up first. The mixing procedure is illustrated in Figures 10-12 and 10-13.

Example   Ordered: 10 units of Novolin Regular and 20 units of Novolin N.
Total units: 30 units
Source: DNA and DNA
Which insulin will you draw up first? *Regular* (see Figure 10-12)

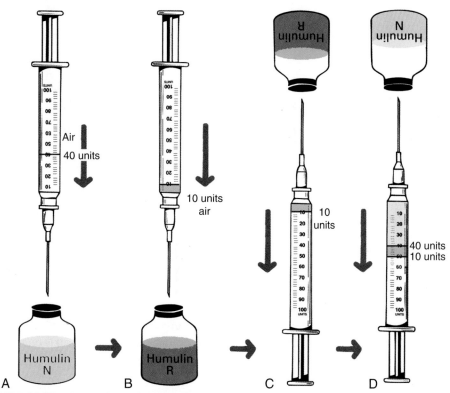

FIGURE 10-12   Order: Give 10 units of Humulin R and 40 units of Humulin N via subcutaneous injection. **A,** Inject 40 units of air into Humulin N first. Do **not** allow needle to touch insulin. Withdraw needle. **B,** Inject 10 units of air into Humulin R. **C,** With needle still in place, invert vial and withdraw 10 units of R. Withdraw needle. **D,** Insert needle into vial of Humulin N, invert vial and withdraw 40 units. Total amount in syringe equals 50 units.

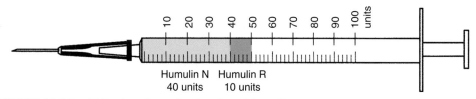

FIGURE 10-13   100-unit syringe showing the mixing of two insulins. Remember: **clear to cloudy when drawing up insulins.**

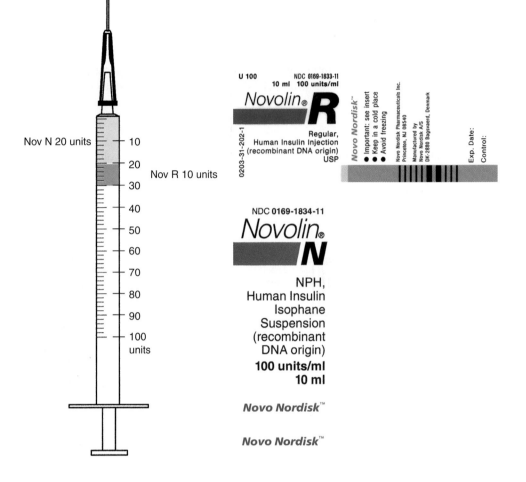

Nov N 20 units

Nov R 10 units

U 100   NDC 0169-1833-11
10 ml   100 units/ml

Novolin® **R**

Regular,
Human Insulin Injection
(recombinant DNA origin)
USP

0203-31-202-1

Novo Nordisk™
● Important: see insert
●●● Keep in a cold place
● Avoid freezing

Novo Nordisk Pharmaceuticals Inc.
Princeton, NJ 08540

Manufactured by
Novo Nordisk A/S
DK-2880 Bagsvaerd, Denmark

Exp. Date:

Control:

NDC 0169-1834-11
Novolin®
N

NPH,
Human Insulin
Isophane
Suspension
(recombinant
DNA origin)
100 units/ml
10 ml

Novo Nordisk™

Novo Nordisk™

Insulin will not stay separated as pictured in the syringe.

⊖ *CLINICAL ALERT*

Draw up regular (clear) insulin first before N (cloudy) is added (see Figure 10-12).

Regular insulin should not be contaminated with Humulin N or any N insulin. **A multiple-dose vial of regular insulin can be used for IV infusion, and contamination with intermediate-acting insulin could be fatal.**

WORKSHEET 10C | **Mixing Insulin**

Calculate the total number of units in the following problems. Circle the letter of the syringe with the correct amount.

1. Ordered: 10 units of Humalog and 38 units Humulin N $\frac{1}{2}$ hr before breakfast. Total units: _____

   a.

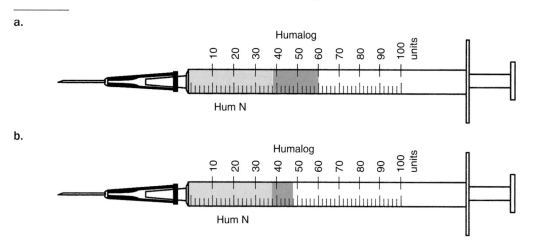

   b.

2. Ordered: Humalog R 14 units and Humulin N 25 units. Total units: _____
   a.

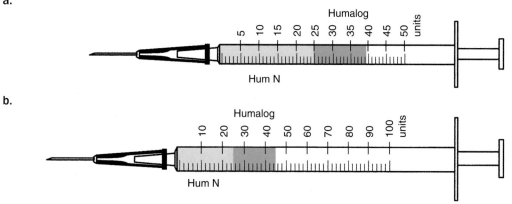

   b.

3. Ordered: Novolin R 8 units and Novolin N 15 units. Total units: _____
   a.

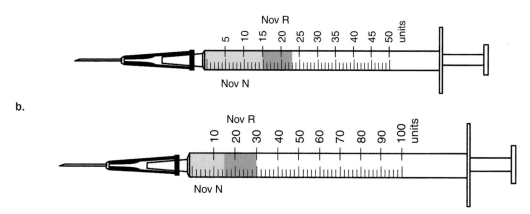

   b.

4. Ordered: Novolin 8 units and Novolin N 30 units. Total units: _____

a.

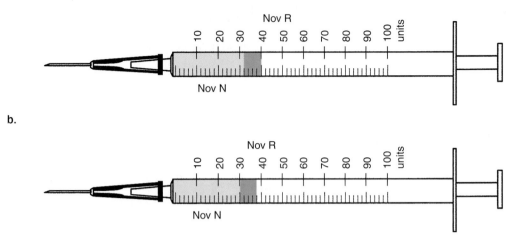

b.

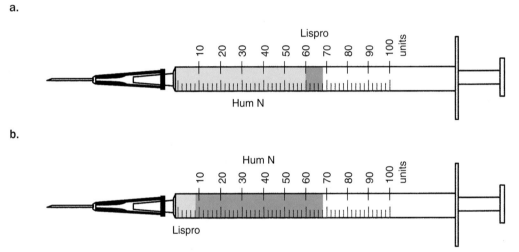

5. Ordered: Lispro insulin 8 units and Humulin N 60 units $\frac{1}{2}$ hr before breakfast.
Total units: _____

a.

b.

Shade in insulin dose on syringe. All orders are for U-100 insulin.

6. Ordered: 15 units of Novolog at 0830 before breakfast. Available: Novolog (aspart). How many units will you administer? When will it peak?

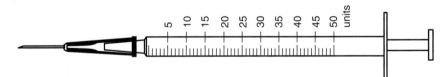

7. Ordered: 10 units of Apidra before meals. Available: Aprida U-100. How many units will you give? When will the action begin (onset)?

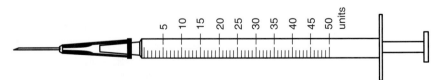

8. Ordered: Fixed combination of 70/30, 44 units daily. Available: Fixed 70/30. How many units will you give? When will it peak? What is the duration?

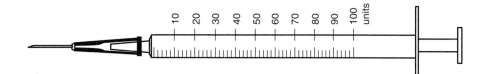

9. Ordered: Novolin R 10 units and Novolin N 40 units subcutaneous every AM $\frac{1}{2}$ before meals. How many total units will you give? What is the duration?

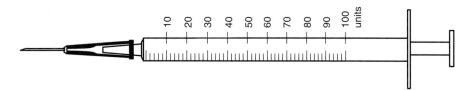

10. Ordered: Humulin R insulin 12 units and Humulin N 30 units every AM before breakfast. How many total units will you give? When will this peak? What is the duration?

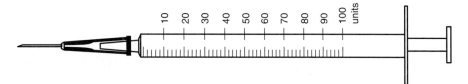

Sliding-Scale Calculations

Insulin administered according to a sliding scale is predicated on the type of diabetes, insulin resistance, weight, age, renal status, and activity level. Blood glucose levels determine how much insulin to give. Blood glucose readings may be taken several times a day to determine daily insulin requirements. **Sliding scales can vary greatly because they are individualized.** Evidence-based computerized medical records information systems used in place of individualized sliding scales result in better glycemic control. The study was completed by the Department of Medicine, University of Washington, Seattle, WA, USA.

Example Ordered: Regular insulin q6hour to follow the sliding scale.

Sliding Scale Blood glucose level

50-80	Treat low BG and retest in 15 min
80-100	10 units
100-150	12 units
150-200	15 units
200-250	17 units
250-300	20 units
300-350	25 units
350-above	Call physician

Repeat blood glucose measurement 4 hr after it peaks.

At 1700 hr, the patient's blood glucose level was 148 mg/dL. How much regular insulin should be given? Shade the amount in the syringe.

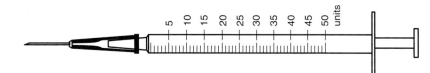

Insulin Infusion Devices

Nurses must understand how to care for patients who are admitted with insulin pumps. It is the nurse's responsibility to ascertain the patient's knowledge of pump management. Patients must be able to manage their diabetes, monitor their blood glucose level four times a day, calculate carbohydrate intake (grams), and determine when a bolus dose is needed. Many times the patient is admitted because of a lack of knowledge or lack of compliance with the regimen. Most hospitals do not keep a supply of insulin pumps or batteries for the pump; therfore, determine if the patient has made arrangements for these supplies.

An insulin pump is a battery-powered pump that delivers a continuous subcutaneous insulin infusion (CSII) (Figure 10-14) that is attached to an infusion set (Figure 10-15) that has a very fine gauge cannula inserted subcutaneously in the abdomen and is attached to the insulin reservoir via tubing. The reservoir can hold either 150 units or more commonly, 300 units of U-100 rapid-acting insulin. Insulin pumps generally take only rapid or short-acting insulin. Buffered and U-400 insulin are used strictly for insulin pumps and must be prescribed by the health care provider. These insulins are not usually kept on the unit. Ketoacidosis can develop quickly if the insulin is interrupted. Because of this significant risk, *the device must not be stopped or disconnected without supplemental insulin coverage.* If the insulin pump has to be disconnected for computerized tomography scans and magnetic resonance imaging tests, the blood sugar level should be checked before disconnecting and after reconnecting the pump. An insulin IV may be needed during the tests.

When using insulin pumps, the blood glucose should be checked before meals and at bedtime. A continuous glucose monitoring system device (Figure 10-16) is an optional device worn by the patient

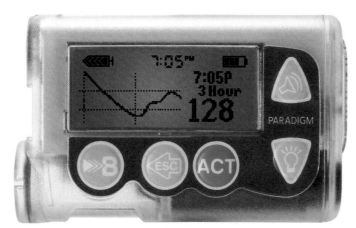

FIGURE 10-14 MiniMed Paradigm® REAL-Time System. (From Medtronic Diabetes, Northridge, CA.)

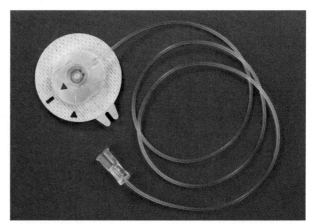

FIGURE 10-15 Quick-set® Infusion Sets. (From Medtronic Diabetes, Northridge, CA.)

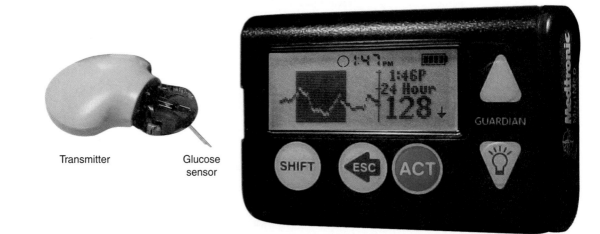

Transmitter   Glucose sensor

Reservoir

FIGURE 10-16 Guardian® REAL-Time System. (From Medtronic Diabetes, Northridge, CA.)

to transmit glucose levels to the insulin pump. It is programmed to take blood glucose levels every 5 minutes. The blood glucose value is sent to the insulin pump where the number is displayed.

The patient will program the pump according to the basal rate set by the health care provider and the patient. If the basal rate is set correctly, the blood glucose will not fluctuate between meals. Basal rates are specific to each patient. They are set in units per hr. See Table 10-2, Basal Rates, (page 248) Insulin Units Based on Required CHO Intake and Weight.

Insulin Dosage Based on Carbohydrate Intake

Because blood glucose levels fluctuate during the day, insulin doses should also fluctuate rather than being a constant dose every day. In order to keep the blood glucose level as close to the desired range as possible, carbohydrate intake must be calculated for each meal based on current blood glucose levels. This technique produces a more constant glucose level, which will help to minimize the detrimental effects of wide variations in blood glucose levels during the day. However, blood glucose levels must be taken before each meal and at bedtime. Usually, an insulin pump is used. If the carbohydrate ratio is high, the insulin pump can provide a bolus dose.

The health care provider will set a daily dose of long-acting insulin, Lantus, is used to cover blood glucose levels outside of meal times individualized parameters for each patient, depending on metabolic needs, such as exercise. The best type of diabetes management is the carbohydrate ratio technique, which is the closest way of replacing insulin made by the pancreas. A high level of compliance is needed for successful management. Rapid-acting insulin is used in the carbohydrate intake-to-weight ratio. See Table 10-2, page 248.

remember Blood glucose levels should be checked before meals for optimal diabetes control.

Example Based on blood glucose level (BGL) and carbohydrate (CHO) intake.
- Desired blood glucose level is 130 mg/dL
- Order: Give 1 unit of insulin for every 20 mg/dL above 130 mg.
  - Give 1 unit of insulin for every 10 g of CHO consumed.

Lunch	CHO
• $\frac{3}{4}$ cup of potato salad	21 g
• 2 slices of whole wheat bread	42 g
• 2 slices of Swiss cheese	2 g
• 2 slices of ham	2 g
• Mustard	1 g
• 1 12 oz can of Pepsi	42 g
• Total	109 g CHO

Step 1 Desired BGL is 130 mg/dL. The BSL before lunch was 145 mg/dL. The difference between 130 and 145 is 15. The order states to give 1 unit of insulin for each 15 mg/dL above the desired 130 mg/dL. Therefore, 1 unit of insulin is required to treat the blood glucose level.

R & P Formula
15 mg : 1 unit :: 15 mg: x units
$15x = 15$
$x = 1$ unit

Easy Method
Divide the BGL difference by the order.
15 divided by 15 = 1 unit

Step 2 Total CHO for lunch is 109 g
Order: give 1 unit of insulin for each 10 g of CHO consumed.

R & P Formula

10 g : 1 unit :: 109 g : x units

10x = 109

x = 10.9 = 11 units

Round to nearest whole number

Easy Method

Divide the total grams of CHO by the order.

109 divided by 10 = 10.9 = 11 units

Give: 1 unit because the blood glucose level is above 15 g and give 11 units for the amount of CHO consumed. Give a total of 12 units of insulin.

Answers on page 406

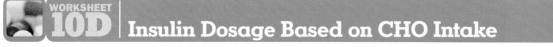

WORKSHEET 10D | Insulin Dosage Based on CHO Intake

Use the following order to answer questions 1, 2, and 3. Round answers to the nearest whole number. Calculate the total number of insulin units required on the basis of the BGL and the CHO intake.

Ordered: BGL of 130 mg/dL is desired.

Give 1 unit of insulin for each 10 mg above 130 mg.

Give 1 unit of insulin for every 8 g of CHO consumed.

1. Breakfast   BGL is 150 mg/dL
    $\frac{3}{4}$ cup Total cereal   CHO = 23 g
    8 oz low-carb milk   3 g
    $\frac{1}{2}$ cup blueberries   1 g
    1 slice wheat toast   21 g
    1 pat butter   0 g
    1 cup black coffee   0 g
    Total units _____

2. Lunch   BGL is 135 mg/dL
    8 oz yogurt   CHO = 25 g
    $\frac{1}{3}$ cup dried cranberries   33 g
    2 apple slices   1 g
    5 grapes   1 g
    5 saltines   11 g
    Plain iced tea   0 g
    Total units_____

3. Dinner   BGL is 145 mg/dL
    1 pork chop   CHO = 0 g
    $\frac{3}{4}$ cup mashed potatoes   34 g
    $\frac{3}{4}$ cup broccoli   0 g
    8 oz plain iced tea   0 g
    Total units_____

    Bedtime snack   BGL is 145 mg/dL
    $\frac{3}{4}$ cup lowfat ice cream   CHO = 15 g

    Total units_____

Use the following order to calculate the total insulin units in questions 4 and 5.

Ordered: The desired BGL is 140 mg/dL
        Give 1 unit of insulin for every 10 mg above 140 mg/dL.
        Give 1 unit of insulin for every 10 g of CHO consumed.

4. Breakfast   BGL is 135 mg/dL
    2 eggs   CHO = 1 g
    2 slices wheat toast   42 g
    2 slices bacon   0 g
    2 cups black coffee   0 g
    Total units _____

5. Lunch   BGL is 160 mg/dL
    4 oz hamburger patty   CHO = 0 g
    1 hamburger bun   28 g
    $\frac{1}{2}$ cup cole slaw   20 g
    1 small serving fries   45 g
    Total units _____

Answers on page 406

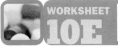 **WORKSHEET 10E** | **Insulin Dosage Based on Blood Glucose and CHO Intake**

Calculate the insulin requirements in questions 1, 2, and 3. The BGL readings and CHO requirements are based on the following orders. **Mark each syringe** with the total dose required.

Ordered: Give 1 unit of insulin for every 20 mg BGL above 160 mg/dL.
        Give 1 unit of insulin for every 15 g of CHO consumed.

1. BGL is 190 mg/dL; 98 g of CHO were consumed.
    How many total units of insulin are required?

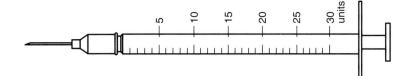

2. BGL is 210 mg/dL; 118 g of CHO were consumed.
    How many total units of insulin are required?

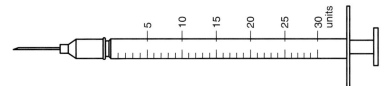

3. BGL is 180 mg/dL; 40 g of CHO were consumed. How many total units of insulin are required?

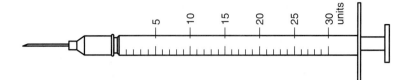

Calculate the total insulin requirements in questions 4 through 7. The BGL reading and CHO requirements are based on the following orders. Mark each syringe with the total dose required.

Ordered: Give 1 unit of insulin for every 30 mg BGL above 150 mg/dL.
            Give 1 unit of insulin for every 10 g of CHO consumed.

4. BGL is 240 mg/dL; 58 g of CHO were consumed. How many total units of insulin are required?

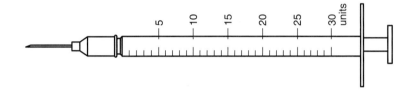

5. BGL is 180 mg/dL; 120 g of CHO were consumed. How many total units of insulin are required?

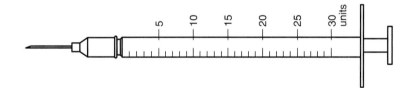

6. BGL is 260 mg/dL; 58 g of CHO were consumed. How many total units of insulin are required?

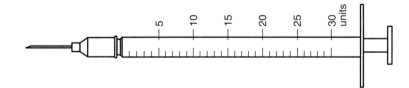

7. BGL is 160 mg/dL; 28 g of CHO were consumed. How many total units of insulin are required?

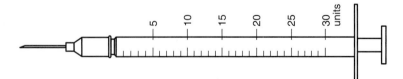

Calculate the total insulin requirements for questions 8, 9, and 10. The BGL and CHO requirements are based on the following orders. Mark each syringe with the total dose required.

Ordered: Give 1 unit of insulin for every 20 mg BGL above 130 mg/dL.

Give 1 unit of insulin for every 8 g of CHO consumed.

8. BGL is 140 mg/dL; 45 g of CHO were consumed. How many total units of insulin are required?

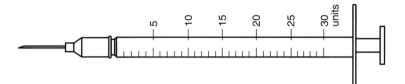

9. BGL is 160 mg/dL; 80 g of CHO were consumed. How many total units of insulin are required?

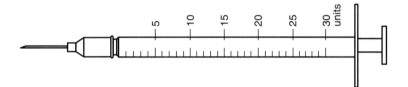

10. BGL is 120 mg/dL; 85 g of CHO were consumed. How many total units of insulin are required?

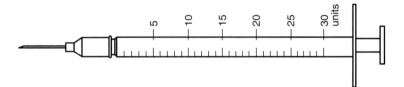

Estimating Insulin-to-Carbohydrate Ratio

This formula is based on estimates of insulin needs according to CHO intake and weight. It is a simple formula that gives estimates for categories of weight based on Table 10-2. Also given is the kilogram ratio for the same number of pounds. Table 10-2 is used to compute all of the problems on Worksheet 9F.

Example Breakfast = 44 CHO. The patient's weight is 165 lb. Refer to Table 10-2. The ratio is 1 unit of insulin to 11 g of CHO consumed.

R & P Method
1 unit : 11 CHO :: x units : 44 CHO
$11x = 44$
$x = 4$ units of R insulin

Total grams of CHO (Divided by) unit-to-CHO Ratio = Insulin Needs

or   44 (divided by) 11 = 4 units

Basal Rates

Weight in Pounds	Weight in Kg	Unit: grams of CHO
100-109	45.5-49.5	1:16
110-129	50-58.6	1:15
130-139	59-63.2	1:14
140-149	63.6-67.7	1:13
150-159	68.2-72.3	1:12
160-169	72.7-76.8	1:11
170-179	77.3-81.4	1:10
180-189	81.8-85.9	1:9
190-198	86.4-90	1:8
200-239	90.9-108.6	1:7
240+	109.1+	1:6

Answers on page 407

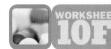

WORKSHEET 10F | Insulin Dosage Based on CHO Intake and Weight

Calculate the insulin requirements for the following CHO intake related to the patient's weight. Refer to Table 10-2 above. Use either method shown in the example.

1. The patient ate 26 g CHO for breakfast. She weighs 142 lb. How many units of R are required?

2. The patient weighs 83 kg and ate 80 g CHO for lunch. How many units of R are required?

3. The patient ate 18 g CHO for lunch. She weighs 108 lb. How many units of R are required?

4. The patient consumed 90 g CHO for dinner and weighs 240 lb. How many units of R are required?

5. The patient weighs 162 lb. The total CHO intake during a 24-hour period was 160 g. How many units of R has the patient received in 24 hours?

6. The patient's total CHO intake during 24 hours was 145 g. How many units of R did she receive? The patient weighs 100 kg.

7. The physician calls at 1500 hours and wants to know how many total units of R his patient has received for the day. You calculate the following: breakfast included 45 g CHO, and he ate half of the CHO plus three quarters of his lunch, which had 72 g CHO. The patient weighs 190 lb. How many total units of R has the patient received?

8. You estimate that the patient ate half of his carbohydrates for lunch. The total CHO on his lunch menu was 50 g. His weight is 81 kg. How many units of R should he receive?

9. The patient weighs 70 kg. He has consumed 44 g CHO for breakfast, 72 g CHO for lunch, and 48 g CHO for dinner. His bedtime snack had 15 g CHO. What is the total amount of CHO the patient has consumed? What is the total amount of R he requires for the day?

10. Breakfast included 38 g CHO. The patient ate half of the CHO on the tray. Lunch included 50 g of CHO, and she ate one quarter of the CHO on the tray. Dinner included 48 g CHO, and she ate one third of the CHO. She weighs 112 lb. What is the total amount of CHO the patient has consumed? What is the total amount of R she requires for the three meals?

IV Insulin

During acute phases of illness, regular insulin is given by the IV route to ensure a controlled supply of medication that will vary depending on laboratory monitoring. A piggyback infusion is always administered with an IV-controlled infusion device. Discard the first 2 to 3 mL of combined infusion through IV tubing to prevent the insulin from binding to the tubing.

RULE Begin the problem with the known amount of medication in the total solution.

The pharmacy standard insulin drip: 100 units Human Regular in 100 mL of NS.

Example   Ordered: Regular human insulin 5 units/hr IV drip. Pharmacy has delivered 100 mL 0.9% NS with 100 units of regular human insulin.
- How many mL/hr will infuse 5 units/hr?
- For how many hours will the IV infuse?

KNOW   WANT TO KNOW

Step 1:   100 units : 100 mL $::$ 5 units : x mL
$100x = 100 \times 5 = 500$
$100x = 500$
$x = 5$ mL/hr = 5 units of insulin

PROOF	$100 \times 5 = 500$
	$100 \times 5 = 500$

HAVE   WANT TO HAVE

Step 2:   5 mL : 1 hr $::$ 100 mL : x hr
$5x = 100$
$x = 20$ hr

PROOF	$20 \times 5 = 100$
	$1 \times 100 = 100$

⊘ CLINICAL ALERT
Only **clear regular** insulin can be used intravenously. Discard if cloudy (Figure 10-17).

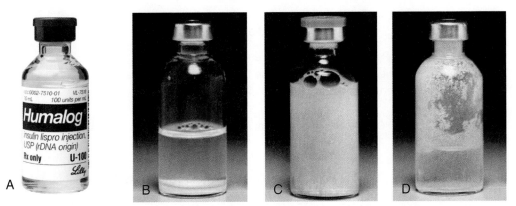

FIGURE 10-17   **A,** Regular and Humalog (lispro), Novolog (aspart), and Aprida (glulisine) should always look clear. **B,** Insulin at the bottom of the bottle; do not use if insulin stays on the bottom of the bottle after gentle rolling. **C,** Clumps of insulin; do not use if there are clumps of insulin in the liquid or on the bottom of the vial. **D,** Bottle appears frosted; do not use if particles of insulin are on the bottom or sides of the bottle and give it a frosty appearance. (Copyright Eli Lilly and Company. All rights reserved. Used with permission.)

Answer questions 1 through 3 using Figure 10-18.

1. The patient's BMBG level is 310 mg/dL at 0820 hr.
   a. At what rate will you set the IV infusion device?
   b. At 0920 hr the BMBG is 270 mg/dL. What will be the rate for the IV infusion device?

2. The patient's blood glucose level is 235 mg/dL at 0400 hr.
   a. At what rate will you set the infusion rate?
   b. In 1 hour, the BMBG level is 270 mg/dL. What will be the new IV rate?
   c. At 0600 hr the physician called and inquired about the BMBG level. He asked how many units of insulin the patient had received since the IV was started. What will you tell the physician?

3. Your patient is receiving insulin IV. The standard rate of 100 units in 100 mL of NS is sent from the pharmacy. The BMBG q1h is as follows: 350 mg/dL, 330, 270, 210, 190, 165, 145, 120, 120 mg/dL. How many total units has the patient received?

4. The pharmacy has sent 50 mL of NS with 100 units of insulin. The order is for 5 units/hr until the BMBG level is stable at 130 mg/dL.
   a. At how many mL/hr will you set the IV infusion device?
   b. It took 16 hours for the BMBG level to stabilize at 130 mg/dL. How many total units of insulin did the patient receive during the 16 hours?

5. Ordered: 100 units Human Regular insulin in 50 mL of NS to be infused at 3 mL/hr until the blood glucose level is stable at 120 mg/dL.
   a. How many units/hr will be delivered?
   b. If it took 8 hours for the blood glucose level to stabilize at 120 mg/dL, how many total units of insulin did the patient receive?

For Problems 6 through 10, calculate the following:
· mL/hr necessary to infuse the ordered amount via an infusion device
· length of time the IV is to infuse

6. Ordered: Humulin R IV at 10 units/hr. Available: 150 mL of 0.9% NS with 100 units Humulin (lispro) R insulin.

7. Ordered: Humulin R in 50 mL to infuse at 8 units/hr. Available: 50 mL 0.9% NS with 50 units Humulin R insulin.

BG (mg/dL)	Std. Infusion Rate (units/hour)	☐ Stress Infusion Rate (units/hour)	☐ Customized (units/hour)
<80	0.2	0.2	_____
80-100	0.5	1.0	_____
101-140	1.0	2.0	_____
141-180	1.5	3.0	_____
181-220	2.0	4.0	_____
221-260	2.5	5.0	_____
261-300	3.0	6.0	_____
301-340	4.0	8.0	_____
>340	5.0	10.0	_____

FIGURE 10-18   Standard Insulin Infusion Chart. (Modified from Scottsdale Healthcare, Scottsdale, AZ.)

8. Ordered: Humulin R in 50 mL to infuse at 15 units/hr. Available: 50 mL 0.9% NS with 75 units Humulin R insulin.

9. Ordered: 120 units Humulin R insulin IV at 10 units/hr. Available: 100 mL of NS 0.9% with 120 units Humulin R insulin.

10. Ordered: 150 units Humulin R insulin IV at 12 units/hr. Available: 150 mL of NS 0.9% with 150 units Humulin R insulin.

Oral Diabetes Medications

Oral diabetes medications (ODMs) are used to treat persons with type 2 diabetes. They are taken alone or in combination with insulin. Blood glucose levels determine the strength of oral medication needed. ODMs are *not* insulin. Some ODMs stimulate the pancreas to produce insulin and other ODMs make more effective use of the insulin that is produced.

There are seven main classes of oral medications for the treatment of type 2 diabetes and combinations thereof:

- Sulfonylureas (SUL-fah-nil-YOO-ree-ahs) stimulate your pancreas to make more insulin. These are sometimes used in conjunction with insulin injections
- Biguanides (by-GWAN-ides) decrease the amount of glucose made by your liver.
- Alpha-glucosidase inhibitors (Al-fa gloo-KOS-ih-dayss in-HIB-it-ers) slow the absorption of the starches you eat.
- Thiazolidinediones (THIGH-ah-ZO-li-deen-DYE-owns) make you more sensitive to insulin.
- Meglitinides (meh-GLIT-in-ides) stimulate your pancreas to make more insulin.
- D-phenylalanine (dee-fen-nel-AL-ah-neen) derivatives help your pancreas make more insulin quickly.
- DPP-IV Inhibitors boost incretin gut hormone production to help lower blood glucose levels.
- Combination oral medicines put together different kinds of pills.

Answers on page 409

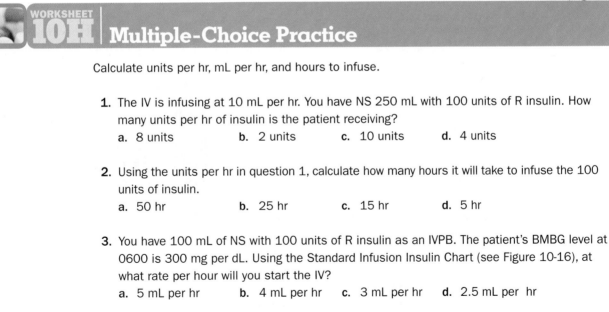

WORKSHEET 10H | **Multiple-Choice Practice**

Calculate units per hr, mL per hr, and hours to infuse.

1. The IV is infusing at 10 mL per hr. You have NS 250 mL with 100 units of R insulin. How many units per hr of insulin is the patient receiving?
   a. 8 units   b. 2 units   c. 10 units   d. 4 units

2. Using the units per hr in question 1, calculate how many hours it will take to infuse the 100 units of insulin.
   a. 50 hr   b. 25 hr   c. 15 hr   d. 5 hr

3. You have 100 mL of NS with 100 units of R insulin as an IVPB. The patient's BMBG level at 0600 is 300 mg per dL. Using the Standard Infusion Insulin Chart (see Figure 10-16), at what rate per hour will you start the IV?
   a. 5 mL per hr   b. 4 mL per hr   c. 3 mL per hr   d. 2.5 mL per hr

4. Ordered: 30 units of R insulin to be infused over 12 hr.
   Available: 50 mL NS with 30 units of insulin. How many units/hr will be infused?
   a. 1.5 units   b. 2.5 units   c. 5 units   d. 4 units

   At how many mL per hr will you set the infusion device?
   a. 4 mL per hr   b. 12 mL per hr c. 41 mL per hr d. 8 mL per hr

5. Ordered: 10 units of R insulin per hr IVPB.
   Available: 500 mL NS with 100 units of R insulin.
   At what rate will you set the IV infusion device?
   a. 50 mL per hr **b.** 25 mL per hr **c.** 100 mL per hr **d.** 5 mL per hr

6. The type of insulin that is used for infusions is
   a. Humulin N **b.** Levemir
   c. Humulin R **d.** Lantus

7. Ordered: 15 units of Lantus (glargine) subcutaneous.
   What is the length of effectiveness of the insulin?
   a. 12 hr **b.** 4 hr **c.** 36 hr **d.** 24 hr

8. Ordered: Humulin N 20 units subcutaneous at 0730.
   When will it peak?
   a. 4-5 hr **b.** 4-10 hr **c.** 1-3 hr **d.** 3-4 hr

9. Lantus (glargine) is the preferred insulin because it:
   a. peaks in 15 minutes **b.** has a duration of 16 hr
   c. is absorbed quickly **d.** is peakless

10. Lantus (glargine) is usually given subcutaneously:
    a. at breakfast **b.** at bed time **c.** at midday **d.** anytime

Critical Thinking Exercises

Analyze the following scenario.

1. Mr. Johnson's blood glucose level was 350 mg/dL. The orders on his chart read: Give 10 units of Humalog stat and check the BMBG in 1 hour. The nurse gave the insulin at 1400 hr. After the change of shift, at 1430 hr, Mr. Johnson was incoherent. On checking the Diabetes Flow Sheet (Figure 10-19) the nurse found that Mr. Johnson had been given 1 mL (100 units) of Humalog.

   Ordered:

   Given:

   Error(s):

   Discussion
   What would be your immediate action?
   How did this error occur?
   How could this error have been prevented?
   Do you think the nurse should have known the safe dosage range?
   What were the potential injuries to the patient?
   How can a safety issue like this be reconciled?

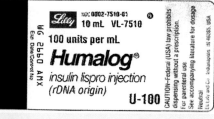

Frequent Blood Glucose Monitoring/Insulin Drip Record

Normal Blood Glucose M 75-110 mg/dL F 65-105 mg/dL

DATE 12/5/12

Time	Glucose (mg/dL)	Intervention Insulin (units/h) or other	Ketones S/M/L/Neg	Initial
00 __ __				
01 __ __				
02 __ __				
03 __ __		IV Insulin Drip Started		
04 _1_ _5_	350	5.0		JB
05 _1_ _5_	303	4.0		JB
06 _1_ _5_	310	4.0		JB
07 _1_ _5_	270	3.0		JB
08 _1_ _5_	180	1.5		JB
09 _1_ _5_	165	1.5		JB
10 _1_ _5_	150	1.5		JB
11 __ __				
12 _1_ _5_	140	1.0		JB
13 _1_ _5_	130	1.0		JB
14 __ __				
15 _1_ _5_	135	1.0		JB
16 __ __				
17 _1_ _5_	140	1.0		JB
18 __ __		Converted to Subcutaneous Insulin		
19 __ __				
20 __ __				
21 __ __				
22 __ __				
23 __ __				
Insulin Total Daily Dose (TDD)				

DATE

Time	Glucose (mg/dL)	Intervention Insulin (units/h) or other	Ketones S/M/L/Neg	Initial
00 __ __				
01 __ __				
02 __ __				
03 __ __				
04 __ __				
05 __ __				
06 __ __				
07 __ __				
08 __ __				
09 __ __				
10 __ __				
11 __ __				
12 __ __				
13 __ __				
14 __ __				
15 __ __				
16 __ __				
17 __ __				
18 __ __				
19 __ __				
20 __ __				
21 __ __				
22 __ __				
23 __ __				
Insulin Total Daily Dose (TDD)				

DATE

Time	Glucose (mg/dL)	Intervention Insulin (units/h) or other	Ketones S/M/L/Neg	Initial
00 __ __				
01 __ __				
02 __ __				
03 __ __				
04 __ __				
05 __ __				
06 __ __				
07 __ __				
08 __ __				
09 __ __				
10 __ __				
11 __ __				
12 __ __				
13 __ __				
14 __ __				
15 __ __				
16 __ __				
17 __ __				
18 __ __				
19 __ __				
20 __ __				
21 __ __				
22 __ __				
23 __ __				
Insulin Total Daily Dose (TDD)				

Initial	Signature	Initial	Signature	Initial	Signature
JB	J Booth				

Original in Medical Chart   **Copy to Pharmacy**

NOTE: IV insulin should always be used with an infusion device, never via gravity feed.

FIGURE 10-19 Diabetes Flow Sheet. (Modified from Scottsdale Healthcare, Scottsdale, AZ.)

2. Mrs. B. was admitted to the surgical unit through the emergency department with a diagnosis of diabetic ulceration on right ankle. She has used an insulin pump for over 1 year and said it works well for her as she is able to be more ambulatory and free from giving herself multiple daily injections. At the time of admission she did not have any diabetic supplies to care for the insulin pump. At 1100 hr she asked the nurse to fill the reservoir on her insulin pump. The nurse checked the order, which read: Fill reservoir with 3 mL of U-100 insulin PRN. After filling the reservoir, the nurse then inserted the reservoir into Mrs. B.'s infusion device. After the change of shift at 1600 hr the evening nurse noticed that Mrs. B. looked flushed. Her skin was warm and dry, and her reflexes were slow. The nurse took her vitals and found: B/P 90/75, respirations 14, pulse 60 and weak. The nurse detected a fruity odor to her breath. The reservoir on the insulin device showed 2.5 mL left. The nurse then tested Mrs. B.'s blood glucose and found it to be 400 mg/dL.

Discussion:
What would be your immediate action?
What error occurred?
Was the order specific?
Should the nurse have known the type of insulin to put in the reservoir?
How can this type of error be remediated to ensure patient safety?

3. After a shoulder replacement Mr. H., who is a type I diabetic, just returned to the surgical unit in your care. He has an IV with 100 units of insulin in 100 mL of 0.9% normal saline infusing at 4 units/hr and heparin IV infusing with 1000 units of heparin in 250 mL infusing at 10 mL/hr. The PACU nurse transferred the MAR and stated that Mr. H. had been given a 5000 unit bolus dose of heparin and 10 mg morphine 10 minutes ago. Upon taking the vitals, the assigned nurse noticed Mr. H.'s blood glucose has escalated to 300 mg/dL, probably due to the stress of surgery. After contacting the physician by phone, he ordered a bolus of 20 units of insulin and then a recheck of the blood glucose in 1 hour. The nurse wrote the order and had it checked by the supervisor, who initialed it as being a correct order. The assigned nurse proceeded to give the 20 units into the IV port as a bolus dose.

After 1 hour, the nurse checked the blood glucose and found it to be 380 mg/dL. The nurse contacted the supervisor and the physician. The two nurses analyzed the situation and realized that the assigned nurse had given a bolus dose of 20 units of heparin in place of the insulin.
What would be your first action?
Insulin is a high-alert drug; therefore, what preventative measures should have been followed?
What are the potential serious consequences for the patient?

CHAPTER 10 Final

1. Ordered: Humalog insulin 15 units stat. Available: Humalog insulin.
   - How many units will you give?
   - Which syringe will give a precise measurement? Shade in correct amount.

   a.

   b.

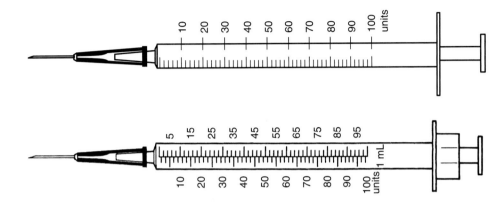

2. The blood glucose level is 280. How many units of Regular insulin will you give subcutaneously? Use the sliding scale on page 241.

3. Ordered: Novolin R 16 units with Novolin N insulin 30 units at 0700. Shade in the amount of regular insulin. Shade in the amount of N insulin and label.

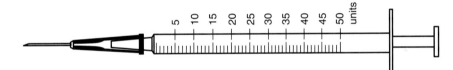

4. Ordered: Humalog 18 units before breakfast at 0930.
   - How many units will you give?
   - Which syringe is easier to read?

   a.

   b.

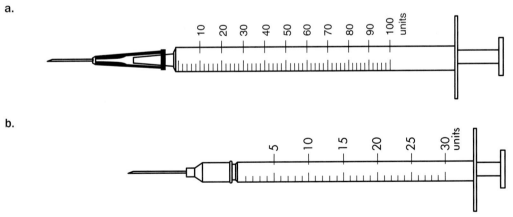

5. Ordered: Glucophage 850 mg tab and Novolin N 15 units before breakfast. How many total units will you give? Shade in the correct amount.

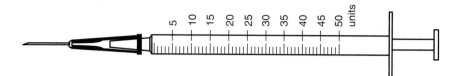

6. Ordered: 10 units per hr Novolin R insulin IV. Available: 500 mL 0.9% saline with 250 units Novolin R regular insulin.
   - How many mL per hr will deliver 10 units per hr?
   - How many hours will the IV infuse?

7. Ordered: 6 units per hr Novolin R IV. Available: 100 units Humulin R insulin in 250 mL of 0.9% saline.
   - How many mL per hr will infuse 6 units of insulin?
   - How many hours will the IV infuse?

8. Ordered: 8 units per hr Novolin R IV. Available: 250 mL NS with 100 units insulin.
   - How many mL per hr will infuse 8 units of insulin?
   - How many hours will the IV infuse?

9. Ordered: 7 units per hr Novolin R IV. Available: 200 mL NS with 100 units Novolin R.
   - How many mL per hr will infuse 7 units per hr?
   - How many hours will the IV infuse?

10. Ordered: Humulin R 9 units per hr IV. Available: 500 mL NS IV solution with 100 units Humulin R.
    - How many mL per hr will infuse 9 units per hr?
    - For how many hours will the IV infuse?

evolve Refer to the Advanced Calculations section of Drug Calculations, version 4 on Evolve for additional practice problems.

Anticoagulants

Objectives
- Compare the actions of oral, subcutaneous, and intravenous anticoagulants.
- Measure a dose in a tuberculin syringe.
- Measure subcutaneous heparin using various concentrations.
- Titrate intravenous heparin for bolus dose, units/kg, units/hr, and mL/hr.
- Calculate the length of time to infuse.
- Analyze medication errors using critical thinking.

Introduction **Various concentrations of subcutaneous heparin sodium, Fragmin, Lovenox, and Arixtra are measured with a tuberculin syringe. Titrated heparin sodium for intravenous drip and titrated Fragmin are calculated for bolus and prophylactic regimens. An example of a flow chart, or medical administration record (MAR), is shown.**

▶ Injectable Anticoagulants

Heparin sodium injection, USP, is a drug used to interrupt the clotting process. It affects the ability of the blood to coagulate, thereby preventing clots from forming. It is used to treat deep vein thrombosis (DVT) and pulmonary embolism (PE); for cardiac surgery; during hemodialysis, myocardial infarction (MI), and disseminated intravascular coagulation (DIC); and prophylactically for immobilized patients. It may be given in therapeutic doses or in small, diluted doses to maintain the patency of IV or intraarterial (IA) lines.

Because it is inactive orally, heparin sodium is administered intravenously or subcutaneously. If administered intramuscularly, the drug produces a high level of pain and may cause hematomas. The orders for heparin are highly individualized and are based on the weight of the patient and coagulation values. Heparin comes in various strengths, including 1000, 5000, 10,000, 20,000, and 50,000 units/mL. Heparin also comes in 10 and 100 units/mL for IV patency flushes. The vial must be checked carefully before administration. Heparin is fast-acting.

Figure 11-1 shows heparin injection sites. Figure 11-2 demonstrates how subcutaneous heparin injections are documented.

Check laboratory values for clotting times before administering heparin. Heparin therapy must not be interrupted and is incompatible with other medications.

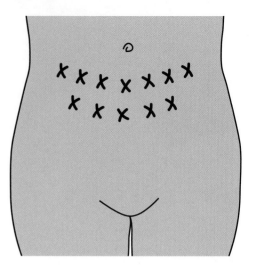

FIGURE 11-1 Subcutaneous injection sites. The abdominal sites are better for absorption of heparin.

				HT :			
ADM. DX :				WT :	**M A R**	**MEDICATION ADMINISTRATION RECORD**	
DIET :				ALLERGIES:			
Start Date/Time	Stop Date/Time	RN/ LPN	Medication		0731-1530	1531-2330	2331-0730
12/13/12		NB	Heparin sodium 5,000 units subcut		0800 RLQ		
		NB	Heparin sodium 5,000 units subcut		1400 LLQ		
		KR	Heparin sodium 5,000 units subcut		2000 RLQ		

Order Date	RN INIT.	Date/Time To Be Given	One Time Orders and Pre-Operatives Medication-Dose-Route	Actual Time Given	Site Codes			Dose Omission Code	
					Arm	LA	RA	A = pt absent	
					Deltoid	LD	RD	H = hold	
					Ventrogluteal	LVG	RVG	M = med absent	
					Gluteal	LG	RG	N = NPO	
					Abdomen	LUQ	RUQ	O = other	
					Abdomen	LLQ	RLQ	R = refused	
								U = unable to tolerate	
					INIT	Signature	INIT	Signature	
					NB	Nancy Berg RN			
					KR	Kay Rae RN			

FIGURE 11-2 Sample MAR. Modified from Scottsdale Healthcare, Scottsdale, AZ.

Heparin has a half-life of 1 to 6 hours. To maintain a therapeutic level in the blood, heparin is usually given as a continuous IV drip during hospitalization. The heparin level is titrated on the basis of partial thromboplastin time (PTT) levels, which are taken every 6 hours to correlate with the half-life of heparin. Heparin can be counteracted with protamine sulfate.

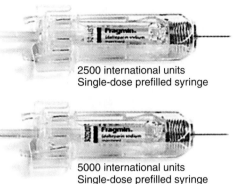

2500 international units
Single-dose prefilled syringe

5000 international units
Single-dose prefilled syringe

FIGURE 11-3 Fragmin single-dose prefilled syringes. Used with permission from Pfizer, Inc.

⊖ CLINICAL ALERT

▶ Heparin is a high-alert medication that carries a risk of causing serious injury if the wrong dosage is administered. It can be confused with insulin as both are measured in units; therefore, have another nurse verify the order and amount before administering heparin, Fragmin, Lovenox, or Arixtra.

Lovenox (enoxaparin) and Fragmin (dalteparin) (Figure 11-3) are low-molecular-weight anticoagulants. They are prescribed for the prevention and treatment of DVT and PE and also after knee and hip surgery. Lovenox and Fragmin have a longer half-life than heparin, and because of their low level of activity in the blood, there is a reduced need for PTT tests because the two drugs have more predictable peaks and durations of action. The preferred sites for low-molecular-weight anticoagulants are the "love handles," or anterolateral abdominal wall.

⊖ CLINICAL ALERT

Anticoagulant dosages require two licensed nurses to verify dosage for accuracy.

⊖ CLINICAL ALERT

Lovenox and Fragmin should never be given in the deltoid because they may cause large hematomas.

Example   Ordered: Lovenox 30 mg subcutaneous q12h after hip replacement. The pharmacy has sent 40 mg/ 0.4 mL in a prefilled syringe. How many milliliters will be administered? How many milliliters will be discarded?

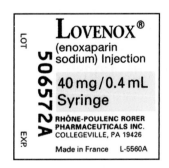

LOT 506572A EXP:

LOVENOX®
(enoxaparin sodium) Injection
40 mg/0.4 mL
Syringe
RHÔNE-POULENC RORER
PHARMACEUTICALS INC.
COLLEGEVILLE, PA 19426
Made in France   L-5560A

HAVE   WANT TO HAVE

40 mg : 0.4 mL :: 30 mg : x mL

$40x = 0.4 \times 30 = 12$

$40x = 12$

$x = 0.3$ mL

0.1 mL will be discarded.

PROOF	$40 \times 0.9 = 12$
	$0.4 \times 30 = 12$

Arixtra (fondaparinux sodium) is a non-heparin anticoagulant made by chemical synthesis and not from animal origin (Figure 11-4). It is a specific inhibitor of the activated factor X (Xa).

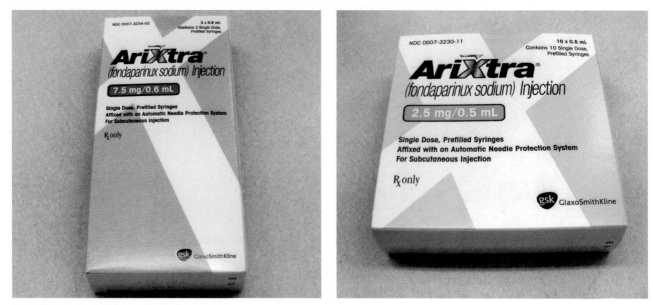

FIGURE 11-4 Arixtra single dose syringes.

Arixtra is used for prophylasis of venous thromboembolism (VTE), such as deep vein thrombosis (DVT), which may lead to pulmonary embolism (PE) in patients undergoing hip fracture surgery, knee replacement or hip replacement surgery, and those at risk for thromboembolitic complications from abdominal surgery.

Warfarin can be administered in conjunction with Arixtra for the treatment of acute DVT when initiated while the patient is hospitalized.

⊖ CLINICAL ALERT

Arixtra is NOT intended for intramuscular use. It CANNOT be used interchangeably with heparin or other low-molecular-weight (LMW) heparinoids such as Lovenox (enoxaparin) and Fragmin (dalteparin).

There is a risk of hemorrhage for patients with impaired renal function and for those who are at increased risk of hemorrhage (thrombocytopenia). If the platelet count falls below 100,000/mm^3, discontinue Arixtra.

Subcutaneous Heparin Injections

Example   Ordered: Heparin 3500 units subcutaneous q6h. Available: Vial containing 5000 units/mL. How many milliliters will the patient receive? Shade in the dose on the tuberculin syringe.

KNOW	WANT TO KNOW
5000 units : 1 mL :: 3500 units : x mL	
5000x = 3500	
x = 0.7 mL	

> **PROOF**
> 5000 × 0.7 = 3500
> 1 × 3500 = 3500

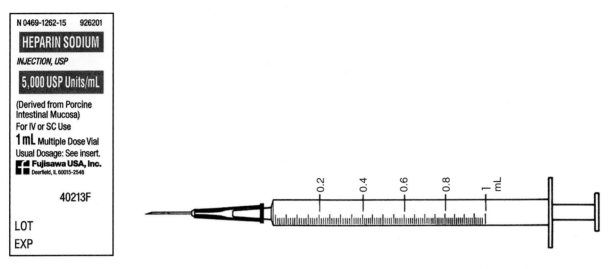

Example Ordered: Fragmin 8000 international units subcutaneous q6h. How many milliliters will you give? Shade in the dose on the syringe.

KNOW

WANT TO KNOW

10,000 international units : 1 mL :: 8000 international units : x mL

$10x = 1 \times 8 = 8$

$x = 0.8$ mL

PROOF

$1 \times 8000 = 8000$

$10,000 \times 0.8 = 8000$

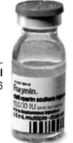

10,000 international units/mL

9.5 mL multidose vial

NDC 0013-2436-06

Used with permission from Pfizer, Inc.

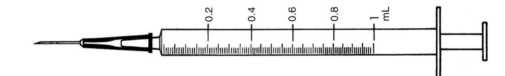

🔄 **CLINICAL ALERT**

Do not substitute insulin syringes for tuberculin syringes. Insulin syringes are calibrated in 100 units per mL and tuberculin syringes are calibrated in tenths per mL.

🔄 **CLINICAL ALERT**

Do not massage the injection site because this increases the incidence of bleeding and hematoma development.

WORKSHEET 11A | **Subcutaneous Injections**

Multidose vials are available in 10, 100, 1000, 5000, 10,000, 20,000, and 50,000 units/mL. Read the labels carefully. Answer the following questions and show your proofs (carry out to nearest hundredth). Shade in doses on syringes.

1. Ordered: Heparin 7000 units subcutaneous. Available: Heparin 10,000 units/mL. How many milliliters will the patient receive?

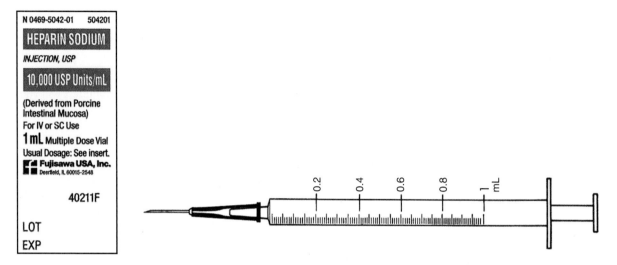

2. Ordered: Heparin 15,000 units subcutaneous q8h. Available: Heparin 20,000 units/mL. How many milliliters will the patient receive?

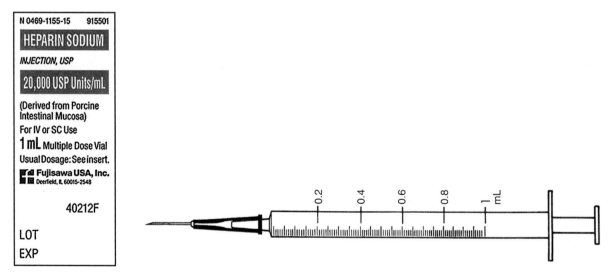

3. Ordered: Heparin 8000 units subcutaneous q8h. Available: Heparin 20,000 units/mL. How many milliliters will the patient receive?

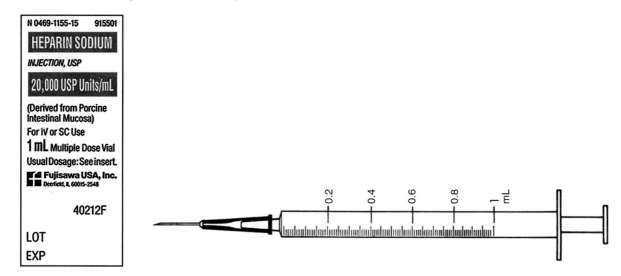

4. Ordered: Heparin 17,000 units subcutaneous stat dose. Available: Heparin 10,000 units/mL and 20,000 units/mL. Which strength will you choose? How many milliliters will the patient receive?

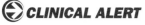

⊖ *CLINICAL ALERT*

The subcutaneous dosage of heparin should not exceed 1 mL.

5. Ordered: Fragmin 7500 units subcutaneous q6hr. Available: Fragmin 10,000 international units/mL. How many milliliters will the patient receive?

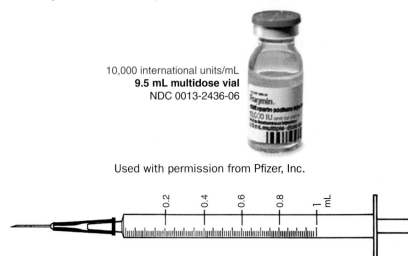

10,000 international units/mL
9.5 mL multidose vial
NDC 0013-2436-06

Used with permission from Pfizer, Inc.

6. Ordered: Heparin 750 units subcutaneous q4h. Available: Heparin 1000 units/mL. How many milliliters will the patient receive?

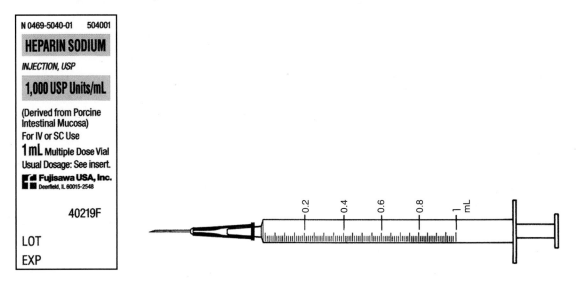

7. Ordered: Heparin 800 units subcutaneous q8hr. Available: Heparin 1000 units/mL in a multi-dose vial. How many milliliters will the patient receive?

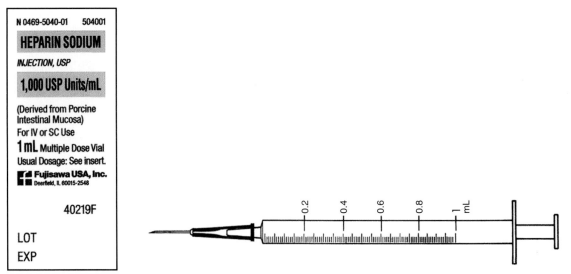

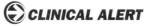

CLINICAL ALERT

Check your patient's chart for allergies. Heparin is made from pork and beef.

8. Ordered: Heparin 3000 units subcutaneous q8h. Available: Heparin 5000 units/mL in a multidose vial. How many milliliters will the patient receive?

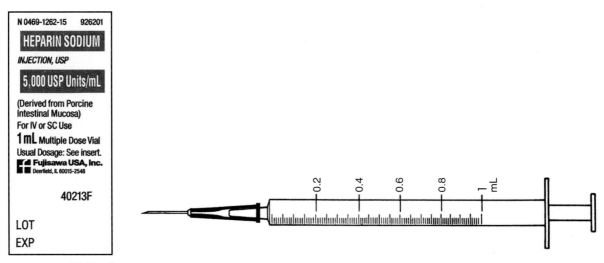

N 0469-1262-15   926201

HEPARIN SODIUM

INJECTION, USP

5,000 USP Units/mL

(Derived from Porcine
Intestinal Mucosa)
For IV or SC Use

1 mL Multiple Dose Vial
Usual Dosage: See insert.
Fujisawa USA, Inc.
Deerfield, IL 60015-2548

40213F

LOT

EXP

IV Flushes

9. Ordered: Heparin flush 5 units after each medication administration to prevent clot formation in the heparin lock. Available: Heparin 10 units/mL. How many units of medication are in the vial? How many milliliters will the patient receive?

HEPFLUSH®-10

*(HEPARIN LOCK FLUSH
SOLUTION, USP)*

10 USP Units/mL

(Derived from Porcine
Intestinal Mucosa)

10 mL Single Dose Vial

N 0469-1700-30   Sterile, Nonpyrogenic   1710

Follow hospital
protocol for saline
and heparin flushes
after medication
administration.

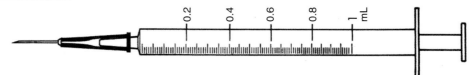

CLINICAL ALERT

Heparin resistance has been documented in elderly patients; therefore, large doses may be ordered.

Symptoms of overdose are nosebleed, bleeding gums, tarry stools, petechiae, and easy bruising. An electric razor should be used for shaving.

IV Flushes

10. Ordered: Heparin flush 50 units q12h for IV site patency. Available: Heparin 100 units/mL. How many milliliters will the patient receive?

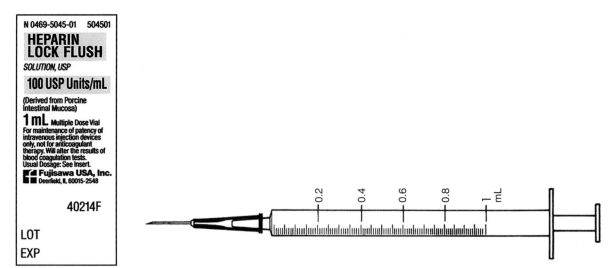

N 0469-5045-01   504501

HEPARIN LOCK FLUSH

SOLUTION, USP

100 USP Units/mL

(Derived from Porcine Intestinal Mucosa)

1 mL Multiple Dose Vial
For maintenance of patency of intravenous injection devices only, not for anticoagulant therapy. Will alter the results of blood coagulation tests.
Usual Dosage: See Insert.
Fujisawa USA, Inc.
Deerfield, IL 60015-2548

40214F

LOT

EXP

IV Flushes

Peripheral lines are flushed with 2 to 3 mL of normal saline using a 5 to 10 mL syringe to reduce pressure on the vein. Heparin locks provide patients with mobility while they are receiving IV medications.

Heparin flushes are used to prevent clot formation in the central line. Central lines are used for access to large veins. Hyperosmolarity solutions can be used without causing vein damage. Heparin flushes come in prefilled 12 mL syringes with 5 mL of 10 units/mL of heparin. Heparin flushes are also available in prefilled 12 mL syringes with 10 mL of 100 units/mL of heparin. Multiple dose vials of various strengths are also available.

⊖ CLINICAL ALERT

Heparin IV flushes are available in many different strengths and multiple-dose vials. READ LABELS CAREFULLY. Hospital protocol will determine the amount to administer.

Polypharmacy

▶ Many people who take prescription drugs also take over-the-counter (OTC) medication. Researchers from the University of Chicago found that about 91% of older adults use at least one medication, and nearly 30% have at least five prescriptions. The study also indicated that many of these older people are taking anticoagulants or antiplatelet agents, which puts them at high risk for adverse drug reactions. It is imperative that all OTC and prescription drugs be charted and the physician notified.

IV Heparin

When intermittent or continuous IV therapy is used, blood should be drawn for a PTT and a hematocrit level to determine the course of therapy. Therapeutic anticoagulant dosage is regulated according to the results of the PTT and the patient's weight.

Pharmacies are standardizing IV heparin preparations in concentrations of 25,000 units/500 mL and 25,000 units/250 mL. Dispensing charts indicating mL/hr and units/hr are available for each concentration. This will reduce overdosing and underdosing. Protamine sulfate is the antagonist for heparin. It is the nurse's responsibility to have protamine sulfate available.

WORKSHEET
11B

IV Heparin Calculations: mL/hr and Hours to Infuse

Answer the following questions and show your proofs (carry out to the nearest hundredth). The heparin will be administered with an infusion device.

Example Ordered: Heparin 1400 units/hr IV. Available: 500 mL of NS with 25,000 units of heparin sodium.

a. How many mL/hr will deliver 1400 units/hr?
b. How many hours will it take to infuse?

KNOW   **WANT TO KNOW**
500 mL : 25,000 units :: x mL : 1400 units
250x = 500 × 14 = 7000
250x = 7000
   x = 28/mL/hr. Set infusion pump to deliver 28 mL/hr.

> **PROOF**
> 500 × 1400 = 7000
> 250 × 28 = 7000

KNOW   **WANT TO KNOW**
28 mL : 1 hr :: 500 mL : x hr
28x = 1 × 500 = 500
28x = 500
  x = 17.85 hr   60 × 0.85 = 51   The IV will take 17 hr 51 minutes to infuse.

> **PROOF**
> 500 × 1 = 500
> 28 × 17.85 = 499.8 = 500

1. Ordered: Heparin sodium 1000 units/hr IV. Available: 1 L of 0.9% saline with 20,000 units of heparin.
   a. How many mL/hr will deliver 1000 units?
   b. How many hours will it take to infuse the bag?

2. Ordered: Heparin sodium 20,000 units IV in 12 hr. Pharmacy has sent 1000 mL of 0.9% normal saline with 20,000 units heparin sodium.
   a. At how many mL/hr should the IV infuse?
   b. How many units/hr will infuse?
   c. The shift reports that 250 mL have been infused. How many hours remain for the infusion?

3. Ordered: Heparin 1500 units/hr IV. Pharmacy has sent 1 L 0.9% saline with 20,000 units of heparin.
   a. How many mL/hr will deliver 1500 units?
   b. How many hours will it take to infuse this bag?

4. Ordered: Heparin 10,000 units in 15 hr. Pharmacy has sent 1000 mL NS with 10,000 units of heparin. The infusion was started at 0830.
   a. How many units/hr will the patient receive?
   b. How many mL/hr will be infused?
   c. The 0700 hr shift reports that 300 mL have been infused. When will the infusion finish? How many hours remain for the infusion?

5. Ordered: Heparin 1200 units/hr. Available: 500 mL NS with 10,000 units of heparin.
   a. How many mL/hr will infuse 1200 units/hr?
   b. How many hours will it take to infuse this bag?

6. Ordered: Heparin 2500 units/hr IV. Available: 50,000 units per 1000 mL 0.9% NS.
   a. How many mL/hr will deliver 2500 units/hr?
   b. How many hours will it take to infuse?

7. Ordered: Heparin 1500 units per hr IV. Available: 25,000 units per 500 mL.
   a. How many mL per hr will deliver 1000 units per hr?
   b. How many hours will it take to infuse?

8. Ordered: Heparin 1300 units per hr IV. Available: 500 mL with 25,000 units of heparin sodium.
   a. How many mL per hr will deliver 1300 units per hr?
   b. How long will it take to infuse?

9. Ordered: Heparin 1800 units per hr IV. Your patient is on fluid restrictions; therefore the pharmacy has sent a concentrated solution of 25,000 units/250 mL of NS.
   a. How many mL per hr will deliver 1800 units per hr?
   b. How many hours will it take to infuse?

10. Ordered: Heparin 1000 units per hr. Your patient is on fluid restrictions. The pharmacy has sent 20,000 units per 250 mL of NS.
    a. How many mL per hr will deliver 1000 units per hr?
    b. How many hours will it take to infuse?

Answers on page 415

WORKSHEET 11C | IV Heparin Calculations Titrated to Kilograms

All intravenous anticoagulants are based on the PTT results. Loading (bolus) doses are individualized and are titrated to weight in kilograms. Hospital protocol is usually standardized for each institution. It is important that the nurses know what the protocol standards are and where they are located. Protocols and literature may vary, but the loading doses are usually between 70 and 100 units per kg. Infusion rates for heparin sodium also vary but are usually between 15 and 25 units per kg per hr.

Example Ordered: IV heparin loading dose to infuse at 18 units per kg per hr. The patient weighs 210 lb. Available: 20,000 units of heparin sodium in 1000 mL of D5W.
At what rate will you set the IV infusion pump?

Change 210 lb to kg.   210 divided by 2.2 = 95.45 = 96 kg
Multiply units per hr by the patient's weight in kg. $18 \times 96 = 1728$ units per hr.

Ratio and Proportion Method

KNOW   WANT TO KNOW
18 units : 1 kg :: x units : 96 kg
$x = 18 \times 96 = 1728$
$x = 1728$ units per hr

PROOF
$18 \times 96 = 1728$
$1 \times 1728 = 1728$

KNOW   WANT TO KNOW
20,000 units : 1000 mL :: 1728 units : x mL
$20,000 x = 1000 \times 1728 = 1728000$
$20x = 1728$

PROOF
$1 \times 1728 = 1728$
$20 \times 86.4 = 1728$

   $x = 86.4$ mL per hr = 86 mL per hr. Set infusion pump to deliver 86 mL/hr.

1. Ordered: Heparin sodium 70 units per kg bolus loading dose. Infusion rate to run at 20 units per kg per hr. Available: 1000 mL D5W with 25,000 units of heparin. The patient weighs 176 lb.
   a. Calculate the loading dose.
   b. Calculate the units per hr based on weight.
   c. Calculate the mL per hr.

2. Ordered: 80 units per kg of heparin as a loading dose. Set infusion rate to deliver 1500 units per hr. Available: 1000 mL NS with 30,000 units of heparin. The patient weighs 160 lb.
   a. Calculate the loading dose.
   b. Calculate the mL per hr.

CLINICAL ALERT
Always have protamine sulfate available as an antidote for heparin.

3. Ordered: Heparin sodium 90 units per kg. Infuse at 25 units per kg per hr. Available: 1000 mL 0.45% NS with 25,000 units of heparin. The patient weighs 210 lb.
   a. How many units is the loading dose?
   b. How many units per hr will the patient receive?
   c. At what rate will you set the mL per hr?

4. Ordered: Loading dose of 75 units per kg; then infuse at 20 units per kg per hr. Available: 1000 mL 0.9% NS with 50,000 units of heparin. The patient weighs 300 lb.
   a. Calculate the loading dose.
   b. How many units per hr will the patient receive?
   c. At what rate will you set the infusion device?

5. Ordered: Loading dose of heparin 75 units per kg. Infuse at 17 units per kg per hr. Available: 1000 mL D5W with 20,000 units of heparin. The patient weighs 185 lb.
   a. How many units is the loading dose?
   b. How many units per hr will the patient receive?
   c. At what rate will you set the infusion device?

6. Ordered: Loading dose of 65 units per kg. Set the infusion to run at 15 units per kg per hr. Available: 500 mL 0.45% NS with 30,000 units of heparin. The patient weighs 145 lb.
   a. How many units is the loading dose?
   b. How many units per hr will infuse?
   c. At what rate will you set the infusion device?

7. Ordered: Bolus dose of heparin at 80 units per kg. Titrate infusion to run at 1000 units per hr. Available: 1000 mL D5W with 25,000 units of heparin. The patient weighs 120 kg.
   a. Calculate the number of units for the loading dose.
   b. Calculate mL per hr to infuse 1000 units per hr.

8. Ordered: A bolus dose of heparin at 70 units per kg. Run the infusion at 18 units per kg per hr. Available: 1000 mL D5W with 30,000 units of heparin. The patient weighs 194 lb.
   a. How many units will you give as the bolus dose?
   b. How many units per hr will infuse?
   c. At what rate will you set the infusion device?

9. Ordered: A loading dose of heparin at 95 units per kg. Pharmacy has sent 1000 mL 0.9% NS with 20,000 units of heparin. Run the infusion at 20 units per kg per hr. The patient weighs 136 kg.
   a. How many units is the loading dose?
   b. How many units per hr will infuse?
   c. At what rate will you set the infusion device?

10. Ordered: Heparin 100 units/kg bolus dose. Infuse at 18 units per kg per hr. Available: 1000 mL 0.45% NS with 35,000 units of heparin. The patient weighs 108 kg.
    a. How many units is the loading dose?
    b. How many units per hr will infuse?
    c. At what rate will you set the infusion device?

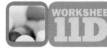 **WORKSHEET 11D** | **Dosing Guidelines**

Directions:

Use the Dosing Guidelines for (DVT-PE) Treatment Chart (Table 11-1) to figure the units per hour for the IV rate for a patient who weighs 70 kg. The standard infusion bag holds 25,000 units per 250 mL (100 units per mL).

Table 11-1 Dosing Guidelines for (DVT-PE) Treatment Chart

(Based on Raschke1 nomogram)
Obtain baseline APTT, prothrombin time (PT), CBC, platelet count. Check for contradictions to heparin therapy.

Patient name: **Location:**
Height: 70 inches   **Weight:** 70 kg   **Dosing weight:** 70 kg

Standard infusion bag concentration: 25000 units/ 250 ml (100 units/ml). Also, all infusion rates below are rounded to the nearest **100** units.

Initial bolus dose (80 units/kg): 5600 units
Initial infusion rate (18 units/kg/hr): 1300 units/hr (13 ml/hr)

APTT (seconds)§	Dose Change Units/kg/hr	Additional action	Next APTT
< 35 (1.2 × mean normal)	**Increase** by 4 units/kg/hr (300 units) or 3 ml/hr	Rebolus with 80 units/kg (5600 units)	6 hours
35 to 45 (1.2 to 1.5 × mean nml)	**Increase** by 2 units/kg/hr (100 units) or 1 ml/hr	Rebolus with 40 units/kg (2800 units)	6 hours
46 to 70 (1.5 to 2.3 × mean nml)	No change	—	6 hours*
71 to 90 (2.3 to 3.0 × mean nml)	**Decrease** by 2 units/kg/hr (100 units) or 1 ml/hr	—	6 hours
> 90 (> 3 × mean nml)	Decrease by 3 units/kg/hr (200 units) or 2 ml/hr	Stop infusion 1 hour	6 hours

*Repeat APTT every 6 hours during the first 24 hours; thereafter, monitor APTT once every morning, unless it is outside therapeutic range.
§The Therapeutic range in seconds should correspond to a plasma heparin level of 0.2 to 0.4 IU/ml by protamine sulfate or 0.3 to 0.6 IU/ml by amidolytic assay.

1. Calculate the initial bolus dose of 80 units per kg for the patient who weighs 70 kg.

2. Calculate the units per hour.

3. Calculate the infusion rate.

The 6 hour APTT is 30. Rebolus with 80 units per kg (5600 units) and increase the rate by 4 units per kg.

4. a. Calculate the increased units per hour.
    b. What is the new units per hour rate?

5. Calculate the new infusion rate.

The 6 hour APTT is 40. Increase the IV rate by 2 units per kg per hour.
Rebolus with 40 units per kg.

6. Calculate the bolus dose.

7. a. Calculate the units per hour increase.
   b. What is the new units per hour rate?

8. Calculate the new infusion rate.

The 6 hour APTT is 55 = no change
The 6 hour APTT is 85 = decrease the rate by 2 units per kg per hour.

9. a. Calculate the decrease units per hour.
   b. What is the new units per hour rate?

10. Calculate the new infusion rate.

The 6 hour APTT is 95 = decrease the rate by 3 units per kg per hour.

11. a. Calculate the decreased units per hour.
    b. What is the new units per hour rate?

12. Calculate the new infusion rate.

13. What will be your next action?

Oral Anticoagulants

Warfarin (Coumadin), (Figure 11-5), is used as prophylaxis after an episode of thrombolytic complications and for atrial fibrillation to prevent blood coagulation. The drug inhibits the activity of vitamin K, which is required for the activation of clotting factors. Patients receiving heparin therapy are converted to an oral anticoagulant in the hospital while still receiving heparin injections. The level of warfarin in the blood is monitored by the laboratory value of the international normalized ratio (INR). The INR is a standardized measurement of the prothrombin time (PTT). The INR should be maintained at 2 to 3 for best results, depending on the illness being treated. Dosing for all anticoagulants is individualized. The antidote for warfarin is vitamin K, plasma, or whole blood. Foods high in vitamin K should be avoided until the INR level has been stabilized. Compliance to daily dose and diet restrictions is essential.

When discharging a patient who will be going home on Coumadin (warfarin), it is extremely important that the patient is knowledgeable about medications that can potentiate the anticoagulation

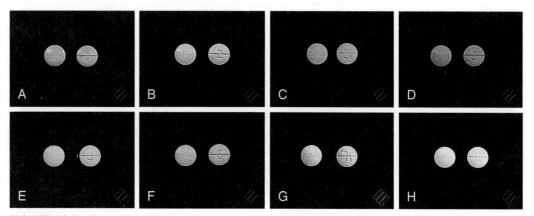

FIGURE 11-5 Examples of Coumadin tablets. **A**, 1 mg, **B**, 2 mg, **C**, 2.5 mg, **D**, 3 mg, **E**, 4 mg, **F**, 6 mg, **G**, 7.5 mg, **H**, 10 mg. From Mosby's Drug Consult 2007, St Louis, 2007, Mosby.

effect of Coumadin. A list of these medications is available from the pharmacist. Also, there are medications that can inhibit the effect of the Coumadin and over-the-counter medications that can increase the effects of the anticoagulant.

Because of the potential harmful effects of anticoagulants, it is a medication that deserves special protocols for use and compliance with the blood testing regimen. The importance must be stressed for all PT/INR tests be taken at the scheduled times. Signs and symptoms of bleeding or clotting must be reported immediately.

▶ Patients taking Coumadin are at increased risk for medication interactions. Always tell the health care provider all medications including over-the-counter medications you are taking.

Clopidogrel (Plavix) is an antiplatelet agent that blocks the formation of blood clots by preventing the clumping of platelets. Plavix is used for the prevention of heart attacks, unstable angina, recent stroke, or peripheral vascular disease. As with warfarin, there are many drug interactions associated with the efficacy of this drug. Atorvastatin (Lipitor) may potentiate the action of Plavix. A proton pump inhibitor (PPI) may subject the patient to another heart attack. The only PPI found to be safe for patients taking Plavix is pantoprazole (Protonix).

Missed doses: Warfarin and Plavix are usually taken once a day. If a dose is missed at the patient's usual dosing time, he or she should take it as soon as possible afterward. If it is missed closer to the 24-hour period, then the patient should resume his or her regular dose the next day. DO NOT DOUBLE THE DOSE.

Acetylsalicylic acid (aspirin) is also an antiplatelet agent that prevents the formation of blood clots. A low dose of aspirin is prescribed for concurrent use along with Warfarin, as these two drugs work in different ways. Warfarin prevents clotting of blood, and Aspirin prevents clumping of platelets that can form blood clots.

▶ CAUTION: There are many over-the-counter and prescribed medications that can adversely affect the efficacy of Warfarin/Coumadin and Clopidogrel/Plavix. A list of medications and foods that interact with Coumadin and Plavix must be discussed with the patient prior to discharge. It is essential that the patient understand the necessity of compliance.

Answers on page 419

WORKSHEET 11E | Multiple-Choice Practice

1. Ordered: Fragmin subcutaneous. Titrate to 120 international units per kg q12h × 5 days. The patient weighs 185 lb. How many international units of Fragmin will you administer for each dose?
   a. 5800 international units
   b. 1800 international units
   c. 10,080 international units
   d. 6400 international units

2. Refer to question 1. Available: 25,000 IU per mL multidose vial of Fragmin. How many milliliters of Fragmin will you give?
   a. 2.2 mL
   b. 0.4 mL
   c. 4.4 mL
   d. 0.2 mL

3. Ordered: Fragmin subcutaneous q12h titrated to kg. Titrate Fragmin to 120 international units per kg subcutaneous. The patient weighs 132 lb. How many kilograms does the patient weigh?
   a. 50 kg
   b. 120 kg
   c. 60 kg
   d. 45 kg

   How many international units of Fragmin will you prepare?
   a. 7000 international units
   b. 5000 international units
   c. 83,000 international units
   d. 7200 international units

4. Refer to question 3. How many milliliters of Fragmin will you give?
   Available: 10,000 IU per mL multidose vial.
   a. 0.7 mL
   b. 0.5 mL
   c. 1 mL
   d. 1.2 mL

5. Ordered: Administer a bolus of heparin sodium IV. The hospital protocol is 80 units per kg. The patient weighs 160 lb. How many units will you give?
   a. 5840 units   b. 6620 units   c. 4320 units   d. 2420 units

6. Ordered: IV heparin to infuse at 18 units per kg per hr. Available: 1000 mL D5W with 20,000 units heparin. The patient weighs 175 lb. How many units per hr will the patient receive?
   a. 1220 units per hr   b. 880 units per hr   c. 1280 units per hr   d. 1440 units per hr

   At what rate will you set the infusion device?
   a. 110 mL per hr   b. 85 mL per hr   c. 68 mL per hr   d. 72 mL per hr

7. Ordered: Heparin drip at 40 units per kg. Available: 25,000 units of heparin in 1000 mL of D5W. The patient weighs 75 kg. At what rate will you set the infusion device?
   a. 100 mL per hr   b. 120 mL per hr   c. 75 mL per hr   d. 82 mL per hr

8. Ordered: Heparin IV drip at 500 units/hr. Available: 500 mL 0.9% NS with 10,000 units of heparin. At what hourly rate will you set the infusion?
   a. 50 mL per hr   b. 75 mL per hr   c. 100 mL per hr   d. 25 mL per hr

9. Ordered: Fragmin subcutaneous titrated to 120 international units per kg q12h × 8 days. Begin treatment at 0800 hr. The patient weighs 220 lb. How many kg does the patient weigh?
   a. 100 kg   b. 120 kg   c. 110 kg   d. 60 kg

   How many international units of Fragmin will the patient receive per dose?
   a. 10,000 international units   b. 15,000 international units
   c. 8,000 international units   d. 12,000 international units

10. Refer to question 9. Available: Fragmin 10,000 international units per mL and Fragmin 25,000 international units per mL multidose vials. Which multidose vial will you use? How many mL will you give?
    a. 1 mL   b. 0.75 mL   c. 0.48 mL   d. 0.66 mL

Critical Thinking Exercises

Analyze the following scenarios.

1. Mrs. Smith, a 76-year-old woman, was recuperating after abdominal surgery. The physician wrote the following order: 2000 units heparin subcut stat. The nurse administered a 1 mL dose taken from a multidose vial labeled 20,000 units/mL. Later that day, the physician re-duced the heparin order. He wrote: *Reduce heparin to 1000 units q8h.* While the nurse is preparing the 1000-unit dose from the multidose vial of 20,000 units/mL, she realizes the error when the first dose of heparin was administered.

   Order:

   Given:

   Error(s):

   Potential injuries:

   Preventive measures:

Discussion

What factors contributed to the error?
How many units of heparin did Mrs. Smith receive for the first dose?
How was the patient's safety jeopardized?
What medication should always be on hand when a patient is receiving heparin?
What safety measures should have been implemented?
How can this type of error be reconciled?

2. Mr. G., an 80-year-old man, was admitted with a diagnosis of pulmonary embolism. He was given a bolus dose of 80 units of heparin and then was started on an IV drip of 25,000 units of heparin in 500 mL of D5W for 3 days. He has an order to start Coumadin 10 mg daily 72 hours before being discharged. Mr. G.'s discharge orders are for Coumadin (Warfarin) 10 mg daily and blood tests for INR status once a week for the first 2 weeks. As the discharge nurse, what precautions will Mr. G. need to be aware of while taking Coumadin?

Discussion:

What types of food might interfere with the desired effects of Coumadin?
What safety precautions should Mr. G. be aware of concerning possible bleeding?
What are some of the OTC medications that could enhance the effect of Coumadin?
What is the need for INR blood tests every week for the first 2 or 3 weeks?
How do you think that noncompliance with diet, medications, life style, and blood testing could interfere with the patient's safety?

3. A 68-year-old woman who had a hip replacement just returned to the general surgery floor. The woman is a type 1 diabetic. The physician wrote a new order that read: Start IV drip with 500 units of insulin in 1 liter of NS. Infuse over 24 hr. Heparin 250 units subcut q6h.

The nurse charted on the MAR: 500 units of heparin subcut. 250 units of insulin R added to the liter of NS. The nurse on the next shift noticed that the wrong medication and the wrong amount of heparin and insulin were charted for the IV and the subcut injection.

Order:

Given:

Discussion:

What factors contributed to the error?
What measures could be implemented for patient safety?
Why is it important to have another licensed nurse check the order?
What hospital protocols should be addressed to remediate these types of errors?
Do you think that the first nurse was aware of the error?

Final

1. Ordered: Heparin 4000 units subcutaneous for prophylaxis of cerebral thrombosis. Available: 5000 units/mL. How many milliliters will the patient receive?

2. Ordered: Heparin 2500 units q4h subcutaneous to prevent thrombi from recurring. Available: 10,000 units/mL vial. How many milliliters will the patient receive?

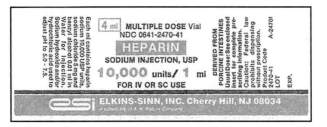

3. Ordered: Heparin 2000 units q4h subcutaneous for venous stasis. Available: 5000 units/mL and 10,000 units/mL. Which vial will you choose? If a tuberculin syringe is used, how many milliliters will the patient receive?

4. Ordered: Heparin 7000 units subcutaneous q8h before initiating a heparin infusion for a venous thromboembolism. Available: 5000, 10,000, and 20,000 units/mL. Which one will you choose? How many milliliters will the patient receive?

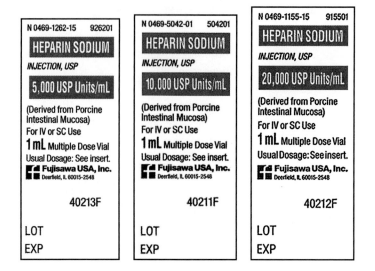

5. Ordered: Heparin 800 units subcutaneous every 4 hours as a prophylaxis for immobility. Available: Heparin 1000 units per mL. How many milliliters will the patient receive?

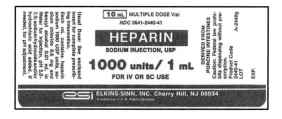

6. Ordered: 700 units per hr IV to infuse. Available: 20,000 units/500 mL. How many mL/hr will provide 700 units/hr? For how many hours will the IV infuse?

7. Ordered: 1500 units per hr IV for hyperlipemia. Available: 25,000 units/500 mL. How many mL/hr will provide 1500 units/hr? For how many hours will the IV infuse?

8. Ordered: Heparin 25,000 units IV in 24 hr for peripheral arterial embolization. Available: 1000 mL with 25,000 units of heparin sodium. How many mL/hr will give 25,000 units in 24 hr? How many units/hr will infuse?

9. Ordered: Heparin 35,000 units IV in 24 hr for atrial fibrillation. Available: 1000 mL 0.9% NS with 35,000 units of heparin sodium. How many mL/hr will the patient receive? How many units/hr will the patient receive?

10. Ordered: Heparin 2000 units per hr IV for pulmonary emboli. Available: Heparin 20,000 units in 1000 mL 0.9% NS. How many mL/hr will be delivered via the infusion device? For how long will the IV infuse?

Refer to the **Advanced Calculations** section of **Drug Calculations Companion, version 4** on Evolve for additional practice problems.

Children's Dosages

12

Objectives

- Calculate 24-hour drug doses and divided doses for specific weights.
- Calculate safe dose ranges in mg/kg, mcg/kg, and square meters of body surface area (BSA).
- Calculate reconstituted pediatric drug doses and small-volume IV flow rates for children.
- Evaluate orders and safe dose range calculations.
- Make a decision:
  Give medication (within therapeutic range).
  Hold medication and clarify promptly (overdose or underdose).
- Analyze medication errors using critical thinking.

Introduction

The trend for increased medication administration safety is to customize all dose orders based on body weight or body surface area and condition, along with other safeguards. Powerful high-alert drugs and most drugs for at-risk populations such as infants and children, adults who are extremely frail, and people who are underweight or overweight often require several steps for safe administration. This chapter will focus on customized dosing of pediatric medication orders to provide practice with smaller fractional amounts of medication and ounce to pound to kg weight conversion, but the principles, skills, and steps for calculation apply to adults as well.

Dosages Based on Body Weight and Surface Area

Infants and children have special medication needs because of their smaller size and weight as well as larger body surface area (BSA) per kilogram of body weight. They have varying capabilities of drug absorption, digestion, distribution, metabolism, and excretion. It is very important for the nurse to check current references for pediatric medication orders and to double-check safe dose ranges (SDRs) to prevent errors and injury. Minute doses that require scrupulous mathematics may be ordered. Pediatric and intensive care nurses use written pediatric drug guidelines and calculators to determine weights and verify SDRs.

The two methods currently used for calculating safe pediatric doses are based on (1) *body weight* in mg/kg or mcg/kg and (2) *body surface area* in square meters (m^2) using a scale called a *nomogram*.

mg/kg Method (Weight-Based Dosing)

The most *frequently* used calculation method for customized dosing is *mg per kg*. References usually state the safe amount of drug in mg per kg for a 24-hour period to be given in one or more divided doses. You may also see *mcg per/kg* cited for therapeutic doses when very small amounts of medication are to be given.

Steps to Solving mg/kg Problems

Step 1   *Estimate* the weight in kilograms by dividing the pounds in half*; then *calculate* the weight in kilograms using 2.2 lb = 1 kg equivalency (divide pounds by 2.2). Use a calculator.
     a. If the weight is in pounds, convert the pounds directly into kilograms (one-step calculation).
     b. If a weight is in pounds and ounces, convert the ounces to the nearest tenth of a pound and *add* this to the total pounds. Then convert the total pounds into kilograms to the nearest tenth (two-step calculation). (Refer to page 279 for kilogram-to-pound conversions and page 13 for rounding instructions.)

Step 2   *Calculate* the safe dose range (SDR) using a calculator and current safe dose recommendations found in the drug literature or drug handbook for this weight child in mg per kg or mcg per kg.

Step 3   *Compare* and *evaluate* the 24-hr ordered dose with the recommended SDR. Be sure the comparisons are for the *same* frequency!

Step 4   If safe, *calculate* the actual dose to be administered using written ratio and proportion. If the ordered dose is *less* than or *more* than the SDR, hold the medication and clarify promptly.

Shortcut Steps

1. Weight in kg
2. SDR
3. Compare with order
4. Calculate dose if safe to give

 RULE   All pediatric medication administration begins with an accurate weight (Step 1) and a calculation of the SDR (Step 2).

Example   Ordered: EryPed (erythromycin ethylsuccinate suspension) 150 mg po q6h for an infant with an infection. The infant weighs 15 lb, 6 oz today. The literature states that the SDR is 30 to 100 mg per/kg per day in four divided doses for severe infections.

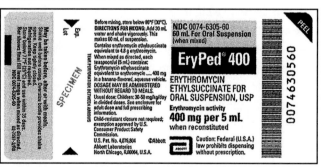

Step 1   **Estimate** the infant's weight.
     a. *Pounds to kilograms:* 15 lb ÷ 2 = 7.5 kg
     Calculate the actual weight.
     b. **Two-step** conversion because ounces are involved.
        Ounces to pounds: 6 oz ÷ 16 = 0.37 lb. Add part of pound to total pounds. The infant thus weighs 15.4 lb.
        Pounds to kilograms: 15.4 lb ÷ 2.2 = 7 kg (close to estimate)

*Estimation helps prevent major math errors; it must be followed by calculation and verification.

Step 2   The **SDR** recommended for children more than 1 month of age is 30 to 100 mg/kg per day po in four divided doses.

Low-range calculation: 30 mg × 7 kg = 210 mg (low SDR) per day ÷ 4   = 52.5 mg/dose
High-range calculation: 100 mg × 7 kg = 700 mg (high SDR) per day ÷ 4   = 175 mg/dose

Step 3   **Compare and evaluate:** The **SDR** recommended for this child's weight is 210 to 700 mg total q24h in four divided doses.
Ordered: 150 mg q6h   or   150 mg × 4 or 600 mg total in 24 hr.

Step 4   **Decision:** Give medication. Administering 600 mg for the day is within the SDR of 210 to 700 mg in four divided doses.
Calculate the individual dose (write out and prove).

KNOW   WANT TO KNOW
400 mg : 5 mL ∷ 150 mg : x mL

$\dfrac{\cancel{400}}{\cancel{400}}\,x = \dfrac{750}{400}$ (5 × 150)

x = 1.87 or 1.9 mL

PROOF
400 × 1.87 = 748
5 × 150 = 750

ANSWER
Give 1.9 mL

HINT   Review and analyze the logic of these four steps.

⊜ *CLINICAL ALERT*

Avoid two potential errors when converting pounds and ounces to kilograms. First, ounces must be converted to part of a pound *before* converting total pounds to kilograms; for example, 6 oz does not convert to 0.6 lb. Second, 15.4 lb does not equal 15.4 kg.

Don't forget the second step—convert the total pounds to kilograms.

Answers on page 420

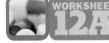

WORKSHEET 12A | Calculator Practice

RULE   Calculators are used in pediatric and adult care units for long division and multiplication problems. Dividing ounces by 16 will give the pound equivalent in the first step of two-step problems. Dividing or multiplying by 2.2 will give pound and kilogram equivalents.

1.   Estimate the weights, then use a calculator to convert from pounds to kilograms or kilograms to pounds. Round to the *nearest* tenth.* Double-check all work.

   a. 14 lb (1 or 2 steps?)
   Estimate:
   Actual:

   c. 10 lb
   Estimate:
   Actual:

   e. 10 kg
   Estimate:
   Actual:

   b. 12 lb, 2 oz (1 or 2 steps?)
   Estimate:
   Actual:

   d. 14 kg
   Estimate:
   Actual:

*For rounding instructions, refer to page 13.

2.   Calculate the 24-hr total dose in milligrams.
   a. 150 mg q8h
   c. 400 mcg q4h
   e. 750 mcg q12h

   b. 200 mg q6h
   d. 50 mg tid

3. Calculate the unit dose.
   a. 1 g in 4 equally divided doses
   b. 750 mg divided tid
   c. 2 g in 4 to 6 equally divided doses
   d. 16 g a day in 2 to 4 divided doses
   e. 500 mg in 4 divided doses

4. Calculate the SDR in milligrams for the following weights. Note that the answers will only be in milligrams or micrograms because *x*, the unknown, is a *dosage* measurement not a weight measurement. You want to know how many milligrams a day and milligrams per dose are safe for this patient. (2.2 lb = 1 kg)

   SDR PER KG; WEIGHT

   a. 10 mg/kg; weight is 5 kg
   b. 5 to 8 mg/kg; weight is 7.3 kg
   c. 6 to 8 mg/kg; weight is 8 lb
   d. 3 to 6 mg/kg; weight is 5 lb, 8 oz
   e. 200 to 400 mcg/kg; weight is 4 lb, 6 oz

   SDR FOR THIS WEIGHT

   _____ safe total mg/day
   _____ SDR for the day in mg
   _____ SDR for the day in mg
   _____ SDR for the day in mg
   _____ SDR for the day in mg

5. Ordered: Drug X, 50 mg tid. SDR: 2 to 3 mg/kg given in three divided doses. Child's weight is 18 kg.
   a. SDR for 24 hr
   b. SDR per dose
   c. Total ordered dose for day and per dose
   d. Evaluation and decision: Safe or unsafe to give? Why?

Answers on page 421

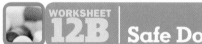

WORKSHEET 12B | **Safe Dose Range (SDR) Practice**

For each problem, use a calculator to determine the child's weight in kilograms to the *nearest* tenth, calculate the SDR, and compare it with the order. If the total dose for 24 hours is excessive, the unit dose is automatically excessive. Evaluate the order and make a decision.

1. Give medication (within SDR for unit dose and 24-hr dose).
2. Hold and clarify promptly (overdose or underdose).

1. Weight: 20 lb
   SDR in literature: 2 to 4 mg per kg per day
   Ordered: 50 mg daily
   a. Estimated weight in kg:
   b. Actual weight in kg:
   c. SDR for this child:
   d. Dose ordered:
   e. Evaluation and decision:

2. Weight: 33 lb
   SDR in literature: 100 to 200 mcg per kg per day in divided doses
   Ordered: 0.5 mg tid
   a. Estimated weight in kg:
   b. Actual weight in kg:
   c. SDR for this child:
   d. Dose ordered:
   e. Evaluation and decision:

3. Weight: 25.4 lb
   SDR in literature: 10 to 30 mg per kg per day in divided doses
   Ordered: 100 mg tid
   a. Estimated weight in kg:
   b. Actual weight in kg:
   c. SDR for this child:
   d. Dose ordered:
   e. Evaluation and decision:

4. Weight: 85 lb
   SDR: 10 to 15 mg/kg/day in 4 to 6 divided doses
   Ordered: 100 mg q6h
   - a. Estimated weight in kg:
   - b. Actual weight in kg:
   - c. SDR for this child:
   - d. Dose ordered:
   - e. Evaluation and decision:

5. Weight 5 lb
   SDR: 10 to 20 mcg/kg/day
   Ordered: 0.03 mg four times daily
   - a. Estimated weight in kg:
   - b. Actual weight in kg:
   - c. SDR for this child:
   - d. Dose ordered:
   - e. Evaluation and decision:

BSA Method (mg/m²)

The term "body surface area" refers to the total area exposed to the outside environment. The estimated BSA in square meters (m²) is derived from height and weight measurements by using a mathematical formula. It is considered the most reliable way to calculate therapeutic dosages.

This method may be used to calculate safe dosages of antineoplastic drugs, of new drugs, and of drugs for special populations such as infants, children, frail elderly patients, and patients with cancer. It may also be used to double-check medication orders for safe dosage.

Example Child weighs 33 lb (15 kg) and has a BSA of 0.55 m².

ORDERED: 20 mg/kg	vs **ORDERED:** 20 mg/m²	vs **ORDERED** 20 mg/lb
20 mg : 1 kg ::	20 mg : 1 m² ::	20 mg : 1 lb ::
x mg : 15 kg	x mg : 0.55	x mg : 33 lb
$x = 20 \times 15 = 300$ mg	$x = 20 \times 0.55 = 11$ mg	$x = 20 \times 33 = 660$ mg

As seen, the doses calculated range from 11 mg to 660 mg and, depending on the unit of measurement, reflect extremely large differences. This illustrates the need to check not only the numbers but also the units of measurement.

The West nomogram in Figure 12-1 allows the user to plot the *estimated* square meters of BSA by using height and weight measurements.

Although the pharmacy usually supplies BSA calculations, the nurse has the option of estimating safe dosages easily and rapidly by using a mathematical formula and a calculator and entering the patient's height and weight data.

Calculating BSA (m²) Using a Mathematical Formula

There are two formulas for calculating BSA (m²), and both use height and weight dimensions.

A. Formula using only metric system   B. Formula using only pounds and inches

$$\sqrt{\frac{\text{Weight (kg)} \times \text{Height (cm)}}{3600}} = \text{m}^2 \text{ BSA} \qquad \sqrt{\frac{\text{Weight (lb)} \times \text{Height (in)}}{3131}} = \text{m}^2 \text{ BSA}$$

Note the differences in the divisors. The formulas must be used exactly as shown.

Directions: Use a calculator. Use the metric formula. Determine the BSA in square meters for a child with a weight of 20 kg and a height of 95 cm.

Step 1 Multiply the kilograms by centimeters first and *divide* the result by 3600 ($20 \times 95 = 900/3600 = 0.527$)

Step 2 Obtain the *square root* of 0.527 by pushing the square root button. *Round* your answer to the *nearest* hundredth.

$$\frac{20 \times 95}{3600} = 0.527 \qquad \sqrt{0.527} = 0.725 = 0.73 \text{ m}^2$$

Compare this answer with the West nomogram (see Figure 12-1). Create a straight line between 20 kg and 95 cm and read the result in the surface area (SA) column on the nomogram. Take care to plot the height and weight on the metric graph—the outside columns. When reading the results (m²) columns, be sure to note the value of each calibrated line on the scale at the intersection point.

You may use either the nomogram or the formula. The formula method is more accurate, and if you have a calculator on hand, it is faster.

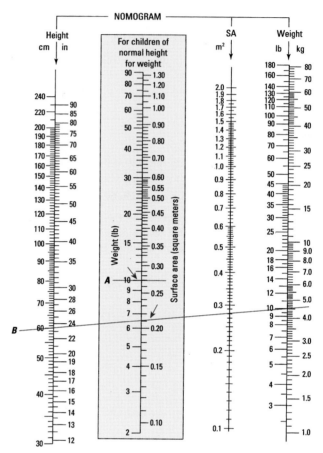

FIGURE 12-1   West nomogram for estimation of body surface area (BSA). **A,** The estimated BSA in square meters for children of normal height for weight is determined by reading the m² at the alignment point with the child's weight in pounds in the highlighted column. The red line denoted by the arrow reveals that an infant weighing 10 lb has an approximate BSA of 0.27 m². **B,** The BSA in square meters for children who are *under*weight or *over*weight (refer to pediatric standard growth charts and development grids for normal height and weight ranges for pediatric groups) is determined by connecting the child's plotted weight in the left column and plotted height in the right column with a straight line and reading the intersection point on the SA (surface area) column, as indicated by the arrow on the red line. This illustrates an estimated BSA of 0.28 m² for an infant of 60 cm height weighing 4.5 kg. Reading the SA column requires that height and weight be plotted in the same system of measurement metric or pounds/inches. (Nomogram modified with data from Berhrman RE, Kleigman RM, Jenson HB: Nelson textbook of pediatrics, ed 18, Philadelphia, 2007, Saunders.)

A square meter is slightly larger than a square yard. Visualize a square meter or a square yard of skin. As seen on the nomogram, a child of 90 lbs has only about 1 square meter of BSA (1 m²). Use one of the formulas to calculate your own BSA.

⊜ CLINICAL ALERT

Nurses are not usually expected to calculate BSA. The pharmacy provides the BSA calculations. Nurses *do* have a critical responsibility to distinguish the difference in a medication order and dosage based in mg/**lb** or mg/**kg** of weight and an order based on mg/**m²** of BSA (e.g., 20 mg/kg vs 20 mg/m² vs 20 mg/lb).

Comparing BSA-Based (mg/m²) Dosages with mg/lb and mg/kg Orders

Use the West nomogram (page 282), highlighted section for children of normal height and weight, to obtain the BSA (m²) based on weight.

Calculate the dose to be given based on the mg/m² and dose ordered.

	WT in lb	BSA in m²	DOSE ORDERED	DOSE TO BE GIVEN
1.	4 lb	0.15	10 mg/m²	10 × 0.15 = 1.5 mg
2.	6 lb	_____	15 mg/m²	_____
3.	10 lb	_____	5 mg/m²	_____

Calculate the dose for the same-weight children in mg/lb measurements, as illustrated in Problem 4.

	WT in lb	DOSE ORDERED	DOSE TO BE GIVEN
4.	4 lb	10 mg/lb	4 × 10 = 40 mg
5.	6 lb	15 mg/lb	_____
6.	10 lb	5 mg/lb	_____

Calculate the dose to be given in mg/kg measurements, as illustrated in Problem 9. Divide lb by 2.2 to obtain kg.

	WT in kg (to nearest tenth)	DOSE ORDERED	DOSE TO BE GIVEN
7.	4 lb = 1.8 kg	10 mg/kg	10 × 1.8 = 18 mg
8.	6 lb = _____ kg	2 mg/kg	

9. Using a calculator, obtain the BSA in m² (to the nearest hundredth for a child with a height of 60 cm and a weight of 100 kg using the appropriate BSA formula on page 281: _____

10. Using a calculator, obtain the BSA in m² for a child with a height of 30 in and weight of 35 lb using the appropriate BSA formula on page 281: _____

⊖ *CLINICAL ALERT*

Consider the patient safety implications when mg/m², mg/lb, and mg/kg are erroneously interchanged. This mistake has resulted in serious errors. The nurse must understand the differences among these three terms and focus to ensure that the correct values are being used when calculating the dose.

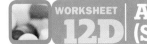

Additional Children's Safe Dose Range (SDR) Practice

Estimate and calculate weights and doses. Evaluate the order. If dose is within the SDR, calculate and prove the answer.

1. Weight: 26 lb
   SDR: 1 to 2 g/day in 4 divided doses
   Ordered: 500 mg q6h
   a. SDR for this child: b. Dose ordered:
   c. Evaluation and decision:

2. Weight: 44 lb, normal weight for height
   SDR: 5 to 8 mg/m^2* daily
   Ordered: 4 mg daily
   a. SDR for this child: b. Dose ordered:
   c. Evaluation and decision:

3. Weight: 19 lb
   SDR: 0.1 to 0.3 mg/kg/day in 2 divided doses
   Ordered: 2500 mcg bid
   a. Estimated weight in kg: b. Actual weight in kg:
   c. SDR for this child: d. Dose ordered:
   e. Evaluation and decision:

4. Weight: 9 lb
   SDR 1 to 5 mcg/kg/day
   Ordered: 0.01 mg daily
   a. Estimated weight in kg: b. Actual weight in kg:
   c. SDR for this child: d. Dose ordered:
   e. Evaluation and decision:

5. Weight: 14 lb
   SDR: 0.02 to 0.05 mg/kg/day
   Ordered: 150 mcg bid
   a. Estimated weight in kg: b. Actual weight in kg:
   c. SDR for this child: d. Dose ordered:
   e. Evaluation and decision:

   *For BSA conversion, refer to West nomogram on page 282.

⊘ CLINICAL ALERT

Estimating the weight in kg before doing the actual calculation is a safety check for calculation errors. Estimating approximate doses of medicines is also a valuable safety check. Estimation can alert you to major math errors. Verify your estimate with calculations.

FIGURE 12-2 **A,** Acceptable devices for measuring and administering oral medication to children (clockwise): measuring spoon, plastic syringes, calibrated nipple, plastic medicine cup, calibrated dropper, hollow-handled medicine spoon. **B,** Prefilled oral syringe. **C,** Calibrated droppers. **A,** From Wong DL et al: Wong's nursing care of infants and children, ed 7, St Louis, 2005, Mosby. **C,** From Macklin D, Chernecky C, Infortuna H: Math for clinical practice, ed 2, St Louis, 2011, Mosby.

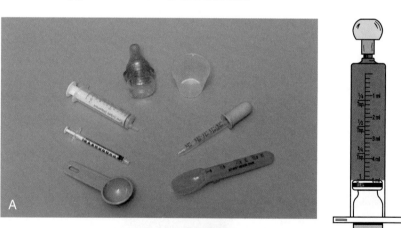

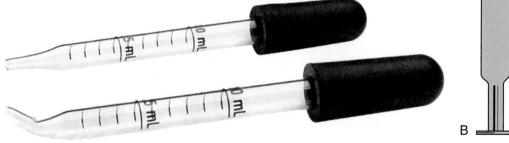

WORKSHEET 12E | Children's Oral Medications

These medications can be given to infants and children with a dropper or in a pre-prepared oral medication syringe (Figure 12-2). Small amounts may be given to an infant in a nipple. You may need to prepare and administer these medications using an oral syringe (without a needle).

For each problem, use a calculator to determine the child's weight in kilograms or pounds if required, calculate the SDR, and compare it with the order. Evaluate the order and make a decision:

1. Give medication (within SDR for unit dose and 24-hr dose).

2. Hold and clarify promptly (overdose or underdose).

◉ CLINICAL ALERT

If a nipple is used to deliver medication, rinse the nipple with water first so that the medicine will flow rather than stick to the nipple. Family may be very helpful by holding the child or by giving the oral medication or something pleasant-tasting following the medication.

For decisions 1 and 2 only, calculate the medication amount to be administered using *written ratio and proportion*. Prove your work. Do *not* calculate overdose or underdose orders. Hold them and clarify promptly.

1. Ordered: Tylenol (acetaminophen children's elixir) 160 mg po for a 4-year-old child who weighs 14 kg today. Label: 80 mg per $\frac{1}{2}$ tsp.

   a. Estimated weight in lb: b. Actual weight in lb:

   c. SDR for this child: d. Dose ordered:

   e. Evaluation and decision: f. Amount to be given in mL if applicable:

Drug Facts (continued)

- use only enclosed dosing cup designed for use with this product. Do not use any other dosing device.
- if needed, repeat dose every 4 hours while symptoms last
- do not give more than 5 times in 24 hours
- do not give for more than 5 days unless directed by a doctor
- this product does not contain directions or complete warnings for adult use

Weight (lb)	Age (yr)	Dose (tsp or mL)
under 24	under 2 years	ask a doctor
24-35	2-3 years	1 tsp or 5 mL
36-47	4-5 years	1 1/2 tsp or 7.5 mL
48-59	6-8 years	2 tsp or 10 mL
60-71	9-10 years	2 1/2 tsp or 12.5 mL
72-95	11 years	3 tsp or 15 mL

Attention: use only enclosed dosing cup specifically designed for use with this product. Do not use any other dosing device.

Other information

- each teaspoon contains: sodium 3 mg
- store at 20°-25°C (68°-77°F)
- do not use if printed neckband is broken or missing

Inactive ingredients anhydrous citric acid, butylparaben, carboxymethylcellulose sodium, carrageenan, D&C red no. 33, FD&C blue no. 1, flavor, glycerin, high fructose corn syrup, hydroxyethyl cellulose, microcrystalline cellulose, propylene glycol, purified water, sodium benzoate, sorbitol solution

Questions? Call 1-800-910-6874

*This product is not manufactured or distributed by the Tylenol Company, owner of the registered trademark Tylenol®.

094 01 0137 ID209441
Distributed by Target Corporation
Minneapolis, MN 55403
© 2009 Target Brands, Inc.
All Rights Reserved Shop Target.com

NDC 11673-130-26

children's acetaminophen
oral suspension

80 mg per ½ teaspoon
(160 mg per 5 mL)
fever reducer/pain reliever

Compare to active ingredient in Children's Tylenol® Oral Suspension*

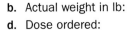 see new warnings information

alcohol free
ibuprofen free
aspirin free

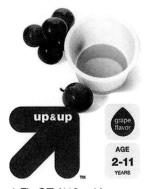

up&up

grape flavor

AGE **2-11** YEARS

4 FL OZ (118 mL)

2. Ordered: Clindamycin HCl pediatric solution 300 mg q8h po. The child weighs 66 lb today. The SDR is 10 to 30 mg/kg/day in 3 to 4 divided doses.

   a. Estimated weight in kg:

   b. Actual weight in kg:

   c. SDR for this child:

   d. Dose ordered:

   e. Evaluation and decision:

   f. Amount to be given in mL if applicable:

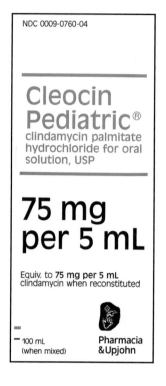

NDC 0009-0760-04

Cleocin Pediatric®
clindamycin palmitate hydrochloride for oral solution, USP

75 mg per 5 mL

Equiv. to **75 mg per 5 mL** clindamycin when reconstituted

100 mL (when mixed)

Pharmacia &Upjohn

⊖ CLINICAL ALERT

Differentiate elixirs and concentrated drops from oral suspensions. Elixirs contain alcohol for flavoring. Suspensions contain solids that must be dispersed in the liquid by shaking or stirring. Concentrated drops contain a greater amount of drug in a smaller volume of liquid than ordinary drops. They need to be gently shaken prior to administration.

⊖ CLINICAL ALERT

Avoid mixing medicines in essential foods such as formula or milk. A changed taste may result in long-term refusal of that food. Water, applesauce, or sherbet may be used to mix the medications if the diet allows. The medicine may be followed immediately with formula, juice, or a popsicle as the diet permits.

3. Ordered: Tegretol (carbamazepine) oral suspension 0.25 g po tid. The SDR for maintenance in a child over 12 years of age is 400 to 800 mg/day in 3 to 4 divided doses.

    a. SDR for this child:

    b. Dose ordered in mg:

    c. Evaluation and decision:

    d. Amount to be given if applicable:

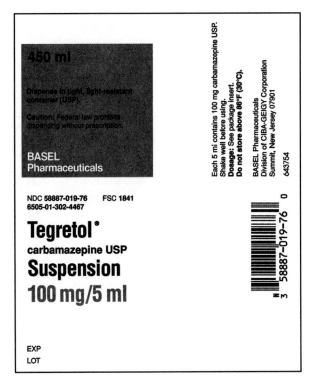

450 ml

Dispense in tight, light-resistant container (USP).

Caution: Federal law prohibits dispensing without prescription.

BASEL
Pharmaceuticals

NDC 58887-019-76   FSC 1841
6505-01-302-4467

Tegretol°

carbamazepine USP
Suspension
100 mg/5 ml

EXP
LOT

Each 5 ml contains 100 mg carbamazepine USP. Shake well before using.
Dosage: See package insert.
Do not store above 86°F (30°C).

BASEL Pharmaceuticals
Division of CIBA-GEIGY Corporation
Summit, New Jersey 07901

643754

3 58887-019-76 0

4. Ordered: Leucovorin calcium 5 mg q6h po. The child weighs 24 lb and has normal weight and height. The SDR according to the literature is 10 mg/m^2 q6h for 72 hr. For BSA calculation, refer to the West nomogram on page 282. The BSA is determined by pounds, not kilograms.

    a. SDR for this child:

    b. Dose ordered:

    c. Evaluation and decision:

    d. Amount to be given if applicable:

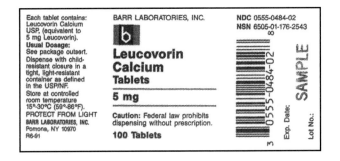

Each tablet contains: Leucovorin Calcium USP, (equivalent to 5 mg Leucovorin).
Usual Dosage:
See package outsert. Dispense with child-resistant closure in a tight, light-resistant container as defined in the USP/NF.
Store at controlled room temperature 15°-30°C (59°-86°F).
PROTECT FROM LIGHT
BARR LABORATORIES, INC.
Pomona, NY 10970
R6-91

BARR LABORATORIES, INC.

ⓑ

Leucovorin Calcium
Tablets

5 mg

Caution: Federal law prohibits dispensing without prescription.

100 Tablets

NDC 0555-0484-02
NSN 6505-01-176-2543

0555-0484-02

SAMPLE

Exp. Date:

Lot No.:

5. Ordered: Amoxil 180 mg q8h po for a child who weighs 27 lb. The SDR is 40 mg/kg/day in 3 divided doses.
   a. Estimated weight in kg:
   b. Actual weight in kg:
   c. SDR for this child:
   d. Dose ordered:
   e. Evaluation and decision:
   f. Amount to be given in mL if applicable:

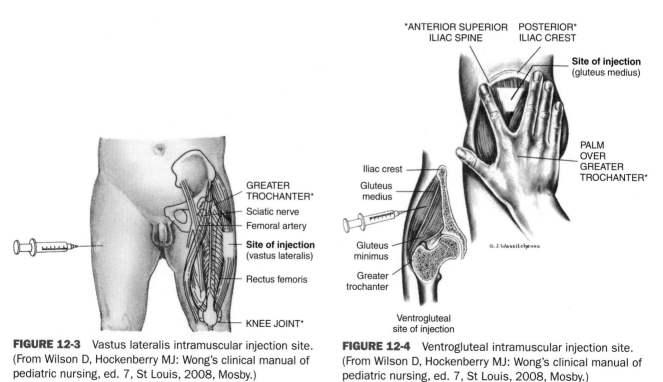

AMOXIL®
125mg/5mL

125mg/5mL
NDC 0029-6008-23

AMOXIL®
AMOXICILLIN
FOR ORAL
SUSPENSION

Directions for mixing: Tap bottle until all powder flows freely. Add approximately 1/3 total amount of water for reconstitution [total=78 mL]; shake vigorously to wet powder. Add remaining water; again shake vigorously. Each 5 mL (1 teaspoonful) will contain amoxicillin trihydrate equivalent to 125 mg amoxicillin.
Usual Adult Dosage: 250 to 500 mg every 8 hours.
Usual Child Dosage: 20 to 40 mg/kg/day in divided doses every 8 hours, depending on age, weight and infection severity. See accompanying prescribing information.

100mL
(when reconstituted)

NSN 6505-01-153-3862
Net contents: Equivalent to 2.5 grams amoxicillin. Store dry powder at room temperature. **Caution:** Federal law prohibits dispensing without prescription.
SmithKline Beecham Pharmaceuticals
Philadelphia, PA 19101

3 0029-6008-23 1

LOT
EXP.

Keep tightly closed.
Shake well before using.
Refrigeration preferable but not required.
Discard suspension after 14 days.

SB SmithKline Beecham

9405793-E

Multiple subcutaneous and intramuscular injections are not ordered for pediatric patients because of limited sites and potential emotional and physical trauma. Nevertheless, some vaccines, analgesics, and other single-dose medicines are given using this route. The technique must be practiced in a clinical lab setting under supervision.

- The vastus lateralis can be used from birth to adulthood but is a *preferred injection* site for babies younger than 7 months (Figure 12-3).
- The ventrogluteal muscle is an *alternate site* for children over 7 months and for adults (Figure 12-4).

*ANTERIOR SUPERIOR
ILIAC SPINE

POSTERIOR*
ILIAC CREST

Site of injection
(gluteus medius)

Iliac crest

Gluteus
medius

PALM
OVER
GREATER
TROCHANTER*

GREATER
TROCHANTER*

Sciatic nerve

Femoral artery

Site of injection
(vastus lateralis)

Rectus femoris

Gluteus
minimus

Greater
trochanter

KNEE JOINT*

Ventrogluteal
site of injection

G. J. Wassilchenko

FIGURE 12-3 Vastus lateralis intramuscular injection site. (From Wilson D, Hockenberry MJ: Wong's clinical manual of pediatric nursing, ed. 7, St Louis, 2008, Mosby.)

FIGURE 12-4 Ventrogluteal intramuscular injection site. (From Wilson D, Hockenberry MJ: Wong's clinical manual of pediatric nursing, ed. 7, St Louis, 2008, Mosby.)

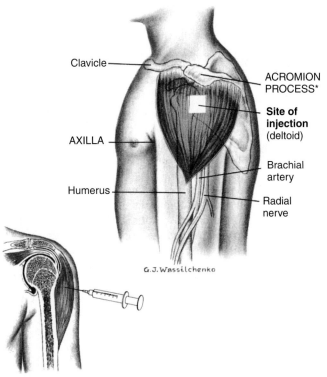

FIGURE 12-5 Deltoid intramuscular injection site. (From Wilson D, Hockenberry MJ: Wong's clinical manual of pediatric nursing, ed. 7, St Louis, 2008, Mosby.)

- The deltoid site may be used for small-volume, non-irritating medications, 0.5 to 1 mL, in older children and adults with *well-developed* deltoid muscles (Figure 12-5).
- Needle lengths and gauges and fluid amounts are much smaller for pediatric patients.
- The dorsogluteal site is not a recommended injection site because of the dangers both in children and adults of damaging the sciatic nerve and striking blood vessels.

Answers on page 424

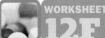 WORKSHEET 12F | **Children's Subcutaneous and Intramuscular Medications**

For each problem, use a calculator to determine the child's weight in kg to the nearest tenth, calculate the SDR, and compare it with the order. Evaluate the order and make a decision:

1. Give medication (within SDR for unit dose and 24-hr dose).
2. Hold and clarify promptly (overdose or underdose).

For decisions 1 and 2 only, calculate the medication amount to be administered using *written ratio and proportion*. Double-check and prove your work. Do *not* calculate overdose orders.

1. Ordered: Codeine 10 mg IM stat for a child in pain who weighs 44 lb. The SDR is 0.5 mg per kg q4-6h IM.
   a. Estimated weight in kg:
   b. Actual weight in kg:
   c. SDR for this child:
   d. Dose ordered:
   e. Evaluation and decision:
   f. Volume to be administered to the nearest hundredth of a mL if applicable:

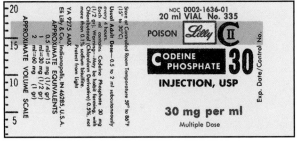

2. Ordered: Morphine sulfate 5 mg IM stat for a child who weighs 55 lb, 8 oz. The SDR is 0.1 to 0.2 mg/kg q4h.
   a. Estimated weight in kg:
   b. Actual weight (1 or 2 steps?):
   c. SDR for this child:
   d. Dose ordered:
   e. Evaluation and decision:
   f. Volume to be administered if applicable:

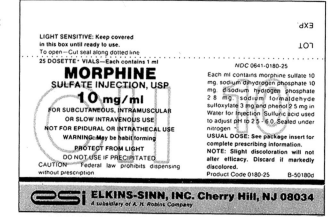

3. Ordered: Atropine sulfate 0.2 mg subcutaneous preoperatively for a child who weighs 17 lb, 9 oz. The SDR for a child weighing 7 to 9 kg is 0.2 mg, 30 to 60 min before surgery.
   a. Estimated weight in kg:
   b. Actual weight (1 or 2 steps?):
   c. SDR for this child:
   d. Dose ordered:
   e. Evaluation and decision:
   f. Volume to be administered if applicable:

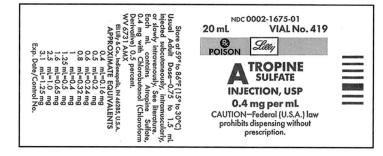

4. Ordered: Ampicillin sodium 500 mg IM q12h for a 7 lb baby with septicemia. SDR is 100 to 200 mg/kg/day in two divided doses.
   a. Estimated weight in kg:
   b. Actual weight (1 or 2 steps?):
   c. SDR for this child:
   d. Dose ordered:
   e. Evaluation and decision:
   f. Volume to be administered if applicable:

5. Ordered: Robinul 0.16 mg IM 60 minutes before anesthesia induction. Child's weight: 88 lb. SDR: 0.004 mg per kg IM.
   a. Estimated weight in kg:
   b. Actual weight (1 or 2 steps?):
   c. SDR for this child:
   d. Dose ordered:
   e. Evaluation and decision:
   f. Volume to be administered if applicable:

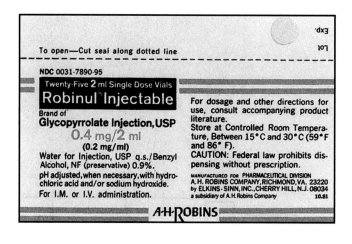

Children's IV Medications: Reconstitution, Dilution, and Flow Rate Information

Hospital pharmacies and pediatric drug references provide directions for dilution and rates of administration of IV medications for children. The volumes are smaller than those for adults. After determining that the ordered dose is within the SDR, the nurse may have to dilute the medication in a prescribed ratio, withdraw the ordered amount, then further dilute it using a compatible IV solution, and administer it directly or by an infusion pump in a volume-control device. Devices used to administer IV medications to children are shown in Figure 12-6. Volume control devices help prevent fluid and/or drug overdoses.

Example Ordered: Antibiotic 1 g q6h IV. Supplied: A powdered form of antibiotic that requires reconstitution. Pediatric directions from pharmacy: *Dilute to 100 mg/mL, withdraw ordered amount, then further dilute to 30 mL, and administer over 20 min.*
The label reads 2 g.

Step 1 Dilute to 100 mg/mL.
The label reads 2 g. (Change to milligrams for dilution: 2 g = 2000 mg.)

KNOW   WANT TO KNOW
100 mg : 1 mL :: 2000 mg : x mL

$$\frac{\cancel{100}}{\cancel{100}} x = \frac{2000}{100}$$

$x = 20$ mL
Reconstitute antibiotic with 20 mL compatible solution.*

PROOF
100 × 20 = 2000
1 × 2000 = 2000

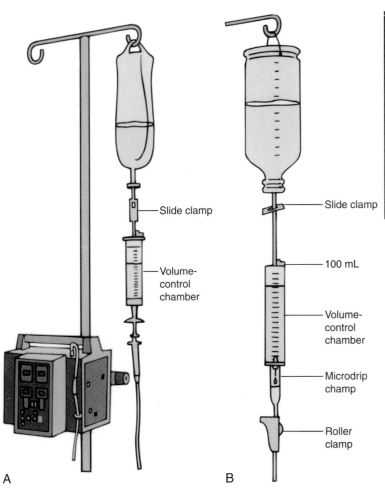

Slide clamp

Volume-
control
chamber

A

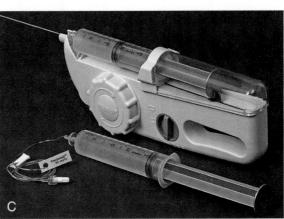

C

Slide clamp

100 mL

Volume-
control
chamber

Microdrip
champ

Roller
clamp

B

FIGURE 12-6 **A,** Electronic infusion pump with volume-control device. **B,** Gravity infusion with microdrip tubing (60 gtt/mL delivered through a needle) and volume-control device. Electronic infusion devices with volume-control devices are preferred for the administration of IV fluids to infants and children. If one of these is not available, microdrip (60-drop factor) tubing should be used with a volume-control device to prevent fluid or drug overload. Small volumes to be delivered IV within a short period may be administered directly through a syringe or a syringe pump. **C,** Freedom 60-syringe infusion pump. This portable reusable manual infusion uses standard 60 mL syringes and can be filled from 1 to 60 mL. It offers flow rates with rate-controlled tubing from 0.5 to 1200 mL per hr. It does not permit free flow. C, From Repro-Med Systems, Inc., Chester, NY.

Step 2 Withdraw ordered amount (1 g).

KNOW   WANT TO KNOW

2 g : 20 mL ∷ 1 g : x mL

$2x = 20$

$x = 10$ mL $= 1$ g

| PROOF |
| $2 \times 10 = 20$ |
| $20 \times 1 = 20$ |

| ANSWER |
| 10 mL |

Step 3 Place the medication in a volume-control device, adding a compatible IV solution to 30 mL. Set the flow rate. Consult a procedure book for use of volume-control devices.
Flow rate:

KNOW   WANT TO KNOW

30 mL : 20 min ∷ x mL : 60 min

$\frac{\cancel{20}}{\cancel{20}} x = \frac{1800}{20}$

$x = 90$ mL

| PROOF |
| $30 \times 60 = 1800$ |
| $20 \times 90 = 1800$ |

| ANSWER |
| Set rate at 90 mL/hr |
| for 20 min |

▮▮▮▮RULE To *estimate* hourly IV flow rates for amounts to be delivered in less than 60 minutes by a pump: for **10** minutes, multiply the volume by 6 because there are six 10-minute periods in an hour; for **15** minutes, multiply the volume by 4; for **20** minutes, multiply the volume by 3; and for **30** minutes, multiply the volume by 2. This will work only for 10-, 15-, 20-, and 30-minute orders.

To *calculate* the setting for mL/hr on a pump for medications to be delivered in less than 1 hour, set up a ratio and proportion of milliliters to minutes. The final dilution may be made with an existing IV solution if it is compatible with the medication.

Example To give 10 mL in 15 min with a pump, *estimate* ($10 \times 4 = 40$ mL/hr):

KNOW   WANT TO KNOW

10 mL : 15 min ∷ x mL : 60 min

$\frac{\cancel{15}}{\cancel{15}} x = \frac{600}{15}$

$x = 40$ mL

| PROOF |
| $10 \times 60 = 600$ |
| $15 \times 40 = 600$ |

| ANSWER |
| 40 mL/hr |

*For information and practice reconstituting medications, refer to Chapter 5.

Example Ordered: Antibiotic 250 mg q4h IV.
The label reads: *Mix (dilute) with 4.2 mL sterile water for injection to yield 5 mL of 100 mg/mL.*
Amount of ordered antibiotic to be withdrawn after mixing:

KNOW   WANT TO KNOW

100 mg : 1 mL ∷ 250 mg : x mL

$\frac{\cancel{100}}{\cancel{100}} x = \frac{250}{100}$

$x = 2.5$ mL

| PROOF |
| $100 \times 2.5 = 250$ |
| $1 \times 250 = 250$ |

| ANSWER |
| 2.5 mL |

Directions for pediatric administration: *Further dilute to 25 mL and administer over 30 minutes.*
Total volume to be administered: 25 mL.

Example Flow rate in volume-control device, estimate ($2 \times 25 = 50$ mL/hr):

KNOW   WANT TO KNOW

25 mL : 30 min ∷ x mL : 60 min

$30x = 25 \times 60$ or 1500

$x = 50$ mL

| PROOF |
| $25 \times 60 = 1500$ |
| $30 \times 50 = 1500$ |

| ANSWER |
| 50 mL/hr |

WORKSHEET 12G | Children's IV Medications

For each problem, use a calculator to determine the child's weight in kg if required, calculate the SDR, and compare it with the order. Round oz, lb, and kg to the nearest tenth. Evaluate the order and make a decision:

1. Give medication (within SDR for unit dose 24-hr dose).
2. Hold and clarify promptly (overdose or underdose).

Calculate the medication amount to be administered based on the label provided. Use written ratio and proportion and prove your answer even if you use a calculator to verify it. Calculate the IV pump flow rate in mL/hr if medication is to be administered for more than 5 min. Round ounces and kilograms to the nearest tenth. Enter calculator data twice for verification.

1. Ordered: Luminal sodium 65 mg IV stat for a child with seizures. The child's weight is 62 lb. The SDR for sedation is 1 to 3 mg/kg q24h.
   Directions: Dilute to 3 mL with sterile water for injection.
   a. Estimated weight in kg:
   b. Actual weight in kg:
   c. SDR for this child:
   d. Dose ordered:
   e. Evaluation and decision:
   f. Dose in mL to be withdrawn before dilution:

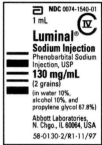

NDC 0074-1540-01
1 mL
Luminal®
Sodium Injection
Phenobarbital Sodium
Injection, USP
130 mg/mL
(2 grains)
(in water 10%,
alcohol 10%, and
propylene glycol 67.8%)
Abbott Laboratories,
N. Chgo., IL 60064, USA
58-0130-2/R1-11/97

2. Ordered: Initial dose of furosemide 25 mg IV stat. The SDR is 1 mg/kg to increase gradually in 1 mg/kg increments to desired response, not to exceed 6 mg/kg. The child weighs 55 lb today.
   a. Estimated weight in kg:
   b. Actual weight in kg:
   c. SDR for this child:
   d. Dose ordered:
   e. Evaluation and decision:
   f. Volume to be administered if applicable:

FUROSEMIDE
INJECTION, USP
40 mg/4 mL
(10 mg/mL)
For IM or IV Use
4 mL Single Dose Vial

N 63323-280-04   Sterile, Nonpyrogenic   28004
Preservative Free
Discard unused portion.
Each mL contains: Furosemide
10 mg; Water for Injection q.s.
Sodium chloride to adjust
isotonicity, pH adjusted with
sodium hydroxide and if
necessary hydrochloric acid.
Usual Dosage: See insert.
PROTECT FROM LIGHT. Do not
use if discolored. Use only if
solution is clear and seal intact.
Store at controlled room
temperature 15°-30°C
(59°-86°F).
Rx only
American
Pharmaceutical
Partners, Inc.
Los Angeles, CA 90024
401736
LOT
EXP

3. Ordered: Garamycin 15 mg IV q8h. The child weighs 13.2 lb today. The SDR is 2-2.5 mg per kg q8h. Directions from the pharmacy say to dilute *to* 50 mL with 0.9% NaCl and administer over 60 min.
   a. Estimated weight in kg:
   b. Actual weight in kg:
   c. SDR for this child:
   d. Dose ordered:
   e. Evaluation and decision:
   f. Amount withdrawn from vial:
   g.

11107672
Rev.11/81
SCHERING
2 ml Multiple Dose Vial NDC-0085-0013-05
Garamycin®   Sterile
PEDIATRIC INJECTABLE
brand of gentamicin sulfate injection, USP
For Parenteral Administration
20 mg Caution: Federal law prohibits dispensing without prescription.
2ml=20mg Schering Pharmaceutical Corporation (PR), Manati, Puerto Rico 00701
An Affiliate of Schering Corporation, Kenilworth, N J 07033

Usual Dose:
See package insert.
Each ml of aqueous solution
contains: gentamicin sulfate, USP
equivalent to 10 mg gentamicin
base; 13 mg methylparaben as preservative and ... sodium bisulfite, and
0.1 mg ... sodium bisulfite, and
0.1 mg edetate disodium.
Store between 2° and 30°C
(36° and 86°F).
Read accompanying
directive, is Carefully.

⊗ CLINICAL ALERT

Many of the antibiotics, particularly the cephalosporins have very similar names, such as ceftizoxime, ceftriaxone, and cephradine. However, the uses and the SDRs are very different!

4. Ordered: Digoxin 0.5 mg IV stat for a child with congestive heart failure. SDR: 0.015 to 0.35 mg per kg. Patient wt: 24 lb, 6 oz. Directions: Administer IV over 5 minutes. Safe to give undiluted. If needed, dilute each mL of drug in 4 mL SW (to permit small amounts of drug to be infused over time). Use a calculator to determine SDR.

LANOXIN®   **2mL**
(digoxin) Injection
(0.5 mg) in 2 mL
[0.25 mg] per mL)
Store at 15° to 25°C (59° to 77°F).
PROTECT FROM LIGHT.
Glaxo Wellcome Inc.
Research Triangle Park, NC 27709
Rev. 1/96

542308

LOT
EXP

a. Estimated weight in kg:
c. SDR for this child:
e. Evaluation and decision:

b. Actual weight in kg:
d. Dose ordered:
f. How many mL of digoxin will you prepare before dilution?

5. Ordered: Geopen (carbenicillin disodium) 2 g IV q6h. The SDR is 50 to 500 mg/kg q24h in divided doses every 4 to 6 hr. Dilute to 200 mg/mL with compatible solution and administer at rate of 1 g/10 min. The child weighs 26 lb.

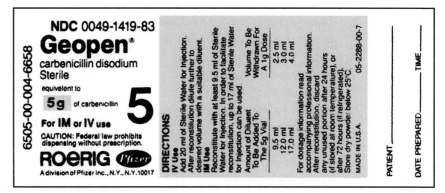

a. Estimated weight in kg:
b. Actual weight in kg:
c. SDR for this child:
d. Dose ordered:
e. Evaluation and decision:
f. Amount withdrawn after reconstitution:
g. Flow rate in mL/hr if applicable:

⊖ CLINICAL ALERT

Pediatric IV flow rates carry a high potential for errors. Consult pediatric IV drug references and pharmacy for pediatric IV dilutions and rates of administration. Note that liquids added to solids result in a higher total volume than just the amount of liquid added. Instructions to dilute **with** x mL result in more volume than instructions to dilute **to** x mL. Dilute to limits a total volume for the mixture. Dilute **with** is just stating the amount of liquid to be added to the solid. When in any doubt about IV dilutions and flow rates, consult the pharmacy and document the verification. The prescriber may have to be contacted too.

WORKSHEET 12H | Children's Dosages

For each problem, use a calculator to determine the child's weight in kilograms to the nearest tenth, calculate the SDR, and compare it with the order. If the total dose for 24 hours is excessive, the unit dose is automatically excessive. Evaluate the order and make a decision:

1. Give the medication (within SDR for unit dose and 24-hr dose).
2. Hold and clarify promptly (overdose or underdose).

Calculate doses less than 1 mL to the nearest hundredth and doses more than 1 mL to the nearest tenth. Double-check your work and show your proof.

1. Ordered: Amoxil 100 mg tid po for a child with otitis media.
   Weight: 33 lb
   SDR: 20 mg/kg in 3 divided doses

a. Estimated weight in kg:

b. Actual weight in kg:

c. SDR for this child:

d. Dose ordered:

e. Evaluation and decision:

f. Amount to be administered if applicable:

2. Ordered: Lufyllin (dyphilline elixir) 75 mg po bid for a child with asthma.
   Weight: 30 kg
   SDR: 5 mg/kg in 2 to 3 divided doses per day

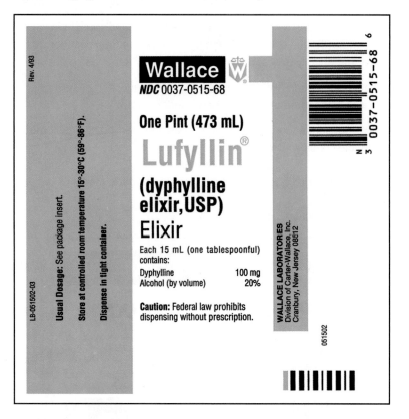

a. SDR for this child:

b. Dose ordered:

c. Evaluation and decision:

d. Amount to be administered to nearest tenth of a mL if applicable:

3. Ordered: Synthroid 0.1 mg IV q AM for a 6-year-old child with hypothyroidism.
   Weight: 49 lb
   SDR: 4 to 5 mcg/kg/day po; IV $\frac{1}{2}$ of po dose

   a. Estimated weight in kg:

   b. Actual weight in kg:

   c. SDR for this child:

   d. Dose ordered:

   e. Evaluation and decision:

   f. Amount to be administered if applicable:

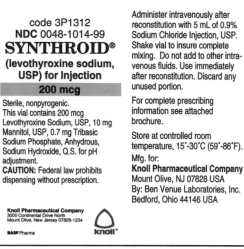

4. Ordered: Morphine sulfate 10 mg IM stat for a child with pain.
Weight: 80 lb
SDR: 0.1 to 0.2 mg per kg

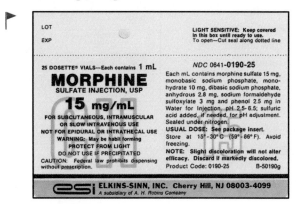

   a. Estimated weight in kg:
   b. Actual weight in kg:
   c. SDR for this child:
   d. Dose ordered:
   e. Evaluation and decision:
   f. Amount to be administered to nearest hundredth of a mL if applicable:

5. Ordered: Deltasone (prednisone) 30 mg per day po for a child with acute asthma.
Weight: 13.6 kg (BSA = 0.6 m^2)
SDR: 40 mg per m^2 day po

   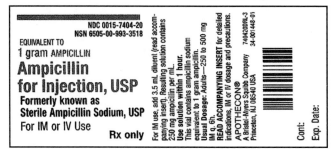

   a. SDR for this child:
   b. Dose ordered:
   c. Evaluation and decision:
   d. Amount to be administered if applicable:

6. Ordered: Ampicillin sodium 0.25 g IV q6h for a child with a kidney infection.
Weight: 22 lb
SDR: 50 to 100 mg per kg per day in 4 divided doses

Directions: Dilute 1 g vial in at least 10 mL of sterile water for injection before further dilutions. Further dilute to 20 mg/mL in D5W. Final concentration should never exceed 30 mg/mL.

   a. Estimated weight in kg:
   b. Actual weight in kg:
   c. SDR for this child:
   d. Dose ordered:
   e. Evaluation and decision:
   f. Amount to be administered if applicable:

7. Ordered: Potassium chloride (KCl) 0.9 mEq to be added to each IV q8h.

Weight: 6 lb

SDR: Up to 3 mEq/kg/24 hr

   a. Estimated weight in kg:

   b. Actual weight in kg:

   c. SDR for this child:

   d. Dose ordered:

   e. Evaluation and decision:

   f. Dose to be added to IV:

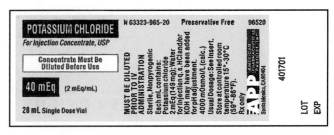

8. Ordered: Rocephin (ceftriaxone sodium) 600 mg IV q12h for a child <u>with an infection by a *Shigella* species.</u>

Weight: 31 lb

SDR: Up to 100 mg per kg per day in 2 divided doses

Directions: Add 9.6 mL sterile water for injection to equal 100 mg/mL. Further dilute to 30 mL with compatible solution over 30 min.

   a. Estimated weight in kg:

   b. Actual weight in kg:

   c. SDR for this child:

   d. Dose ordered:

   e. Evaluation and decision:

   f. Dose to be administered after reconstitution if applicable:

   g. Flow rate in Volutrol:

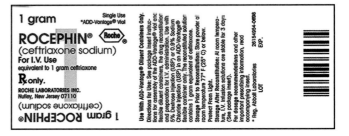

9. Ordered: Acetaminophen drops 20 mg po q4h for a 3-month-old infant with fever. Physician has verified dosage and concentrated drop preparation.

   a. Dose to be administered:

   b. Measuring device to be used:

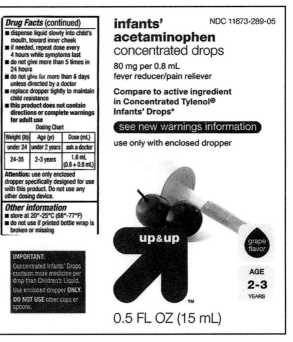

10. Ordered: Vibramycin syrup (doxycycline calcium) 56 mg po q12h day of admission for a child with an infection.

Weight: 28 lb

SDR: Refer to label

a. SDR for this child:

b. Evaluation and decision:

c. Dose to be administered if applicable:

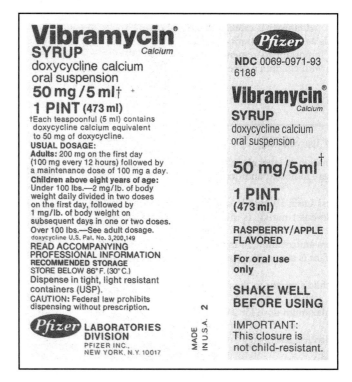

Answers on page 428

WORKSHEET 121 | Multiple-Choice Practice

For the following problems, estimate kilograms, then calculate kilograms to the *nearest* tenth when a pound-to-kilogram conversion is needed and estimate the answers before solving each step.

1. Ordered: 20 mg per kg po daily of Drug Y for a child weighing 50 lb. How many milligrams of the drug will you administer to the child?
   a. 400 mg
   b. 454 mg
   c. 500 mg
   d. 1000 mg

2. Ordered: methotrexate sodium 30 mg per m² po daily maintenance for a child with leukemia. The child's BSA is 1.20 m².* How much medication will you administer?
   a. 1.20 mg
   b. 30 mg
   c. 36 mg
   d. 30.12 mg

3. Ordered: 1.5 tsp of acetaminophen suspension liquid po stat for a child with fever. How many milliliters will you administer?
   a. 5 mL
   b. 7.5 mL
   c. 8 mL
   d. 10 mL

   *Note: Trailing zeros appear in BSA m² measurements. Delete them for math calculations.

4. Ordered: Drug Y 30 mg po stat for a child weighing 25 lb. SDR is 2 to 5 mg per kg. Using the nursing process, what decision will you make regarding this medication order?
   a. Hold and clarify the order promptly. It is an overdose.
   b. Hold and clarify the order promptly. It is an underdose.
   c. Give the medication because the order is within the SDR.
   d. Consult with a supervisor about this order. It is unclear.

5. Ordered: Garamycin 50 mg IV q8h for a 55 lb child with an infection. The SDR is 2 to 2.5 mg per kg q8h. Your decision:
   a. Give the medication. The order is within safe limits.
   b. Hold the medication. Consult with physician. The order is an overdose.
   c. Hold the medication and consult with the physician. The order is an underdose.
   d. Call the pharmacy and clarify the order.

6. Ordered: V-Cillin K 125 mg po daily for a 5.5 lb. child with an infection. The literature states: 40 mg/kg/day in divided doses. Label states: 125 mg per 5 mL. Your decision:
   a. Give the medication. The order is safe.
   b. Hold the medication. Consult with a colleague.
   c. Hold the medication. Consult with physician. The order is an underdose.
   d. Hold the medication and clarify with the physician promptly by telephone. The order is an overdose.

7. Ordered: Phenytoin oral suspension 15 mg bid po for a 6-kg child with seizures. The SDR is 5 mg per kg in 2 to 3 divided doses. Label reads: Dilantin pediatric suspension 30 mg per 5 mL. Your decision:
   a. Hold and clarify the order with the physician. It is an overdose.
   b. The order is safe. Give 2.5 mL.
   c. Clarify the order with an experienced supervisor.
   d. The order is safe. Give 5 mL.

8. Ordered: Synthroid 0.5 mg qAM IV for a child with hypothyroidism. Label reads: Synthroid 200 mcg per 10 mL. What is the amount to be administered?
   a. 2.0 mL
   b. 2.5 mL
   c. 20 mL
   d. 25 mL

9. Ordered: morphine sulfate 5 mg IM preoperatively for a child weighing 58 lb. SDR: 0.1 to 0.2 mg per kg. Calculate weight in kg to the nearest tenth. Your decision:
   a. The order is an overdose. Hold and contact physician.
   b. The order is an underdose. Hold and contact physician.
   c. The order is safe. Give 5 mL.
   d. The order is safe. Give 0.5 mL.

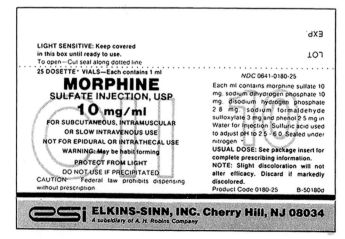

10. Ordered: Ampicillin suspension 250 mg po q8h for a child with an infection. Weight is 30 lb. SDR is 25 to 50 mg per kg per day po in 4 divided doses. The label reads: 125 mg per 5 mL. What is your decision?

   a. The order is safe. Give 10 mL.
   b. The order is an overdose. Hold and contact physician.
   c. The order is an underdose. Hold and contact physician.
   d. Give 5 mL and contact the physician.

Analyze the following scenarios.

1. Baby Louise is in your unit with a diagnosis of congestive heart failure secondary to a congenital heart defect. She weighs 8.4 kg at age 18 months. Her orders include lanoxin 0.05 mg po bid. The orders include temporary fluid restriction to 500 mL per 24-hr period.

   On hand is furosemide oral solution 10 mg/mL. Given this AM by the reporting nurse: 2 mL.

   During report, the nurse tells you that for the past 24 hours the intake exceeded 500 mL by 120 mL because the baby wouldn't take the medicine without a lot of juice. Is there a problem with mathematics? What error in concepts of arithmetic rounding might have led to an error? Which knowledge bases are insufficient?

   Medication error(s) and possible causes:

   Fluid intake error:

   Potential injuries:

   Nursing actions:

   Recommendations for the nurse and for patient safety if you were on a hospital committee studying these incidents:

2. John, a 3-year-old boy weighing 20 kg, has an order for IV anticoagulation. Heparin *25 units per kg per hr* continuous infusion is ordered until the next laboratory checks. Pharmacy supplies a premixed drug concentration (12,500 International Units in 250 mL D5W). Pharmacy instruction is to infuse at 10 mL per hr.

   Nurse A has calculated that the child needs 500 units per hr, that 50 units per mL (12,500 per 250) are in the solution, and that the flow rate should be 50 mL per hr.

   How many units per hr are needed based on John's kg weight? How many units of heparin per mL are there in the solution? How many mL per hour should be infused? Who is correct, the pharmacist or the nurse?

   Potential ADE/sentinel events:

   What would you do if you were Nurse A?

   Recommendations for the agency Patient Safety Committee if you were on the Patient Safety Committee:

   Do you believe that nurses should also double-check the SDR for all drug orders?

3. Note: See web references below. A 10 kg child admitted with hyperglycemia, patient of nurse A, has an order for Regular insulin 0.05 units per kg per hr. The agency requires a second independent nurse check for all high-risk drugs. Nurse A and nurse B agree that the order is safe. Nurse B, the independent check nurse, leaves. Nurse A programs 0.5 units Regular insulin per kg per hr on the IV Smart Pump. An overdose alarm alert sounds. There is also an option on the pump to override the visual and auditory alert and administer the IV. Nurse A needs to decide whether to override or recheck.

How much of an error was programmed?

Why do you think this happened?

Potential ADE from this event?

Under what circumstances do you believe an agency should or should not permit an override of a pump alert?

What sort of procedure should a hospital have for an override?

Do you have any recommendations for nurse B, the independent check nurse?

Web references:
- formularyjournal.modernmedicine.com/...IV.../611706
- www.ihi.org
- www.ismp.org/Newsletters/acutecare/articles/20070419.asp
- http://www.medscape.com/viewarticle/716351
- journals.lww.com/.../The_Use_of_Smart_Pumps_for_Preventing_Medication.6.aspx

Answers on page 431

Use a calculator to determine the child's weight in kilograms (to the nearest tenth) and the SDR for each child. Evaluate the order and make a decision.

1. Give medication (within SDR for unit dose and 24-hr dose).
2. Hold and clarify promptly (overdose or underdose).

If the order is to be carried out, use written ratio and proportion to calculate doses, and show your proof.*

1. Ordered: Cephalexin 200 mg oral suspension po four times daily for Johnny who has a streptococcal infection of the throat and a history of allergy to penicillin. The SDR is 25 to 50 mg per kg per day in 4 divided doses. The child weighs 42 lb today.

   a. Estimated weight in kg:
   b. Actual weight in kg:
   c. SDR for this child:
   d. Dose ordered:
   e. Evaluation and decision:
   f. Dose to be administered if applicable:

   TO PATIENT:
   Shake well before using. Keep tightly closed. Store in refrigerator and discard unused portion after 14 days. Oversize bottle provides shake space.
   TO THE PHARMACIST:
   When prepared as directed, each 5 mL teaspoonful contains Cephalexin Monohydrate equivalent to 125 mg Cephalexin.
   Bottle contains Cephalexin Monohydrate equivalent to 5.0 g of Cephalexin.
   Usual Dose: See package outsert.
   Store at controlled room temperature 15°-30°C (59°-86°F) in dry form.
   Directions for Preparation: Important — water must be added in divided amounts. At the time of dispensing add 120 mL of water to the dry mixture in the bottle in two portions. Shake well after each addition.
   BARR LABORATORIES, INC.
   Pomona, NY 10970
   R11-90

   BARR LABORATORIES, INC.
   NDC 0555-0525-23

   Cephalexin
   for Oral
   Suspension, USP

   125 mg per 5 mL

   Caution: Federal law prohibits dispensing without prescription.

   0555-0525-23   SAMPLE

   200 mL (when mixed)

   Exp. Date:
   Lot No.:

2. Johnny's mother returns to the office with him 3 days after the initial visit because he has a generalized pruritic rash. His practitioner changes his antibiotic order to erythromycin oral suspension 175 mg four times daily po. The SDR is 30 to 50 mg per kg per day divided q6h. Johnny still weighs 42 lb.

   a. Actual weight in kg:
   b. SDR for this child:
   c. Dose ordered:
   d. Evaluation and decision:
   e. Dose to be administered:

   TO PATIENT:
   Shake well before using.
   Keep tightly closed. Store in refrigerator and discard unused portion after ten days. Oversize bottle provides shake space.
   TO THE PHARMACIST:
   When prepared as directed, each 5 mL teaspoonful contains erythromycin ethylsuccinate equivalent to 200 mg of erythromycin in a cherry-flavored suspension.
   Bottle contains erythromycin ethylsuccinate equivalent to 8 g of erythromycin.
   Usual Dose: See package outsert.
   Store at room temperature in dry form.
   Child-Resistant closure not required; Reference: Federal Register Vol.39 No.29.
   DIRECTIONS FOR PREPARATION: Slowly add 140 mL of water and shake vigorously to make 200 mL of suspension.
   BARR LABORATORIES, INC.
   Pomona, NY 10970
   R11-90

   BARR LABORATORIES, INC.
   NDC 0555-0215-23
   NSN 6505-00-080-0653

   Erythromycin Ethylsuccinate
   for Oral
   Suspension, USP

   200 mg of erythromycin activity per 5 mL reconstituted

   Caution: Federal law prohibits dispensing without prescription.

   0555-0215-23   SAMPLE

   200 mL (when mixed)

   Exp. Date:
   Lot No.:

*Calculate amounts *less* than 1 mL to the nearest hundredth and *greater* than 1 mL to the nearest tenth.

3. Also ordered for Johnny's pruritis is Benadryl Allergy Liquid (diphenhydramine HCl) 25 mg po tid and at bedtime × 3 days. Johnny is 8 years old. Read the label and make your decision.
   a. Safe daily dose maximum for this child:
   b. Dose ordered for 24 hr:
   c. Evaluation and decision:
   d. Dose to be administered:

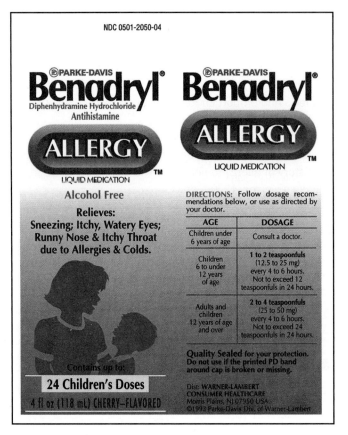

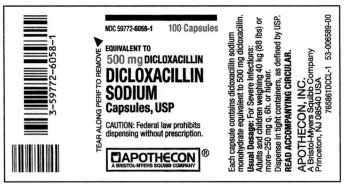

⊜ **CLINICAL ALERT**

Approximately 15% of people, or 1 in 6 persons, with an allergy to penicillin will have an allergy to the cephalosporins.

4. Ordered for Johnny's 8-year-old sister are dicloxacillin sodium capsules 500 mg po q6h for an infection. The SDR is 12.5 to 25 mg/kg/day in divided doses q6h. His sister weighs 32 kg. Read the label and make your evaluation and decision.

   a. SDR for this child:
   b. Dose ordered:
   c. Evaluation and decision:
   d. Dose to be administered if applicable:

5. Karen, age 3, is admitted to the hospital with a compound fracture of the femur incurred during an automobile accident. Ordered: Atropine sulfate 0.3 mg preop IM. The SDR for children weighing 12 to 16 kg is 0.3 mg 30 to 60 min before surgery. Karen weighs 35 lb.

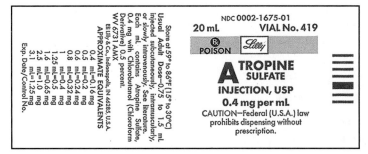

   a. Estimated weight in kg:
   b. Actual weight in kg:
   c. SDR for this child:
   d. Dose ordered:
   e. Evaluation and decision:
   f. Dose to be administered if applicable:

6. Ordered postoperatively for Karen is Amoxil oral suspension 0.5 g tid po. The SDR is 20 to 40 mg/kg in 3 divided doses. Karen weighs 35 lb.

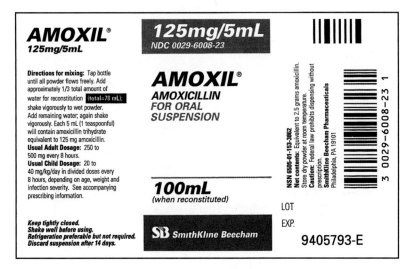

   a. Estimated weight in kg:
   b. Actual weight in kg:
   c. SDR for this child:
   d. Dose ordered:
   e. Evaluation and decision:
   f. Dose to be administered if applicable:

7. Also ordered for Karen is to resume her antiseizure medication, Tegretol chewable tab 0.1 g tid po. SDR: 10 to 20 mg per kg divided in two or three doses.
   a. SDR for Karen's weight: (For weight refer to problem 6.)
   b. Evaluation and decision:
   c. Dose to be administered, if applicable:

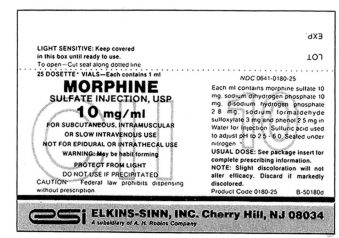

8. Morphine sulfate 5 mg IV q4h prn pain × 48 hr is ordered for Karen. The SDR is 0.05 to 0.1 mg per kg q4h for direct IV. Directions state to dilute with 5 mL of sterile water or sterile saline for injection and administer over 5 min.
   a. Actual weight in kg:
   b. SDR for this child:
   c. Dose ordered:
   d. Evaluation and decision:
   e. Dose before dilution:

9. Ordered: Leucovorin calcium 0.01 g q6h po for a child with toxic effects resulting from an antineoplastic agent. The child weighs 70 lb and has normal height for weight. The SDR for children is up to 10 mg per m^2 q6h for 72 hr. Use the West nomogram* to determine the BSA for this child's weight.
   a. BSA in m^2:
   b. SDR for this child:
   c. Dose ordered:
   d. Evaluation and decision:
   e. Amount to be given if applicable:

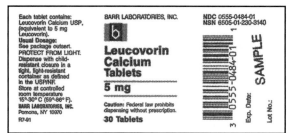

*For the West nomogram, refer to page 282.

10. Ordered for a child with hemophilia: a recommended dose of NovoSeven 90 mcg per kg, IV bolus, q3h until hemostasis is achieved or until the treatment has been judged to be inadequate. The child's weight is 22 kg. Directions: Administer over 2 to 5 minutes slow bolus. This bolus will be administered over 3 minutes with the syringe provided. These are single dose vials that must be discarded 3 hours after reconstitution. Use a calculator for long division and multiplication.

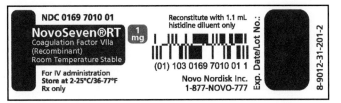

NovoSeven® RT 1 mg

a. Dose in mcg ordered for this child:

b. Equivalent dose in mg:

c. Total mL to be administered:

d. How many vials of medication will the nurse need?

e. Total calibrations to be occupied by the volume (refer to syringe):

f. mL per minute:

g. Indicate the total dose with an arrow on the syringe.

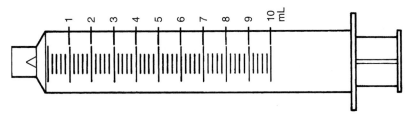

h. How many mL will remain after a. 1 minute; b. 2 minutes; c. 3 minutes?

> ## ⊜ CLINICAL ALERT
>
> Beware of medication orders for "T" and "t" and "tsp" for example, 1 T daily or 1 tsp daily. Teaspoon and tablespoon abbreviations can easily be confused.
>
> Also, dosage strength may vary per teaspoon among infant, child, and adult preparations and may also vary among manufacturers. Call the physician and clarify the specific strength desired in milligrams, milliequivalents or units.

evolve **Refer to the Pediatric Calculations section of Drug Calculations Companion, version 4 on Evolve, for additional practice problems.**

Multiple-Choice Final

Estimate reasonable answers when possible. Round kg to the nearest tenth. Round liquid oral and injection doses to the nearest tenth of a mL. Round IV flow rates to the nearest whole mL. Answers can be found on page 433.

1. Ordered: Cimetidine 0.4 g po daily for a patient with an ulcer. Give:

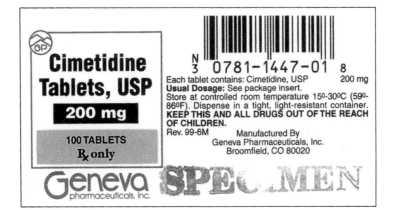

   a. 0.5 tab
   b. 1 tab
   c. 2 tab
   d. 4 tab

2. Ordered: Klonopin (clonazepam) 1 mg po stat for a patient who has seizures. Give:

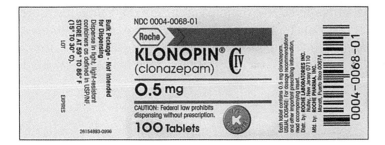

   a. 0.5 tab
   b. 1 tab
   c. 2 tab
   d. 4 tab

3. Ordered: Lanoxin 0.125 mg po daily in the AM for a patient with heart failure. Give:
   a. 0.5 tab
   b. 1 tab
   c. 2 tab
   d. 4 tab

NDC 0173-0249-56

100 Tablets
(10 blisterpacks of 10 tablets each)

UNIT DOSE PACK

LANOXIN® (digoxin)
Tablets

Each scored tablet contains
250 mcg (0.25 mg)

See package insert for Dosage and
Administration.

Store at 25°C (77°F); excursions permitted to
15 to 30°C (59 to 86°F) [see USP Controlled
Room Temperature] in a dry place.

4. Ordered: Famotidine oral suspension 50 mg po bid for a patient with an ulcer. Give to the nearest tenth of a mL:
   a. 4.8 mL
   b. 6.2 mL
   c. 6.3 mL
   d. 6.5 mL

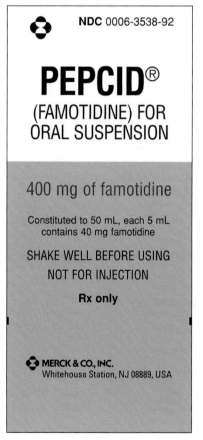

NDC 0006-3538-92

PEPCID®

(FAMOTIDINE) FOR
ORAL SUSPENSION

400 mg of famotidine

Constituted to 50 mL, each 5 mL
contains 40 mg famotidine

SHAKE WELL BEFORE USING

NOT FOR INJECTION

Rx only

◆ MERCK & CO., INC.
Whitehouse Station, NJ 08889, USA

5. Ordered: Naloxone HCl 600 mcg IM stat to reverse effects of a narcotic overdose. Give:

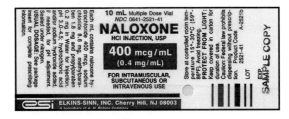

   a. 0.8 mL

   b. 1.1 mL

   c. 1.3 mL

   d. 1.5 mL

6. Ordered: Cipro (ciprofloxacin) 1.5 g po bid for a patient with an infection. Give:

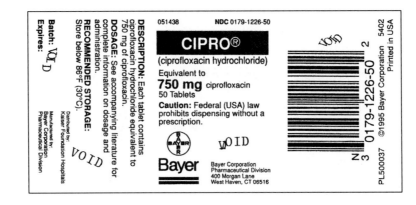

   a. 0.5 tab

   b. 1 tab

   c. 2 tab

   d. 3 tab

7. Ordered: Morphine sulfate 8 mg IM q4h prn for pain. Give:

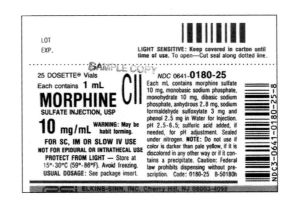

   a. 0.6 mL

   b. 0.8 mL

   c. 1 mL

   d. 1.2 mL

8. Ordered: Glycopyrrolate 0.3 mg IM at 8 AM preoperatively to reduce excessive pharyngeal secretions and protect the heart from vagal stimulation. Give:

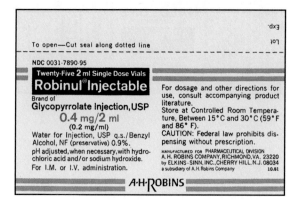

   a. 0.5 mL
   b. 0.7 mL
   c. 1.5 mL
   d. 2 mL

9. The nurse is trying to interpret a prescriber order that is illegible. What is the best action to take?
   a. Ask a staff nurse who works regularly on the floor.
   b. Check to see if something similar has been given before to the patient.
   c. Call the pharmacy.
   d. Call the prescriber.

10. Ordered: Promethazine 20 mg IM stat for a patient with nausea. Give:

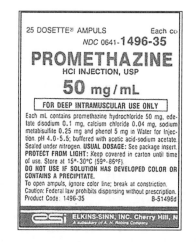

   a. 0.4 mL
   b. 0.5 mL
   c. 0.8 mL
   d. 1.2 mL

11. Ordered: Ativan (lorazepam) 5 mg IM stat for an agitated patient. Give to the nearest tenth of a mL:

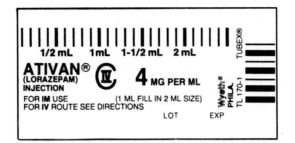

a. 0.8 mL
b. 1.2 mL
c. 1.3 mL
d. 1.4 mL

12. Ordered: 500 mg Claforan IM q8h for a patient with an infection. Available: Claforan (cefotaxime sodium) 1 g IM or IV. Follow the preparation directions. Give 500 mg with the least volume.

Strength	Diluent	Withdrawable Volume	Approx. Concentration
1 g vial (IM)	3.0 mL	3.4 mL	300 mg/mL
2 g vial (IM)	5.0 mL	6.0 mL	330 mg/mL
1 g vial (IV)	10.0 mL	10.4 mL	95 mg/mL
2 g vial (IV)	10.0 mL	11.0 mL	180 mg/mL

How many milliliters will you give the patient?
a. 2.0 mL
b. 1.5 mL
c. 2.5 mL
d. 3.0 mL

13. Ordered: Rocephin 1 g q12h IV for a patient with pneumonitis. Available: ceftriaxone sodium (Rocephin) 1 g for IM or IV use. Directions for IV use: Reconstitute with 5 mL of normal saline solution. Mix well. Further dilute with normal saline to 50 mL and infuse in 20 to 40 minutes. What is the maximum rate in milliliters per hour you could set the infusion device?
a. 150 mL per hr
b. 200 mL per hr
c. 300 mL per hr
d. 400 mL per hr

14. Ordered: Carbenicillin disodium 1 g IM q8h for a patient with bronchitis. Available: carbenicillin disodium 5 g for IM or IV use. Directions for IM use: Use sterile water as diluent for injection. The medication displaces 3 mL. If you reconstitute the carbenicillin disodium using 12 mL of sterile water for injection, how many doses of 1 g will you have?

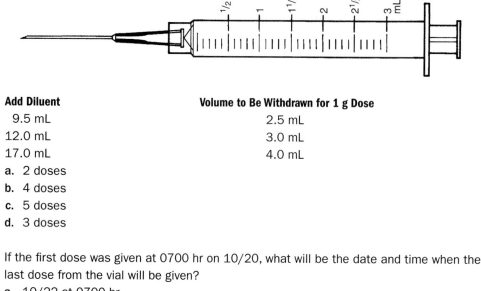

Add Diluent
9.5 mL
12.0 mL
17.0 mL

Volume to Be Withdrawn for 1 g Dose
2.5 mL
3.0 mL
4.0 mL

a. 2 doses
b. 4 doses
c. 5 doses
d. 3 doses

If the first dose was given at 0700 hr on 10/20, what will be the date and time when the last dose from the vial will be given?
a. 10/22 at 0700 hr
b. 10/22 at 2000 hr
c. 10/21 at 2400 hr
d. 10/21 at 1500 hr

15. The IV is infusing at 30 gtt per min. The drop factor is 20 gtt per mL. The IV label reads 500 mL 5% dextrose and 0.45% sodium chloride. The IV had been infusing for $1\frac{1}{2}$ hours when you came on duty. How much longer does the IV have to infuse?

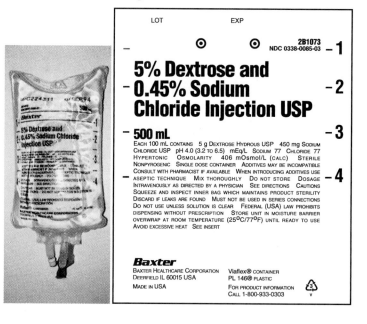

a. 4 hr
b. 50 min
c. 3 hr
d. $3\frac{1}{2}$ hr

16. Ordered: Monocid 600 mg IM. Available: Cefonicid 1 g for reconstitution. How many mL will you administer?

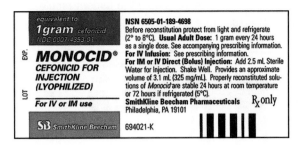

   a. 1.8 mL
   b. 0.7 mL
   c. 1.3 mL
   d. 1.5 mL

17. Ordered: IV of 1000 mL D5W to infuse at 125 mL per hr on admission. The drop factor is 20. How many gtt/min will you set the IV to infuse?
   a. 12 gtt per min
   b. 42 gtt per min
   c. 20 gtt per min
   d. 33 gtt per min

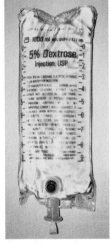

18. Ordered: Ampicillin 1 g IV bid. Available: Ampicillin 1 g for IV use. Directions: Add 4.5 mL of sodium chloride diluent to yield 5 mL. Dilute with normal saline to 50 mL and infuse in 15 minutes. On hand you have a microdrip infusion set. At how many mL/hr will you set the IV?

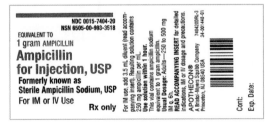

   a. 100 mL per hr
   b. 150 mL per hr
   c. 200 mL per hr
   d. 250 mL per hr

19. The pharmacy standard insulin drip is 100 units of Human Regular in
    250 mL of normal saline. 1 unit = 2.5 mL. Your patient's blood glucose
    level is 218 mg/dL. How many units/hr should the patient receive? Use the following chart
    to determine the correct insulin rate for the IV:

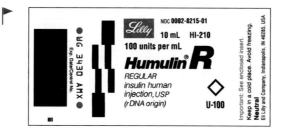

Blood Glucose (BG)/dL	Standard Rate in units/hr
101-140	1.0
141-180	1.5
181-220	2.0
221-260	2.5
261-300	3.0

    a. 1.5 units per hr
    b. 2.5 units per hr
    c. 3.0 units per hr
    d. 2.0 units per hr

    At what rate will you set the IV infusion device?
    a. 3 mL/hr
    b. 4 mL/hr
    c. 5 mL/hr
    d. 6 mL/hr

20. Ordered: Novolin R insulin 15 units per hr IV for a patient having surgery. Available: 250 mL
    of sodium chloride 0.9% with 100 units of Humulin R insulin. At how many mL/hr will you
    need to set the electronic infusion device?

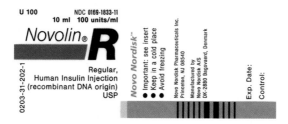

    a. 56 mL per hr
    b. 33 mL per hr
    c. 38 mL per hr
    d. 58 mL per hr

    How many hours will it take to infuse the 250 mL?
    a. 5 hr 30 min
    b. 8 hr
    c. 9 hr 40 min
    d. 6 hr 36 min

21. Ordered: Heparin sodium 10,000 units IV in 15 hr postoperative hip surgery. Available: Pharmacy has sent 1000 mL of normal saline solution with 10,000 units of heparin sodium. At how many mL/hr will you set the IV infusion device?

a. 67 mL/hr
b. 125 mL/hr
c. 83 mL/hr
d. 100 mL/hr

If the IV described above was started at 2000 hr on 10/21, when should it be finished?

a. 10/22 at 0900 hr
b. 10/23 at 0200 hr
c. 10/23 at 1000 hr
d. 10/22 at 1100 hr

22. Ordered: Fragmin 18,000 units subcutaneous for a patient with a deep venous thrombosis (DVT). Available: A 9.5 mL multidose vial of Fragmin. The label reads: 1 mL = 10,000 units. How many milliliters will you give?

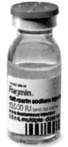

10,000 international units/mL
9.5 mL multidose vial
NDC 0013-2436-06

Used with permission from Pfizer, Inc.

a. 1.8 mL
b. 2 mL
c. 1.5 mL
d. 1.2 mL

23. A blood glucose level (BGL) of 120 mg per dL is desired. Orders for this patient are: Give 1 unit of Regular insulin for every 8 mg above 120 mg per dL. Give 1 unit of Regular insulin for each 8 g of CHO consumed. The BGL is 160 mg per dL. The amount of CHO consumed is 64 g. How many total units of insulin will the patient receive?

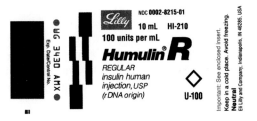

a. 10 units
b. 13 units
c. 24 units
d. 28 units

24. Ordered: IV heparin to infuse at 20 units per kg per hr. Available: 1000 mL D5W with 25,000 units of heparin sodium. The patient weighs 80 kg. How many units per hour will the patient receive on the electronic infusion device?
   a. 160 units
   b. 1600 units
   c. 1620 units
   d. 1640 units

   At how many mL per hr will you set the infusion device?
   a. 58 mL/hr
   b. 48 mL/hr
   c. 66 mL/hr
   d. 64 mL/hr

25. Ordered: 90 units per kg of heparin for a loading dose. Set the infusion to run at 1200 units per hr. Available: 500 mL NS with 25,000 units of heparin. The patient weighs 177 lb. How many units will you give as the loading dose?
   a. 5700 units
   b. 6900 units
   c. 7000 units
   d. 7240 units

   At how many mL per hr will you set the infusion device?
   a. 84 mL per hr
   b. 60 mL per hr
   c. 64 mL per hr
   d. 24 mL per hr

26. The patient has a TPN solution for nutritional therapy with 8.5% amino acids in 375 mL. The total volume (TV) is 1500 mL. How many grams of protein will the patient receive? Use the following formula for calculating the amino acids.

   Step 1:   % × mL = g per L

   Step 2:   g per L × TV per L × g per bag

   a. 8.5 g per bag
   b. 47.8 g per bag
   c. 478 g per bag
   d. 31.8 g per bag

27. Ordered: A maintenance dose of Methotrexate 30 mg per m^2 po twice a week for a child with lymphocytic leukemia. Child's weight is 30 lb, which is normal height for weight (per nomogram). Using the appropriate column in the West nomogram on page 282, calculate the dose.
   a. 12 mg
   b. 15 mg
   c. 18 mg
   d. 20 mg

28. Ordered: Dobutrex HCl to be infused at 2 mcg per kg per min in a solution of 500 mL D5W for a patient with cardiac decompensation. Patient's weight: 110 lb. At how many mL per hr will the IV infusion pump be set?

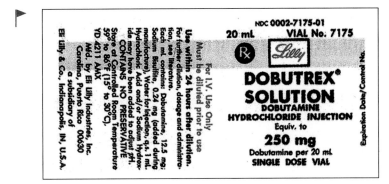

a. 6 mL per hr
b. 8 mL per hr
c. 10 mL per hr
d. 12 mL per hr

29. Ordered: Morphine sulfate 5 mg IV push for a patient in severe pain. Directions: Dilute *to* 5 mL of NS or sterile water for injection and administer over 5 minutes. Identify the correct total dose and mL/minute to inject.

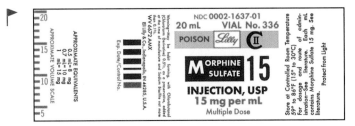

a. Administer 5 mL at 1 mL per min.
b. Administer 5 mL at 0.4 mL per min.
c. Administer 6 mL at 0.4 mL per min.
d. Administer 8 mL at 0.03 mL per min.

30. Ordered: A diuretic, Furosemide 15 mg IV, for a child with edema. The child's weight is 14 kg. SDR: 1-2 mg per kg per dose IV every 6 to 12 hours. Your decision:

a. Give 15 mg. The order is within the safe dose range.
b. Hold. Contact the physician promptly and clarify. The order is an underdose.
c. Hold. Contact the physician promptly and clarify. The order is an overdose.
d. Hold. The order is unclear.

Comprehensive Final

Estimate answers and then solve the following problems. Prove your answers. Answers can be found on page 435.

1. Ordered: Lipitor 20 mg po daily for a patient with hypercholesterolemia. How many tablets will be administered?

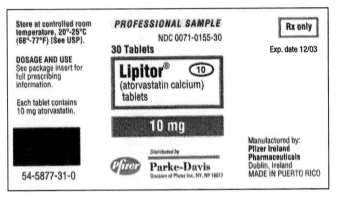

2. Ordered: Cimetidine 0.4 g bid po for a patient with a duodenal ulcer. How many tablets will be administered?

3. Ordered: Carbamazepine chewable tablet 0.2 g daily for a patient with seizures. How many tablets will be administered?

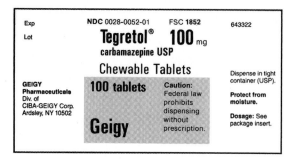

4. Ordered: Diltiazem HCl 0.24 g at bedtime daily for a patient with high blood pressure. How many tablets will be administered?

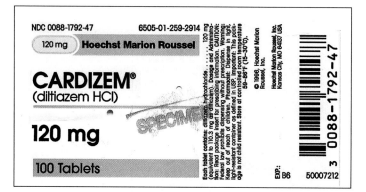

5. Ordered: Aspirin delayed-release tablet 975 mg at bedtime daily for a patient with arthritis. How many tablets will be administered?

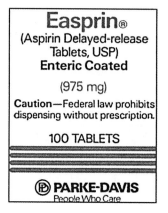

6. Ordered: Isoniazid 0.1 g po for a patient with tuberculosis. How many tablets will be administered?

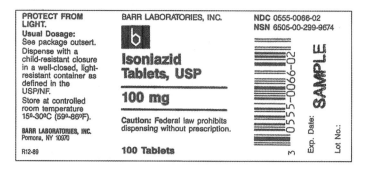

7. Ordered: Fluoxetine hydrochloride oral solution 30 mg po for a patient with anxiety. How many mL will be administered? Shade in the medicine cup with the nearest measurable dose. Mark the syringe provided with the additional amount needed to the nearest measurable dose.

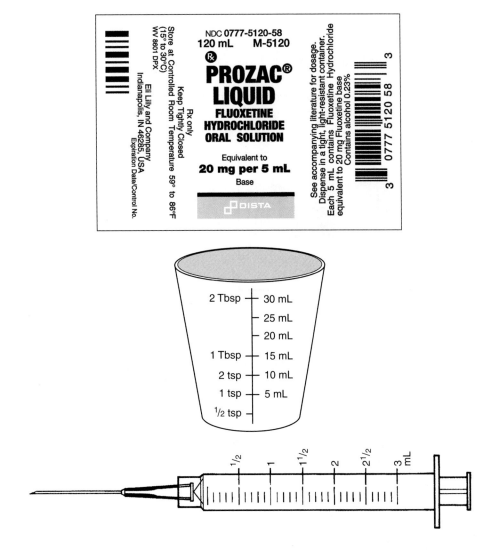

8. Ordered: Morphine sulfate 10 mg IM stat for a patient with pain. How many mL (to the nearest tenth of a mL) will be administered? Mark the syringe provided with the nearest measurable amount.

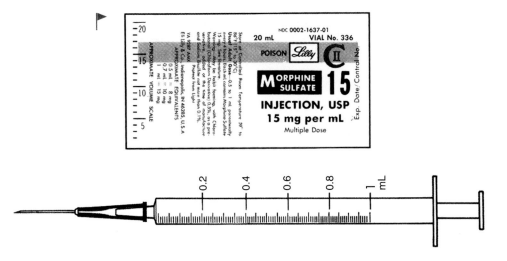

9. Ordered: Morphine sulfate 10 mg q4h prn pain; last administered, according to the MAR, at 0400 hr.

Given: Morphine 10 mg at 0800 hr by Nurse A.

Given: Morphine 10 mg at 0845 hr by Nurse B, a busy staff nurse who covered Nurse A's patient during Nurse A's break.

Error:

Current Actions:

What are some ways this error might have been prevented?

10. Ordered: Codeine phosphate 35 mg IM stat for a patient with pain. How many mL (to the nearest tenth of a mL) will be administered? Mark the syringe provided with the nearest measurable amount.

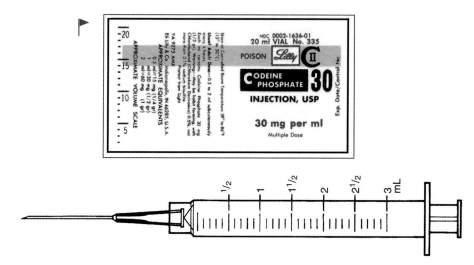

11. Ordered: Atropine sulfate 0.5 mg IV for a patient with an apical pulse 40 beats per minute or below. How many mL (to the nearest tenth of a mL) will be administered? Mark the syringe provided with the nearest measurable amount.

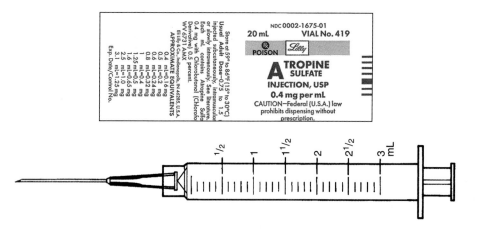

12. Ordered: Pfizerpen 400,000 units IM q8h for a patient with an infection.
    Available: Penicillin G potassium (Pfizerpen) 5 million units for reconstitution.
    Follow the directions on the label to answer the questions.
    a. If you add 18.2 mL of diluent, how many units per milliliter will you have?
    b. How many milliliters will yield 400,000 units?
    c. If you add 8.2 mL of diluent, how many units per milliliter will you have?
    d. Using the 8.2 mL of diluent, how many milliliters will yield 400,000 units?

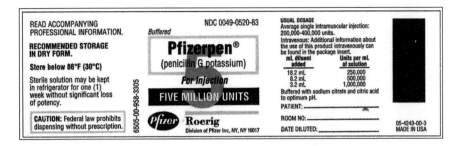

13. Ordered: Cefadyl 1 g IM q6h for a patient with cellulitis.
    a. How much diluent will you add? Shade in the syringe.
    b. How many vials will be used in 24 hr?
    c. How many mL will you give per dose?

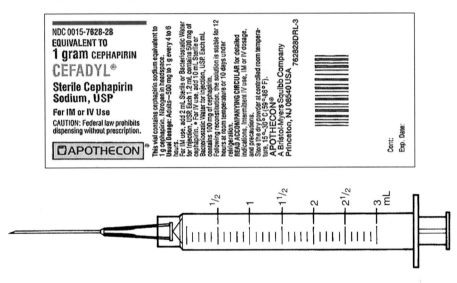

14. Ordered: Cefazolin 250 mg IM q8h for a patient with an infection.
    Available: Ancef 1 g for reconstitution.
    a. How many mL of diluent will you add?
    b. Where will the medication be stored?
    c. How many mL will you give?

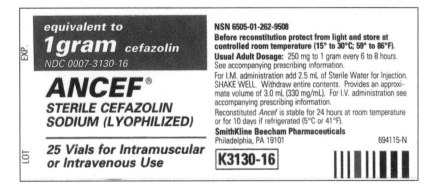

15. Ordered: 2000 mL D5/Ringer's lactate solution to be infused in 24 hr for hydration. The drop factor is 15.

    a. How many gtt/min will be infused via gravity infusion?

    b. How many mL/hr will be infused by an electronic device?

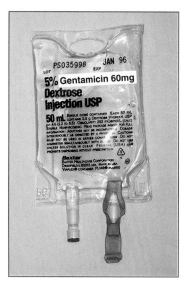

16. Ordered: Gentamicin 60 mg in 50 mL, IVPB for pneumonitis. Infuse in 40 minutes.

    a. At how many milliliters per hr will you set the electronic infusion device?

    b. How many gtt per min will be infused by a microdrip set?

17. Ordered: 1000 mL D5NS followed by 1000 mL D5W, then 500 mL NS to infuse in 24 hr for hydration. The drop factor is 10.

    a. At how many mL/hr will you set the electronic infusion device to deliver 2500 mL in 24 hr?

    b. At how many gtt/min will you regulate the IV?

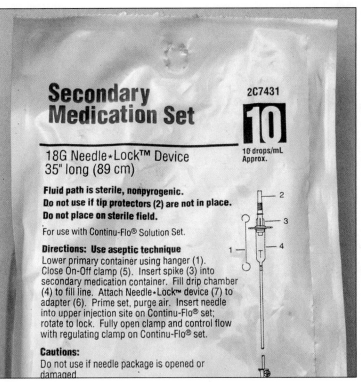

From Macklin D, Chernecky C, Infortuna H: *Math for clinical practice*, ed 2, St Louis, 2011, Mosby.

18. Your patient's blood glucose level (BGL) at 0600 hr is 176 mg per dL. According to the titration schedule, how many units of Lantus will the patient receive? Shade in the amount on the insulin syringe.

Effective Diabetes Management

Logical titration schedule helps
achieve tight control, with low
incidence of severe hypoglycemia

Self-monitored FPG (mg/dL) for 2 consecutive days with no episodes of severe hypoglycemia or PG ≤72 mg/dL	Increase in insulin dose (international units/day)
100-120 mg/dL	2
120-140 mg/dL	4
140-180 mg/dL	6
≥180 mg/dL	8

Treat-to-Target FPG ≤100 mg/dL

Small decreases (2-4 international units/day per adjustment) in dose are allowed in the instance of self-monitored plasma glucose below 56 mg/dL or in the occurrence of a severe hypoglycemic episode.

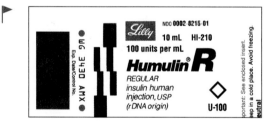

19. Ordered: Humulin R insulin 50 units in 500 mL of 0.9% NS IV to infuse at 7 units per hr. At what rate will you set the IV infusion device?

NDC 0002-8215-01
Lilly
10 mL   HI-210
100 units per mL
Humulin® R
REGULAR
insulin human
injection, USP
(rDNA origin)   U-100

MG 3430 XMA
Exp. Date/Control No.

Important: See enclosed insert.
Keep in a cold place. Avoid freezing.
Neutral

20. Ordered: The patient has consumed 35 g CHO for breakfast, 90 g CHO for lunch, and 25 g CHO for dinner. The patient weighs 270 lb.

How many total units of R has the patient received based on the units-to-CHO ratio chart?

Insulin Units Required Based on CHO Intake and Weight		
Weight in Pounds	**Weight in Kg**	**Unit: grams of CHO**
100-109	45.5-49.5	1:16
110-129	50-58.6	1:15
130-139	59-63.2	1:14
140-149	63.6-67.7	1:13
150-159	68.2-72.3	1:12
160-169	72.7-76.8	1:11
170-179	77.3-81.4	1:10
180-189	81.8-85.9	1:9
190-198	86.4-90	1:8
200-239	90.9-108.6	1:7
240+	109.1+	1:6

21. Ordered: Regular Humulin insulin to infuse at 3 units per hr.

Available: 250 mL NS with 40 units of Humulin R insulin.

a. At how many mL per hr will you set the electronic infusion device?

b. The IV was started at 0830. At what hour will the IV be complete?

22. Ordered: Fragmin injection 8000 units subcutaneous q12h before surgery.

Available: A multidose vial of Fragmin (dalteparin sodium injection).

How many milliliters will you give? Shade in the amount on the syringe.

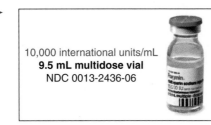

10,000 international units/mL
9.5 mL multidose vial
NDC 0013-2436-06

Used with permission from Pfizer, Inc.

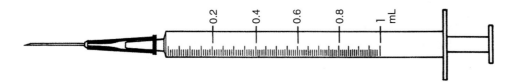

23. Ordered: Heparin sodium 1000 units per hr IV. The pharmacy has sent 1000 mL of 0.9% sodium chloride with 20,000 units of heparin sodium for a patient with a DVT.

    a. At what rate will you set the infusion device?

    b. How long will it take to infuse the 20,000 units?

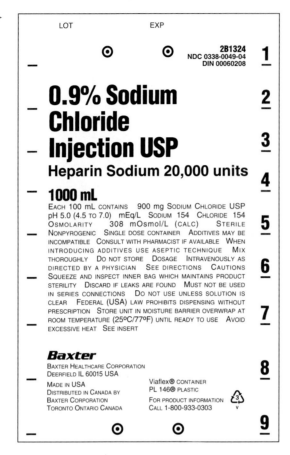

24. Ordered: Loading dose of IV heparin at 82 units per kg per min. Set infusion to run at 18 units per kg per hr. Available: 500 mL D5W with 20,000 units of heparin. The patient weighs 160 lb.

    a. How many units of heparin will you give for the bolus loading dose?

    b. How many units per hr will infuse?

    c. How many hours will it take to infuse?

    d. At what rate will you set the infusion device to deliver 18 units per kg per hr?

25. Calculate the grams of amino acids, dextrose, and lipids per bag the patient on nutritional therapy will receive. Use the following formulas on the TPN label below. The total volume is 1158 mL.

    Step 1:   % × mL = g per L   **Step 2:**   g/L × TV/L = g per bag

    TPN Label

    a. Ordered: Amino acid 5.5% in 300 mL for a patient needing hyperalimentation.

    b. Ordered: Dextrose 10% in 250 mL for a patient needing hyperalimentation.

    c. Ordered: Lipids 10% in 125 mL for a patient needing hyperalimentation.

26. Using the answers from Problem 25, how many kilocalories will the patient receive?

27. The pharmacy has supplied potassium chloride (KCl) 30 mEq in an IV of 500 mL D5W.

    a. How many mEq are there per mL on the available label?

    b. How many mg are there per mL on the available label?

    c. How many mL of KCL would the pharmacy have added to the IV?

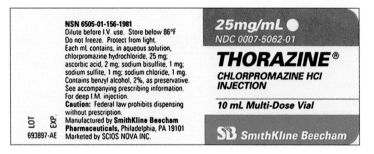

28. Ordered: Thorazine 2 mg IV push. Directions: Dilute each 25 mg (1 mL) with 24 mL of NS for IV injection. Each mL will contain 1 mg. Give at slow rate of 1 mg per min.

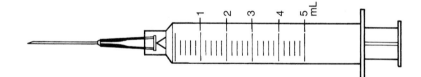

    a. Total milliliters to be injected

    b. Total time in *seconds* to be injected

    c. mL/min to be injected for how many minutes

    d. Seconds to be injected per calibration

29. Ordered: Leucovorin calcium tablets 0.01 g po for a child who has delayed excretion of methotrexate. The SDR is 10 mg/m^2. The child's weight is 70 lb. Refer to the West nomogram on page 282 for the child's body surface area in square meters. How many milligrams are needed? How many tablets will you prepare to the nearest whole tablet?

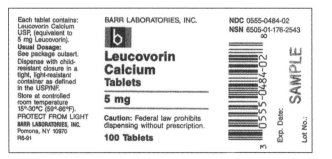

30. Ordered: Dopamine 5 mcg per kg per min. The dopamine is infusing at 30 mL per hr on an infusion device with an IV container of 200 mg per 250 mL D5W. The patient weighs 176 lb.

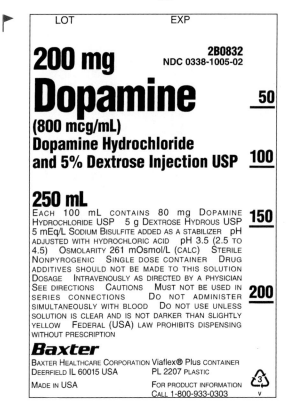

LOT   EXP

200 mg   2B0832
NDC 0338-1005-02

Dopamine   <u>50</u>

(800 mcg/mL)
Dopamine Hydrochloride
and 5% Dextrose Injection USP   <u>100</u>

250 mL
EACH 100 mL CONTAINS 80 mg DOPAMINE   <u>150</u>
HYDROCHLORIDE USP   5 g DEXTROSE HYDROUS USP
5 mEq/L SODIUM BISULFITE ADDED AS A STABILIZER   pH
ADJUSTED WITH HYDROCHLORIC ACID   pH 3.5 (2.5 TO
4.5)   OSMOLARITY 261 mOsmol/L (CALC)   STERILE
NONPYROGENIC   SINGLE DOSE CONTAINER   DRUG
ADDITIVES SHOULD NOT BE MADE TO THIS SOLUTION
DOSAGE   INTRAVENOUSLY AS DIRECTED BY A PHYSICIAN
SEE DIRECTIONS   CAUTIONS   MUST NOT BE USED IN   <u>200</u>
SERIES CONNECTIONS   DO NOT ADMINISTER
SIMULTANEOUSLY WITH BLOOD   DO NOT USE UNLESS
SOLUTION IS CLEAR AND IS NOT DARKER THAN SLIGHTLY
YELLOW   FEDERAL (USA) LAW PROHIBITS DISPENSING
WITHOUT PRESCRIPTION

Baxter
BAXTER HEALTHCARE CORPORATION Viaflex® PLUS CONTAINER
DEERFIELD IL 60015 USA   PL 2207 PLASTIC
MADE IN USA   FOR PRODUCT INFORMATION
CALL 1-800-933-0303

a. How many mcg per hr are ordered?

b. How many mg per hr are ordered?

c. How many mg per mL are contained with solution (to the nearest tenth of a mL)?

d. How many mL per hr should be infusing?

e. Is the flow rate correct?

5 Minute Sample Verbal Communication Hand-off Report

A hand-off report is the transfer and acceptance of patient care responsibilities through effective communication between caregivers at shift change, transfer between units, agencies, or to home, to ensure patient safety.

Many errors, *including medication errors,* have been attributed to inadequate "hand-off" communication. The highlighted areas in the sample report below pertain to key medication-related information for the report.

Additional information would be given for discharge communication to home as well as accompanying written materials about all medications, treatments, and when to make appointments for checkup. Whereas for shift change, only major medication issues are verbally reported, for all physical patient transfers complete medication resolution must be provided in writing for patient safety. Check agency procedures and forms for Hand-Off communication and Medication Resolution.

(Nurse giving report to next caregiver at shift change on a medical-surgical unit)

(Sex, Age, Mental /Emotional status, Main Diagnoses, Date of Admissions and Transfers, Additional Diagnoses, Allergies)

"Mr. G. is a 73-year old moderately hard -of- hearing, alert, oriented x 3 (to person, time, and place) cooperative English-speaking male in no acute distress admitted to ICU with uncontrolled hypertension and acute bronchitis on the 3rd of October and transferred to our unit on the 6th. He also has chronic prostatitis, mild anemia, and an artificial hip replacement as of a year ago which requires use of a cane for stability, and occasional asthmatic episodes controlled with an inhaler. He is allergic to Penicillin and Aspirin, reacts with hives and wheezing, as well as diarrhea from Penicillin, and is a fairly reliable historian. He lives with his daughter so it's best to include her in all teaching, particularly because of the hearing loss.

(Vital Signs)

His vitals signs are all stable today.

(Medications: medication changes, medications due, related orders)

He had a central line removed before transfer here. His main medications are: an intravenous antibiotic piggyback (IVPB) every 6 hr for 24 more hrs for his bronchitis. His next one is due soon at 1700 hrs. He is on digoxin every morning and two new blood pressure meds, one a diuretic in the morning and the other, an ace inhibitor, in the evening. His blood pressure needs to be recorded each shift) and after any complaint of weakness or extreme fatigue. Notify the attending physician if the systolic pressure exceeds 170. Make sure his inhaler is within reach and record his use.

(Labs)

His white blood count is still elevated at 13,000 but has been improving steadily. He is NPO after midnight for fasting blood work and also has a lung function test scheduled. in the morning. His other labs are within normal limits.

Hold the diuretic in the morning until the labs are completed.

(Treatments)

The discontinued central line site needs to be assessed once a day.

He is receiving respiratory therapy every morning beween 0800 and 0900 hrs and wants to bathe before they come.

(Nutrition; and Intake and Output)

He is now tolerating a regular diet well but needs encouragement to drink more fluids.

Since he started on the diuretic, he self-limits fluids to try to reduce urination. The fluid intake and urinary output is to be recorded until discharge. Notify the attending physician if the intake or output drops below 1000 mL per day.

(Activity level: Mobility)

He does need assistance and encouragement getting in and out of bed but does not need assistance walking as long as he has the cane. The doctor wants him to be out of bed most of the day if possible. Bedrails are up at bedtime and a urinal within reach at all times because of the diuretic and urinary frequency.

(Other needs; Discharge planning)

His discharge is tentatively planned for next Monday so special emphasis needs to be given to teaching Mr. G about the new medication regime and need for fluids and activity. He lives with his daughter who visits after work daily. Be sure to include her in all teaching and discharge because day shift doesn't see her often.. A main issue is that he is unhappy about having to take "new pills" so we've already started reinforcing the importance of compliance with him and the daughter. Be sure to get feedback because he does not always mention that he did not hear everything.

Note: Although this seems like a lot of information, the nurse who cares for the patient for a full shift and who has *established a sequential format* for the reporting information, can communicate this information verbally on each assigned patient with ease. It helps to keep a checklist on hand with abbreviated cues (see the sample bold subheadings), to ensure the verbal hand-off report covers all major bases. The receiving nurse refers to the written record for further details. There are many potential variations for reporting, for example, fasting could be included under Intake/Output/Nutrition instead of labs.

Institute for Safe Medication Practices

ISMP's List of *High-Alert Medications*

High-alert medications are drugs that bear a heightened risk of causing significant patient harm when they are used in error. Although mistakes may or may not be more common with these drugs, the consequences of an error are clearly more devastating to patients. We hope you will use this list to determine which medications require special safeguards to reduce the risk of errors. This may include strategies like improving access to information about these drugs; limiting access to high-alert medications; using auxiliary labels and automated alerts; standardizing the ordering, storage, preparation, and administration of these products; and employing redundancies such as automated or independent double-checks when necessary. (Note: manual independent double-checks are not always the optimal error-reduction strategy and may not be practical for all of the medications on the list).

Classes/Categories of Medications
adrenergic agonists, IV (e.g., epinephrine, phenylephrine, norepinephrine)
adrenergic antagonists, IV (e.g., propranolol, metoprolol, labetalol)
anesthetic agents, general, inhaled and IV (e.g., propofol, ketamine)
antiarrhythmics, IV (e.g., lidocaine, amiodarone)
antithrombotic agents (anticoagulants), including warfarin, low-molecular-weight heparin, IV unfractionated heparin, Factor Xa inhibitors (fondaparinux), direct thrombin inhibitors (e.g., argatroban, lepirudin, bivalirudin), thrombolytics (e.g., alteplase, reteplase, tenecteplase), and glycoprotein IIb/IIIa inhibitors (e.g., eptifibatide)
cardioplegic solutions
chemotherapeutic agents, parenteral and oral
dextrose, hypertonic, 20% or greater
dialysis solutions, peritoneal and hemodialysis
epidural or intrathecal medications
hypoglycemics, oral
inotropic medications, IV (e.g., digoxin, milrinone)
liposomal forms of drugs (e.g., liposomal amphotericin B)
moderate sedation agents, IV (e.g., midazolam)
moderate sedation agents, oral, for children (e.g., chloral hydrate)
narcotics/opiates, IV, transdermal, and oral (including liquid concentrates, immediate and sustained-release formulations)
neuromuscular blocking agents (e.g., succinylcholine, rocuronium, vecuronium)
radiocontrast agents, IV
total parenteral nutrition solutions

Specific Medications
epoprostenol (Flolan), IV
insulin, subcutaneous and IV
magnesium sulfate injection
methotrexate, oral, non-oncologic use
opium tincture
oxytocin, IV
nitroprusside sodium for injection
potassium chloride for injection concentrate
potassium phosphates injection
promethazine, IV
sodium chloride for injection, hypertonic (greater than 0.9% concentration)
sterile water for injection, inhalation, and irrigation (excluding pour bottles) in containers of 100 mL or more

Background
Based on error reports submitted to the USP-ISMP Medication Errors Reporting Program, reports of harmful errors in the literature, and input from practitioners and safety experts, ISMP created and periodically updates a list of potential high-alert medications. During February-April 2007, 770 practitioners responded to an ISMP survey designed to identify which medications were most frequently considered high-alert drugs by individuals and organizations. Further, to assure relevance and completeness, the clinical staff at ISMP, members of our advisory board, and safety experts throughout the US were asked to review the potential list. This list of drugs and drug categories reflects the collective thinking of all who provided input.

Institute for Safe
Medication Practices
www.ismp.org

© ISMP 2008

Answer Key

General Mathematics Self-Assessment (page 1)

1. $4\frac{1}{2}$
2. $5\frac{1}{5}$
3. $\frac{25}{3}$
4. $\frac{27}{5}$

5. 88
6. 45
7. $1\frac{1}{30}$
8. $6\frac{19}{24}$

9. $\frac{8}{21}$
10. $4\frac{7}{8}$
11. $\frac{1}{18}$
12. $\frac{1}{3}$

13. $\frac{5}{6}$
14. $\frac{9}{20}$
15. $\frac{1}{30}$
16. $\frac{3}{7}$

17. 0.12
18. 3.016
19. 4.904
20. 28.708

21. 2.96
22. 0.8241
23. 0.1
24. 1.2

25. 33.333
26. 98.095
27. 0.545
28. 9.125

29. 75
30. 0.5
31. $\frac{5}{1000} = \frac{1}{200}$
32. $\frac{5}{100} = \frac{1}{20}$

33. 0.75 75%
34. 0.125 $12\frac{1}{2}$%

	Decimal	Nearest Whole Number	Nearest Hundredth	Nearest Tenth
35.	0.8734	1	0.87	0.9
36.	0.842	1	0.84	0.8
37.	0.553	1	0.55	0.6
38.	0.689	1	0.69	0.7
39.	2.75	3	2.75	2.8

40. $\frac{1}{2}$ (0.5)
41. $\frac{1}{2}$ (0.5)
42. $1\frac{1}{2}$ (1.5)
43. 2

44. 2
45. 2

1 General Mathematics

1. 1 2. 5 3. $3\frac{1}{4}$ 4. $1\frac{5}{9}$

5. $5\frac{2}{3}$ 6. 5 7. $2\frac{1}{4}$ 8. $1\frac{7}{8}$

9. 6 10. $6\frac{5}{6}$

1. $\frac{7}{2}$ 2. $\frac{7}{6}$ 3. $\frac{33}{8}$ 4. $\frac{43}{12}$

5. $\frac{68}{5}$ 6. $\frac{49}{3}$ 7. $\frac{23}{6}$ 8. $\frac{21}{8}$

9. $\frac{63}{6}$ 10. $\frac{377}{3}$

1.
$$\begin{array}{r} \frac{2}{5} \\ +\frac{2}{5} \\ \hline \frac{4}{5} \end{array}$$

2.
$$\begin{array}{r} \frac{4}{5}=\frac{12}{15} \\ +\frac{2}{3}=\frac{10}{15} \\ \hline \frac{22}{15}=1\frac{7}{15} \end{array}$$

3.
$$\begin{array}{r} 6\frac{1}{6}=6\frac{4}{24} \\ +9\frac{5}{8}=9\frac{15}{24} \\ \hline 15\frac{19}{24} \end{array}$$

4.
$$\begin{array}{r} 2\frac{1}{4}=2\frac{2}{8} \\ +3\frac{1}{8}=3\frac{1}{8} \\ \hline 5\frac{3}{8} \end{array}$$

5.
$$\begin{array}{r} 1\frac{3}{4}=1\frac{30}{40} \\ +9\frac{9}{10}=9\frac{36}{40} \\ \hline 10\frac{66}{40}=11\frac{13}{20} \end{array}$$

6.
$$\begin{array}{r} \frac{1}{8}=\frac{9}{72} \\ \frac{1}{4}=\frac{18}{72} \\ +\frac{3}{9}=\frac{24}{72} \\ \hline \frac{51}{72} \end{array}$$

7.
$$\begin{array}{r} \frac{7}{9}=\frac{7}{90} \\ \frac{4}{5}=\frac{72}{90} \\ +\frac{9}{10}=\frac{81}{90} \\ \hline \frac{223}{90}=2\frac{43}{90} \end{array}$$

8.
$$\begin{array}{r} 3\frac{1}{4} \\ +9\frac{3}{4} \\ \hline 12\frac{4}{4}=13 \end{array}$$

9.
$$\begin{array}{r} 8\frac{2}{5}=8\frac{4}{10} \\ 14\frac{7}{10}=14\frac{7}{10} \\ +9\frac{9}{10}=9\frac{9}{10} \\ \hline 31\frac{20}{10}=33 \end{array}$$

10.
$$\begin{array}{r} 2\frac{1}{3}=2\frac{2}{6} \\ +4\frac{1}{6}=4\frac{1}{6} \\ \hline 6\frac{3}{6}=6\frac{1}{2} \text{ v} \end{array}$$

1.
$$\begin{array}{r} \frac{2}{3}=\frac{4}{6} \\ -\frac{1}{2}=\frac{3}{6} \\ \hline \frac{1}{6} \end{array}$$

2.
$$\begin{array}{r} \frac{27}{32} \\ -\frac{18}{32} \\ \hline \frac{9}{32} \end{array}$$

3.
$$\begin{array}{r} 10\frac{2}{5}=10\frac{8}{20} \\ -6\frac{1}{4}=6\frac{5}{20} \\ \hline 4\frac{3}{20} \end{array}$$

4.
$$\begin{array}{r} 7\frac{16}{24}=7\frac{16}{24} \\ -3\frac{1}{8}=3\frac{3}{24} \\ \hline 4\frac{13}{24} \end{array}$$

(Must borrow from the whole number.)

5.
$$\begin{array}{r} 6\frac{3}{10}=6\frac{3}{10} \\ -2\frac{1}{5}=2\frac{2}{10} \\ \hline 4\frac{1}{10} \end{array}$$

6.
$$\begin{array}{r} \frac{7}{8}=\frac{21}{24} \\ -\frac{1}{3}=\frac{8}{24} \\ \hline \frac{13}{24} \end{array}$$

7.
$$\begin{array}{r} 3\frac{5}{8} \\ -1\frac{3}{8} \\ \hline 2\frac{2}{8}=2\frac{1}{4} \end{array}$$

8.
$$\begin{array}{r} 5\frac{3}{7}=4\frac{10}{7} \\ -1\frac{6}{7}=1\frac{6}{7} \\ \hline 3\frac{4}{7} \end{array}$$

(Must borrow from the whole number.)

$$7 = 6\frac{4}{4}$$
$$-1\frac{3}{4} = 1\frac{3}{4}$$
$$\overline{\qquad 5\frac{1}{4}}$$

9.

$$2\frac{7}{8} = 2\frac{7}{8}$$
$$-\frac{3}{4} = \frac{6}{8}$$
$$\overline{\qquad 2\frac{1}{8}}$$

10.

(Must borrow from the whole number.)

WORKSHEET **1E** (page 10)

1. $\frac{1}{5} \times \frac{2}{4} = \frac{2}{20} = \frac{1}{10}$

2. $\frac{1}{5} \times \frac{1}{6} = \frac{1}{30}$

3. $1\frac{3}{4} \times 3\frac{1}{7} = \frac{\overset{1}{7}}{4} \times \frac{22}{\underset{1}{7}} = \frac{22}{4} = 22 \div 4 = 5\frac{1}{2}$

4. $4 \times 3\frac{1}{3} = 4 \times \frac{10}{3} = \frac{40}{3} = 13\frac{1}{3}$

5. $\frac{2}{4} \times 2\frac{1}{6} = \frac{\overset{1}{2}}{4} \times \frac{13}{\underset{3}{6}} = \frac{13}{12} = 1\frac{1}{12}$

6. $5\frac{1}{2} \times 3\frac{1}{8} = \frac{11}{2} \times \frac{25}{8} = \frac{275}{16} = 275 \div 16 = 17\frac{3}{16}$

7. $\frac{3}{5} \times \frac{5}{8} = \frac{15}{40} = \frac{3}{8}$

8. $\frac{5}{6} \times 1\frac{9}{16} = \frac{5}{6} \times \frac{25}{16} = \frac{125}{96} = 125 \div 96 = 1\frac{29}{96}$

9. $\frac{5}{100} \times 900 = \frac{5}{\underset{1}{100}} \times \frac{\overset{9}{900}}{1} = 45$

10. $2\frac{1}{10} \times 4\frac{1}{3} = \frac{21}{10} \times \frac{13}{\underset{1}{3}} = \frac{91}{10} = 9\frac{1}{10}$

WORKSHEET **1F** (page 11)

1. $\frac{1}{5} \div \frac{1}{8} = \frac{1}{5} \times \frac{8}{1} = \frac{8}{5} = 1\frac{3}{5}$

2. $\frac{1}{3} \div \frac{1}{2} = \frac{1}{3} \times \frac{2}{1} = \frac{2}{3}$

3. $\frac{3}{4} \div \frac{1}{8} = \frac{3}{\underset{1}{4}} \times \frac{\overset{2}{8}}{1} = 6$

4. $\frac{1}{16} \div \frac{1}{4} = \frac{1}{\underset{4}{16}} \times \frac{\overset{1}{4}}{1} = \frac{1}{4}$

5. $8\frac{3}{4} \div 15 = \frac{\overset{7}{35}}{4} \times \frac{1}{\underset{3}{15}} = \frac{7}{12}$

6. $\frac{3}{4} \div 6 = \frac{\overset{1}{3}}{4} \times \frac{1}{\underset{2}{6}} = \frac{1}{8}$

7. $2 \div \frac{1}{5} = \frac{2}{1} \times \frac{5}{1} = 10$

8. $3\frac{3}{8} \div 4\frac{1}{2} = \frac{27}{8} \div \frac{9}{2} = \frac{\overset{3}{27}}{\underset{4}{8}} \times \frac{\overset{1}{2}}{\underset{1}{9}} = \frac{3}{4}$

9. $\frac{3}{5} \div \frac{3}{8} = \frac{3}{5} \times \frac{8}{\underset{1}{3}} = \frac{8}{5} = 1\frac{3}{5}$

10. $4 \div 2\frac{1}{8} = \frac{4}{1} \times \frac{8}{17} = \frac{32}{17} = 1\frac{15}{17}$

WORKSHEET **1G** (page 11)

1. $\frac{1}{10}$

2. $\frac{2}{7}$

3. $\frac{1}{20}$

4. $\frac{1}{100,000}$

5. More

6. $\frac{1}{5}$

7. $\frac{1}{150}$

8. $\frac{1}{250}$

9. $\frac{1}{9}$

10. $\frac{1}{200}$

WORKSHEET **1HA** (page 14)

	Nearest Whole Number	Nearest Tenth	Nearest Hundredth
1. 93.489	93	93.5	93.49
2. 25.43	25	25.4	25.43
3. 38.1	38	38.1	38.10
4. 57.8888	58	57.9	57.89
5. 0.0092	0	0	0.01
6. 3.144	3	3.1	3.14
7. 8.999	9	9.0	9.00
8. 77.788	78	77.8	77.79
9. 12.959	13	13.0	12.96
10. 12.959	6	5.8	5.77

WORKSHEET **1HB** (page 14)

1. Six hundredths
2. Ninety-two thousandths
3. Five thousandths
4. One hundred and one hundredth
5. Nine tenths
6. 0.34
7. 0.003
8. 2.017
9. 9.0002
10. 34.1

Round to tenths	Round to hundredths
1. 0.3	**6.** 0.30
2. 4.4	**7.** 4.44
3. 2.8	**8.** 2.75
4. 0.8	**9.** 0.85
5. 6.8	**10.** 6.77

Round to thousandths	Round to ten-thousandths
11. 8.937	**16.** 8.9375
12. 5.626	**17.** 5.6257
13. 10.9	**18.** 10.8976
14. 4.626	**19.** 4.6256
15. 3.739	**20.** 3.7387

WORKSHEET **1IB** (page 16)

Smaller:

1. 0.3	**2.** 0.25
3. 0.125	**4.** 2.07
5. 1.29	

Larger:

6. 0.9	**7.** 0.7
8. 0.58	**9.** 0.25
10. 0.1	

WORKSHEET **1J** (page 17)

$$\begin{array}{r} 0.4 \\ +\,0.7 \\ \hline 1.1 \end{array}$$

1.

$$\begin{array}{r} 5.030 \\ +\,2.999 \\ \hline 8.029 \end{array}$$

2.

$$\begin{array}{r} 1.27 \\ 0.06 \\ +\,4.00 \\ \hline 5.33 \end{array}$$

3.

$$\begin{array}{r} 15.60 \\ 0.19 \\ +\,500.00 \\ \hline 515.79 \end{array}$$

4.

$$\begin{array}{r} 210.79 \\ 2.00 \\ +\,68.41 \\ \hline 281.2\cancel{0}* \end{array}$$

5.

WORKSHEET **1K** (page 17)

$$\begin{array}{r} 2.5 \\ -\,1.25 \\ \hline 1.25 \end{array}$$

1.

$$\begin{array}{r} 0.5 \\ -\,0.25 \\ \hline 0.25 \end{array}$$

2.

$$\begin{array}{r} 0.450 \\ -\,0.367 \\ \hline 0.083 \end{array}$$

3.

$$\begin{array}{r} 108.56 \\ -\,5.40 \\ \hline 103.16 \end{array}$$

4.

$$\begin{array}{r} 1.25 \\ -\,0.75 \\ \hline 0.5\cancel{0}* \end{array}$$

5.

WORKSHEET **1L** (page 18)

$$\begin{array}{r} 0.5 \\ \times\,100 \\ \hline 50.\cancel{0} \end{array}$$

1.   Count 1 decimal place in from the right.

$$\begin{array}{r} 0.25 \\ \times\,2 \\ \hline 0.5\cancel{0} \end{array}$$

2.

3.
$$
\begin{array}{r}
3.14 \\
\times\ 0.002 \\
\hline
0.00628
\end{array}
$$

You do not have to multiply zeros. Count 5 decimal places in from the right, adding zeros where needed.

4.
$$
\begin{array}{r}
2.14 \\
\times\ 0.03 \\
\hline
0.0642
\end{array}
$$

Count 4 decimal places in from the right, adding zeros as needed.

5.
$$
\begin{array}{r}
36.8 \\
\times\ 70.1 \\
\hline
368 \\
2578 \\
\hline
2579.68
\end{array}
$$

_____

*Trailing zeros must be removed from answers.

WORKSHEET **1M** (page 19)

1. $60\overline{)1.35}$ **2.** $20\overline{)15.6}$ **3.** $19\overline{)10.14}$ **4.** $7\overline{)60.5}$

5. $25\overline{)35.9}$

6.
$$
\begin{array}{r}
2. \\
0.25\overline{)0.50} \\
50 \\
\hline
0
\end{array}
$$
ANSWER: 1.6

7.
$$
0.1\overline{)0.5}\ \ \ \ 5.
$$
ANSWER: 5

8.
$$
\begin{array}{r}
0.40 \\
4.8\overline{)2.0\,40} \\
1\,9\,2 \\
\hline
20
\end{array}
$$
ANSWER: 0.4

9.
$$
\begin{array}{r}
0.5 \\
0.5\overline{)0.2\,5} \\
2\,5
\end{array}
$$
ANSWER: 0.5

10.
$$
\begin{array}{r}
3.66 \\
0.12\overline{)0.44\,00} \\
36 \\
\hline
8\,0 \\
7\,2 \\
\hline
80 \\
72 \\
\hline
8
\end{array}
$$
ANSWER: 3.7

WORKSHEET **1N** (page 20)

1.
$$
\begin{array}{r}
3\,3.333 \\
6.0\overline{)200.0\,000} \\
180 \\
\hline
20\,0 \\
18\,0 \\
\hline
2\,00 \\
1\,80 \\
\hline
2\,00 \\
1\,80 \\
\hline
200 \\
180
\end{array}
$$

PROOF
$$
\begin{array}{r}
33.333 \\
\times\ \ \ \ 60 \\
\hline
1999.980
\end{array}
$$

2.
$$
\begin{array}{r}
2.51 \\
6\overline{)15.06} \\
12 \\
\hline
30 \\
30 \\
\hline
06 \\
6 \\
\hline
\end{array}
$$

PROOF
$$
\begin{array}{r}
2.51 \\
\times\ \ 6 \\
\hline
15.06
\end{array}
$$

3.

$$0.87\overline{)79.40\,000}$$

$$\begin{array}{r} 91.264 \\ \hline 78\,30 \\ \hline 1\,10 \\ 87 \\ \hline 23\,0 \\ 17\,4 \\ \hline 5\,60 \\ 5\,22 \\ \hline 380 \\ 348 \end{array}$$

PROOF

$$\begin{array}{r} 91.264 \\ \times\quad 87 \\ \hline 638\,848 \\ 7301\,12 \\ \hline 7939.968 \end{array}$$

4.

$$48\overline{)158.4}$$

$$\begin{array}{r} 3.3 \\ \hline 144 \\ \hline 14\,4 \\ 14\,4 \\ \hline \end{array}$$

PROOF

$$\begin{array}{r} 48 \\ \times\,3.3 \\ \hline 14\,4 \\ 144 \\ \hline 158.4 \end{array}$$

5.

$$0.78\overline{)670.80}$$

$$\begin{array}{r} 860. \\ \hline 624 \\ \hline 46\,8 \\ 46\,8 \\ \hline \end{array}$$

PROOF

$$\begin{array}{r} 860 \\ \times\,78 \\ \hline 6880 \\ 6020 \\ \hline 67080 \end{array}$$

WORKSHEET 1O (page 21)

1. $\dfrac{8}{10} = \dfrac{4}{5}$ **2.** $\dfrac{4}{10} = \dfrac{2}{5}$ **3.** $\dfrac{25}{100} = \dfrac{1}{4}$ **4.** $1\dfrac{32}{100} = 1\dfrac{8}{25}$

5. $4\dfrac{8}{100} = 4\dfrac{2}{25}$ **6.** $\dfrac{5}{10} = \dfrac{1}{2}$ **7.** $\dfrac{75}{100} = \dfrac{3}{4}$ **8.** $\dfrac{2}{10} = \dfrac{1}{5}$

9. $\dfrac{65}{100} = \dfrac{13}{20}$ **10.** $\dfrac{7}{10}$

WORKSHEET 1P (page 21)

1.

$$5\overline{)1.0}$$

$$\begin{array}{r} 0.2 \\ \hline 1\,0 \\ \hline \end{array}$$

2.

$$3\overline{)2.000}$$

$$\begin{array}{r} 0.666 \\ \hline 1\,8 \\ \hline 20 \\ 18 \\ \hline 20 \\ 18 \end{array}$$

3.

$$2\overline{)1.0}$$

$$\begin{array}{r} 0.5 \\ \hline 1\,0 \\ \hline \end{array}$$

4.

$$12\overline{)1.000}$$

$$\begin{array}{r} 0.083 \\ \hline 96 \\ \hline 40 \\ 36 \\ \hline \end{array}$$

5.

$$8\overline{)6.00}$$

$$\begin{array}{r} 0.75 \\ \hline 5\,6 \\ \hline 40 \\ 40 \\ \hline \end{array}$$

WORKSHEET 1Q (page 22)

1. Decimal: 0.5
Percentage: 50%

2. Fraction: $\dfrac{1}{2}$
Decimal: 0.5

3. Fraction: $\dfrac{5}{100} = \dfrac{1}{20}$
Percentage: 5%

4. Decimal: 0.083
Percentage: 8.33%

5. Decimal: 0.003
Percentage: 0.3%

6. Fraction: $\dfrac{1}{10}$
Percentage: 10%

7. Fraction: $\dfrac{250}{100} = \dfrac{5}{2}$
Decimal: 2.5

8. Fraction: $\dfrac{7}{20}$
Percentage: 35%

9. Decimal: 0.8
Percentage: 80%

10. Fraction: $\dfrac{75}{100} = \dfrac{3}{4}$
Decimal: 0.75

1.
$$
\begin{array}{r}
1500 \\
\times\,0.02 \\
\hline
30.0\cancel{0}\,* \\
\end{array}
$$

2.
$$
\begin{array}{r}
240 \\
\times\,1.14 \\
\hline
960 \\
240 \\
240 \\
\hline
273.6\cancel{0}\,* \\
\end{array}
$$

3.
$$
\begin{array}{r}
50 \\
\times\,0.28 \\
\hline
400 \\
100 \\
\hline
14.00\,* \\
\end{array}
$$

4.
$$
\begin{array}{r}
200 \\
\times\,0.09 \\
\hline
18.0\cancel{0}\,* \\
\end{array}
$$

5. $\dfrac{1/2}{100} = \dfrac{1}{2} \div \dfrac{100}{1} = \dfrac{1}{2} \times \dfrac{1}{100} = \dfrac{1}{200} = 200\overline{)1.000}\,^{0.005}$

$$
\begin{array}{r}
9328 \\
\times\,0.005 \\
\hline
46.64\cancel{0}\,* \\
\end{array}
$$

6. $\dfrac{1/3}{100} = \dfrac{1}{3} \div \dfrac{100}{1} = \dfrac{1}{3} \times \dfrac{1}{100} = \dfrac{1}{300} = 300\overline{)1.000}\,^{0.003}$

$$
\begin{array}{r}
900 \\
\hline
100 \\
\end{array}
$$

$$
\begin{array}{r}
930 \\
\times\,0.003 \\
\hline
2.79\cancel{0}\,* \\
\end{array}
$$

7.
$$
\begin{array}{r}
400 \\
\times\,1.20 \\
\hline
8000 \\
400 \\
\hline
480.0\cancel{0}\,* \\
\end{array}
$$

8.
$$
\begin{array}{r}
105.80 \\
\times\,0.05 \\
\hline
5.29\cancel{00}\,* \\
\end{array}
$$

9.
$$
\begin{array}{r}
520 \\
\times\,0.10 \\
\hline
52.0\cancel{0}\,* \\
\end{array}
$$

10.
$$
\begin{array}{r}
40.80 \\
\times\,0.03 \\
\hline
1.224\cancel{0}\,* \\
\end{array}
$$

---

*Trailing zeros must be removed from answers.

1. $2 : 3 :: x : 450$
   $3x = 2 \times 450 = 900$
   $x = 300$ mL of hydrogen peroxide + 600 mL NS = $\frac{2}{3}$ strength solution

2. $1 : 3 :: x : 6$
   $3x = 6$
   $x = 2$ oz of hydrogen peroxide + 4 oz of NS = 6 oz of $\frac{1}{3}$ strength solution

3. $1 : 4 :: x : 500$
   $4x = 500$
   $x = 125$ mL hydrogen peroxide + 375 mL NS = 500 mL $\frac{1}{4}$ strength solution

4. $3 : 4 :: x : 800$
   $4x = 3 \times 800 = 2400$
   $x = 600$ mL hydrogen peroxide + 200 mL NS = 800 mL $\frac{3}{4}$ strength solution

5. $2 : 5 :: x : 120$
   $5x = 2 \times 120 = 240$
   $x = 48$ mL hydrogen peroxide + 72 mL NS = 120 mL $\frac{2}{5}$ strength solution

1. a The other responses can be eliminated quickly because only **a** offers 3 as the whole number.
2. b   3. d   4. a   5. c
6. b   7. b   8. d   9. b
10. a   11. b   12. d   13. d
14. a   15. c   16. a   17. a
18. a   19. c   20. b

1. $6\frac{1}{4}$
2. 4
3. $\frac{51}{5}$
4. $\frac{23}{6}$

5. 20
6. 40
7. $\frac{19}{36}$
8. $10\frac{7}{8}$

9. $\frac{5}{24}$
10. 1
11. $\frac{1}{30}$
12. $\frac{10}{48} = \frac{5}{24}$

13. $\frac{24}{4} = 6$
14. $\frac{3}{4}$
15. $\frac{1}{250}$
16. $\frac{1}{3}$

17. 0.05
18. 2.017
19. 8.009
20. 60.97

21. 3.824
22. 0.1562
23. 0.00001Ø*
24. 3.5

25. 3.3ØØ*
26. 91.264
27. 1.1875
28. 8.0625

29. 12.48
30. 583
31. $\frac{2}{5}$
32. $\frac{57}{200}$

---

*Trailing zeros must be removed from answers.

	Fraction	Decimal to Nearest Tenth	Decimal to Nearest Hundredth	Percentage
33.	$\frac{1}{3}$	0.3	0.33	33%
34.	$\frac{5}{100} = \left(\frac{1}{20}\right)$	0.1	0.05	5%
35.	$\frac{2}{5}$	0.4	0.40	40%
36.	$\frac{22}{100} = \left(\frac{11}{50}\right)$	0.2	0.22	22%
37.	$\frac{1}{8}$	0.1	0.12	12.5%
38.	$\frac{10}{100} = \left(\frac{1}{10}\right)$	0.1	0.10	10%
39.	$\frac{1}{12}$	0.1	0.08	8%
40.	$\frac{1}{200}$	0	0.01	$\frac{1}{2}$%
41.	$\frac{5}{16}$	0.3	0.31	31%
42.	$\frac{15}{100} = \left(\frac{3}{20}\right)$	0.2	0.15	15%
43.	$\frac{1}{4}$	0.3	0.25	25%
44.	$\frac{12}{100} = \left(\frac{3}{25}\right)$	0.1	0.12	12%
45.	$\frac{1}{100}$	0.0	0.01	1%
46.	$\frac{80}{100} = \left(\frac{4}{5}\right)$	0.8	0.80	80%

Fraction	Decimal to Nearest Tenth	Decimal to Nearest Hundredth	Percentage
47. $\frac{1}{200}$	0.0	0.00	0.5%
48. $\frac{33}{100}$	0.3	0.33	33%
49. $\frac{1}{250}$	0	0	$\frac{2}{5}$%
50. $\frac{75}{100} = \left(\frac{3}{4}\right)$	0.8	0.75	75%

2 Ratio and Proportion

WORKSHEET **2A** (page 31)

1. $\frac{2}{4} = \frac{1}{2}$
2. $\frac{6}{8} = \frac{3}{4}$
3. $\frac{2}{500} = \frac{1}{250}$
4. $\frac{6}{1000} = \frac{3}{500}$

5. $\frac{43}{86} = \frac{1}{2}$
6. $\frac{2}{13}$
7. $\frac{8}{10} = \frac{4}{5}$
8. $\frac{1}{10}$

9. $\frac{1}{150}$
10. $\frac{4}{100} = \frac{1}{25}$

WORKSHEET **2B** (page 33)

1. $5 : 300 :: 9 : x$

$5x = 9 \times 300$

$5x = 2700$

$\frac{\cancel{5}}{\cancel{5}}x = \frac{2700}{5} = 2700 \div 5$

$x = 540$

PROOF

$540 \times 5 = 2700$

$9 \times 300 = 2700$

2. $9 : 27 :: 300 : x$

$9x = 27 \times 300 = 8100$

$\frac{\cancel{9}}{\cancel{9}}x = \frac{8100}{9} = 8100 \div 9$

$x = 900$

PROOF

$27 \times 300 = 8100$

$9 \times 900 = 8100$

3. $\frac{1}{2} : x :: 1 : 8$

$1x = \frac{1}{2} \times 8$

$\frac{\cancel{1}}{\cancel{1}}x = \frac{1}{2} \times \frac{8}{1}$

$x = 4$

PROOF

$4 \times 1 = 4$

$\frac{1}{2} \times 8 = 4$

4. $\frac{1}{4} : 500 :: x : 1000$

$500x = \frac{1}{4} \times 1000$

$500x = 250$

$\frac{\cancel{500}}{\cancel{500}}x = \frac{250}{500} = 250 \div 500$

$x = 0.5$

PROOF

$500 \times 0.5 = 250$

$\frac{1}{4} \times 100 = 250$

5. $6 : 24 :: 0.75 : x$

$6x = 24 \times 0.75 = 18$

$6x = 18$

$\dfrac{\cancel{6}}{\cancel{6}} x = \dfrac{18}{6} = 18 \div 6$

$x = \mathbf{3}$

PROOF

$24 \times 0.75 = 18$

$6 \times 3 = 18$

6. $36 : 12 :: \dfrac{1}{100} : x$

$36x = 12 \times \dfrac{1}{100}$

$36x = \dfrac{12}{1} \times \dfrac{1}{100} = \dfrac{3}{25}$

$\dfrac{\cancel{36}}{\cancel{36}} x = \dfrac{^{3/25}}{36} = \dfrac{3}{25} \div 36 = \dfrac{3}{25} \times \dfrac{1}{\underset{12}{\cancel{36}}}$

$x = \dfrac{1}{300}$

PROOF

$36 \times \dfrac{1}{300} = \dfrac{3}{25}$

$12 \times \dfrac{1}{100} = \dfrac{3}{25}$

7. $4 : 120 :: x : 600$

$120x = 4 \times 600 = 2400$

$\dfrac{\cancel{120}}{\cancel{120}} x = \dfrac{240\cancel{0}}{12\cancel{0}} = 240 \div 12$

$x = 20$

PROOF

$600 \times 4 = 2400$

$20 \times 120 = 2400$

8. $0.7 : 70 :: x : 1000$

$70x = 0.7 \times 1000 = 700$

$\dfrac{\cancel{70}}{\cancel{70}} x = \dfrac{700}{70} = 70 \div 7$

$x = 10$

PROOF

$70 \times 10 = 700$

$0.7 \times 1000 = 700$

9. $\dfrac{1}{1000} : \dfrac{1}{100} :: x : 60$

$\dfrac{1}{100}x = \dfrac{1}{1000} \times 60$

$\dfrac{1}{100}x = \dfrac{1}{100\cancel{0}} \times \dfrac{6\cancel{0}}{1} = \dfrac{3}{50}$

$\dfrac{^{1/100}}{^{1/100}} x = \dfrac{^{3/50}}{^{1/100}} = \dfrac{3}{50} \div \dfrac{1}{100} = \dfrac{3}{50} \times \dfrac{100}{1} = \dfrac{300}{50}$

$x = 6$

PROOF

$\dfrac{1}{1000} \times 60 = \dfrac{3}{50}$

$\dfrac{1}{100} \times 6 = \dfrac{3}{50}$

10. $6 : 12 :: \dfrac{1}{4} : x$

$6x = 12 \times \dfrac{1}{4} = 3$

$\dfrac{\cancel{6}}{\cancel{6}} x = \dfrac{3}{6} = 3 \div 6$

$x = 0.5$

PROOF

$12 \times \dfrac{1}{4} = 3$

$6 \times 0.5 = 3$

WORKSHEET 2C (page 33)

1. $\dfrac{1}{2} : \dfrac{1}{6} :: \dfrac{1}{4} : x$

$\dfrac{1}{2}x = \dfrac{1}{6} \times \dfrac{1}{4} = \dfrac{1}{24}$

$\dfrac{^{1/2}}{^{1/2}} x = \dfrac{^{1/24}}{^{1/2}} = \dfrac{1}{24} \div \dfrac{1}{2} = \dfrac{1}{24} \times \dfrac{2}{1}$

$x = \dfrac{1}{12}$

PROOF

$\dfrac{1}{2} \times \dfrac{1}{12} = \dfrac{1}{24}$

$\dfrac{1}{6} \times \dfrac{1}{4} = \dfrac{1}{24}$

2. $15 : 30 :: x : 12$

$30x = 15 \times 12$

$30x = 180$

$\dfrac{\cancel{30}}{\cancel{30}} x = \dfrac{180}{30} = 180 \div 30$

$x = 6$

PROOF

$30 \times 6 = 180$

$15 \times 12 = 180$

3. $15 : x :: 1.5 : 10$

$1.5x = 15 \times 10 = 150$

$\dfrac{\cancel{1.5}}{\cancel{1.5}}x = \dfrac{150}{1.5} = 150 \div 1.5$

$\quad x = 100$

PROOF

$15 \times 10 = 150$

$100 \times 1.5 = 150$

4. $6 : 12 :: 0.25 : x$

$6x = 12 \times 0.25 = 3$

$\dfrac{\cancel{6}}{\cancel{6}}x = \dfrac{3}{6} = 3 \div 6$

$\quad x = 0.5$

PROOF

$12 \times 0.25 = 3$

$6 \times 0.5 = 3$

5. $300 : 5 :: x : \dfrac{1}{60}$

$5x = \dfrac{1}{60} \times 300$

$5x = \dfrac{1}{60} \times \dfrac{300}{1} = 5$

$\dfrac{\cancel{5}}{\cancel{5}}x = \dfrac{5}{5} = 5 \div 5$

$\quad x = 1$

PROOF

$300 \times \dfrac{1}{60} = 5$

$5 \times 1 = 5$

6. $\dfrac{1}{150} : \dfrac{1}{200} :: 2 : x$

$\dfrac{1}{150}x = \dfrac{1}{200} \times 2$

$\dfrac{1}{150}x = \dfrac{1}{200} \times \dfrac{2}{1} = \dfrac{1}{100}$

$\dfrac{1/\cancel{150}}{1/\cancel{100}}x = \dfrac{1/100}{1/150} = \dfrac{1}{100} \div \dfrac{1}{150} = \dfrac{1}{100} \times \dfrac{150}{1} = \dfrac{3}{2}$

$\quad x = 1\dfrac{1}{2}$

PROOF

$\dfrac{1}{150} \times \dfrac{3}{2}\left(1\dfrac{1}{2}\right) = \dfrac{1}{100}$

$\dfrac{1}{200} \times 2 = \dfrac{1}{100}$

7. $1 : 800 :: \dfrac{1}{200} : x$

$1x = \dfrac{1}{200} \times 800$

$1x = \dfrac{1}{200} \times \dfrac{800}{1} = 4$

$\dfrac{\cancel{1}}{\cancel{1}}x = \dfrac{4}{1} = 4 \div 1$

$\quad x = \mathbf{4}$

PROOF

$4 \times 1 = 4$

$\dfrac{1}{200} \times 800 = 4$

8. $7.5 : 12 :: x : 28$

$12x = 7.5 \times 28 = 210$

$\dfrac{\cancel{12}}{\cancel{12}}x = \dfrac{210}{12} = 210 \div 12$

$\quad x = 17.5$

PROOF

$7.5 \times 28 = 210$

$12 \times 17.5 = 210$

9. $\dfrac{1}{1000} : \dfrac{1}{100} :: x : 30$

$\dfrac{1}{100}x = \dfrac{1}{1000} \times 30$

$\dfrac{1}{100}x = \dfrac{1}{1000} \times \dfrac{30}{1} = \dfrac{3}{100}$

$\dfrac{1/\cancel{100}}{1/\cancel{100}}x = \dfrac{3/100}{1/100} = \dfrac{3}{100} \div \dfrac{1}{100} = \dfrac{3}{100} \times \dfrac{100}{1}$

$\quad x = 3$

PROOF

$\dfrac{1}{1000} \times 30 = \dfrac{3}{100}$

$\dfrac{1}{100} \times 3 = \dfrac{3}{100}$

10. $0.4 : 12 :: 10 : x$

$0.4x = 10 \times 12 = 120$

$\dfrac{\cancel{0.4}}{\cancel{0.4}}x = \dfrac{120}{0.4} = 120 \div 0.4$

$\quad x = 300$

PROOF

$10 \times 12 = 120$

$300 \times 0.4 = 120$

1. KNOW   WANT TO KNOW

Bananas : Apples :: x Bananas : Apples

$6 : 9 :: x : 72$

$9x = 6 \times 72 = 432$

$\dfrac{\cancel{9}}{\cancel{9}}x = \dfrac{432}{9}$

   $x = 48$ bananas

PROOF

$6 : 9 :: 48 : 72$

$9 \times 48 = 432$

$6 \times 72 = 432$

2. KNOW   WANT TO KNOW

Scoops : Cups :: x Scoops : Cups

$7 : 8 :: x : 40$

$8x = 40 \times 7 = 280$

$\dfrac{\cancel{8}}{\cancel{8}}x = \dfrac{280}{8}$

   $x = 35$ scoops

PROOF

$7 : 8 :: 35 : 40$

$8 \times 35 = 280$

$7 \times 40 = 280$

remember   Scoops : Cups < Scoops : Cups

Apples : Bananas < Apples : Bananas

Miles : Gallons < Miles : Gallons

3. KNOW   WANT TO KNOW

Scoops : Cups :: x Scoops : Cups

$4 : 6 :: x : 18$

$6x = 72$

$\dfrac{\cancel{6}}{\cancel{6}}x = \dfrac{72}{6}$

   $x = 12$ scoops of cocoa

PROOF

$4 : 6 :: 12 : 18$

$6 \times 12 = 72$

$4 \times 18 = 72$

4. KNOW   WANT TO KNOW

4 pills : 1 day :: x pills : 21 days

$x = 4 \times 21$

$x = 84$ pills

PROOF

$4 : 1 :: 84 : 21$

$4 \times 21 = 84$

$1 \times 84 = 84$

5. KNOW   WANT TO KNOW

Bushes : Trees :: x Bushes : Trees

$8 : 2 :: x : 36$

$2x = 8 \times 36 = 288$

$\dfrac{\cancel{2}}{\cancel{2}}x = \dfrac{288}{2}$

   $x = 144$ bushes

PROOF

$8 : 2 :: 144 : 36$

$8 \times 36 = 288$

$2 \times 144 = 288$

6. KNOW   WANT TO KNOW

Cups : Day :: Cups : x Days

$4 : 1 :: 84 : x$

$4x = 84$

$\dfrac{\cancel{4}}{\cancel{4}}x = \dfrac{84}{4}$

   $x = 21$ days

PROOF

$4 : 1 :: 84 : 21$

$1 \times 84 = 84$

$4 \times 21 = 84$

7. KNOW   WANT TO KNOW

Cups : Loaves :: Cups : x Loaves

$4 : 3 :: 24 : x$

$4x = 24 \times 3 = 72$

$\dfrac{\cancel{4}}{\cancel{4}}x = \dfrac{72}{4}$

   $x = 18$ loaves

PROOF

$4 : 3 :: 24 : 18$

$4 \times 18 = 72$

$3 \times 24 = 72$

8. KNOW   WANT TO KNOW

3 soda : $\dfrac{1}{2}$ fruit juice :: x soda : 2 fruit juice

$\dfrac{1}{2}x = 3 \times 2$

$\dfrac{\cancel{1/2}}{\cancel{1/2}}x = \dfrac{6}{\frac{1}{2}}$ $6 \div \dfrac{1}{2} = 6 \times \dfrac{2}{1}$

   $x = 12$ cups soda

PROOF

$3 : \dfrac{1}{2} :: 12 : 2$

$3 \times 2 = 6$

$\dfrac{1}{2} \times 12 = 6$

9.

KNOW   WANT TO KNOW

4 Tbsp sugar : 1 glass :: x Tbsp sugar : 6 glasses

$x = 6 \times 4$

$x = 24$ tbsp sugar

PROOF

$4 : 1 :: 24 : 6$

$4 \times 6 = 24$

$1 \times 24 = 24$

10.

KNOW   WANT TO KNOW

4 cap : 1 day :: x cap : 14 days

$x = 4 \times 14$

$x = 56$ cap

PROOF

$4 : 1 :: 56 : 14$

$4 \times 14 = 56$

$1 \times 56 = 56$

WORKSHEET 2E (page 35)

1.

KNOW   WANT TO KNOW

200 envelopes : 1 box :: 4000 envelopes : x boxes

$200x = 4000$

$\dfrac{\cancel{200}}{\cancel{200}}x = \dfrac{4\cancel{000}}{2\cancel{00}}$

$x = 20$ boxes

PROOF

$200 \times 20 = 4000$

$1 \times 4000 = 4000$

2.

KNOW   WANT TO KNOW

10 disks : 1 package :: 300 disks : x packages

$10x = 300$

$\dfrac{\cancel{10}}{\cancel{10}}x = \dfrac{30\cancel{0}}{1\cancel{0}}$

$x = 30$ packages

PROOF

$10 \times 30 = 300$

$1 \times 300 = 300$

3.

KNOW   WANT TO KNOW

1 computer : 18 students ::

                   x computers : 1260 students

$18x = 1260$

$\dfrac{\cancel{18}}{\cancel{18}}x = \dfrac{1260}{18}$

$x = 70$ computers

PROOF

$1 \times 1260 = 1260$

$18 \times 70 = 1260$

4.

KNOW   WANT TO KNOW

3 water : 2 apples :: 24 water : x apples

$3x = 48$

$\dfrac{\cancel{3}}{\cancel{3}}x = \dfrac{48}{3}$

$x = 16$ apples

PROOF

$3 \times 16 = 48$

$2 \times 24 = 48$

5.

KNOW   WANT TO KNOW

6 pens : 8 pencils :: x pens : 72 pencils

$8x = 432$

$\dfrac{\cancel{8}}{\cancel{8}}x = \dfrac{432}{8}$

$x = 54$ pens

PROOF

$6 \times 72 = 432$

$8 \times 54 = 432$

6.

KNOW   WANT TO KNOW

1 nurse : 6 patients :: x nurses : 36 patients

$6x = 36$

$\dfrac{\cancel{6}}{\cancel{6}}x = \dfrac{36}{6}$

$x = 6$ nurses

PROOF

$1 \times 36 = 36$

$6 \times 6 = 36$

7.

KNOW   WANT TO KNOW

4 Tbsp : 8 oz water :: x Tbsp : 56 oz water

$8x = 4 \times 56 = 224$

$\dfrac{\cancel{8}}{\cancel{8}}x = \dfrac{224}{8}$

$x = 28$ Tbsp formula

PROOF

$4 \times 56 = 224$

$8 \times 28 = 224$

8.

KNOW   WANT TO KNOW

2 nurses : 12 hr :: x nurses : 72 hr

$12x = 144$

$\dfrac{\cancel{12}}{\cancel{12}}x = \dfrac{124}{12}$

$x = 12$ nurses needed

PROOF

$12 \times 12 = 144$

$2 \times 72 = 144$

9. KNOW   WANT TO KNOW

8 aspirin : 1 day :: x aspirin : 14 days

$x = 8 \times 14$

$x = 112$ Aspirin tablets

PROOF

$8 \times 14 = 112$

$1 \times 112 = 112$

10. KNOW   WANT TO KNOW

5 milliliters : 1 day :: 100 milliliters : x days

$\frac{\cancel{5}}{\cancel{5}} x = \frac{100}{5}$

$x = 20$ Days

PROOF

$5 \times 20 = 100$

$1 \times 100 = 100$

WORKSHEET **2F** (page 36)

1. a. KNOW   WANT TO KNOW

10 diapers : 1 day :: 50 diapers : x days

$\frac{\cancel{10}}{\cancel{10}} x = \frac{50}{10}$

$x = 5$ days

PROOF

$10 \times 5 = 50$

$1 \times 50 = 50$

2. b. KNOW   WANT TO KNOW

10 syringes : 1 package :: 120 syringes : x packages

$\frac{\cancel{10}}{\cancel{10}} x = \frac{120}{10}$

$x = 12$ packages

PROOF

$10 \times 12 = 120$

$1 \times 120 = 120$

3. d. KNOW   WANT TO KNOW

4 tsp : 1 day :: 80 tsp : x days

$\frac{\cancel{4}}{\cancel{4}} x = \frac{80}{4}$

$x = 20$ days

PROOF

$4 \times 20 = 80$

$1 \times 80 = 80$

4. d. KNOW   WANT TO KNOW

3 capsules : 1 day :: x capsules : 21 days

$x = 3 \times 21$

$x = 63$ capsules

PROOF

$3 \times 21 = 63$

$1 \times 63 = 63$

5. b. KNOW   WANT TO KNOW

5 mL : 1 dose :: 30 mL : x doses

$\frac{\cancel{5}}{\cancel{5}} x = \frac{30}{5}$

$x = 6$ doses

PROOF

$5 \times 6 = 30$

$1 \times 30 = 30$

6. b. KNOW   WANT TO KNOW

120 days : 15 depts :: x days : 1 dept

$\frac{\cancel{15}}{\cancel{15}} x = \frac{120}{15}$

$x = 8$ days

PROOF

$120 \times 1 = 120$

$15 \times 8 = 120$

7. a. KNOW   WANT TO KNOW

8 patients : 1 RN :: 240 patients : x RNs

$\frac{\cancel{8}}{\cancel{8}} x = \frac{240}{8}$

$x = 30$ RNs

PROOF

$8 \times 30 = 240$

$1 \times 240 = 240$

8. c. KNOW   WANT TO KNOW

4 oz : 1 portion :: x oz : 20 portions

$x = 4 \times 20$

$x = 80$ oz

PROOF

$4 \times 20 = 80$

$1 \times 80 = 80$

9. c. KNOW   WANT TO KNOW

$15 : 1 hr :: $450 : x hr

$\frac{\cancel{15}}{\cancel{15}} x = \frac{450}{15}$

$x = 30$ hr

PROOF

$15 \times 30 = 450$

$1 \times 450 = 450$

10. a. KNOW   WANT TO KNOW

1 NA : 20 beds :: x NAs : 360 beds

$\frac{\cancel{20}}{\cancel{20}} x = \frac{360}{20}$

$x = 18$ NAs

PROOF

$1 \times 360 = 360$

$20 \times 18 = 360$

1.	15 supervisors	**2.**	25 nurses
3.	800 sheets	**4.**	224 patient discharges
5.	$480	**6.**	30 CNAs
7.	5 supervisors	**8.**	$3000 for 4 weeks
9.	21 interns	**10.**	approximately 40 medication errors
11.	12 tablets	**12.**	28 capsules
13.	10 days	**14.**	64 oz
15.	4 inservice days	**16.**	8 doses
17.	12 people	**18.**	32 RNs
19.	12 guest speakers	**20.**	240 tablets

3 Safe Medication Administration

WORKSHEET 3A (page 43)

Time	Abbreviation (if Applicable)	Time	Abbreviation (if Applicable)
before	a	after	p
before meals	ac	after meals	pc
daily	Write out daily	three times a day	tid
twice a day	bid	every other day	Write out every other day
every day	Write out every day	every 6 hours	q6h
every 4 hours	every 4 hours	every 12 hours	q12h
whenever necessary	prn	as desired, freely	ad lib (fluids and activities only)
immediately, at once	stat	bedtime	Write out bedtime
with	c̄	without	s̄

Route	Abbreviation (if Applicable)	Route	Abbreviation (if Applicable)
by mouth	po	nothing by mouth	NPO
intravenously	IV	intramuscularly	IM
sublingual	SL	subcutaneous	subcut
intradermal	ID	suppository	supp
left eye	Write out left eye	right ear	Write out right ear
nasogastric	NG	per gastrostomy tube	GT

WORKSHEET 3B (page 46)

Metric Measurement Term	Metric Measurement Abbreviation
microgram(s)	mcg
milligram(s)	mg
gram(s)	g
kilogram(s)	kg
milliliter(s)	mL
milliequivalent(s)	mEq
unit	Write out unit
international unit	Write out international unit
liter	L
square meter	m^2

Other Measurement Term	Abbreviation
one-half	Write out one half
teaspoon	tsp.
tablespoon	tbs, Tbsp
pound	lb

WORKSHEET **3C** (page 47)

Term	Recommended Abbreviation
capsule	cap
tablet	tab
fluid	fld
solution	sol
suspension	susp
elixir	elix
teaspoon	tsp
tablespoon	tbs, Tbsp
liquid	liq
ounce	oz
double strength	DS
extended release	XR
long acting	LA
sustained release	SR
controlled release	CR

WORKSHEET **3D** (page 53)

1. a. Lopressor
   b. metoprolol tartrate USP
   c. 50 mg per tab
   d. 1000 tab
   e. 50 mg:1 tab
3. a. Amoxil
   b. 78 mL
   c. 125 mg/5 mL
   d. 100 mL
   e. 125 mg:5 mL
   f. 14 days
5. a. streptomycin sulfate
   b. IM only
   c. 400 mg/mL
   d. 1 g/2.5 mL
   e. Refrigerate 2° to 8° C

2. a. Rifadin
   b. rifampin
   c. 150 mg per cap
   d. 30 cap
   e. 150 mg:1 cap
4. a. tetracycline HCl
   b. 500 mg per tab
   c. 100 cap
   d. 500 mg:1 cap

WORKSHEET **3E** (page 61)

1. Mistaken for "0," "4," or "cc"
2. Periods and "Os can be mistaken for "I" (the letter I or the number 1). Write out "daily." (It is also recommended to write Q.I.D. as "4 times a day.")
3. A decimal point can be missed, which may result in overdoses.
4. All medication-related documents that are handwritten, entered on a computer, and filled in on preprinted forms must abide by The Joint Commission's "Do Not Use" list.
5. The preferred abbreviation is mL. The capital L for milliliter will not be confused with the number 1 as with ml, and cc can be confused with U (units) and aa (of each) if written poorly.
6. The letter "I" can be mistaken for a number 1 if the dose name and dose amount are run together.
7. Large numbers without commas can be easily misread resulting in very large dose errors.

8. 10 mg, with a space between the numbers and the abbreviation.

9. Slashes have been mistaken as the number 1 in front of the dose.

10. x3d meant to mean times 3 days has been misinterpreted as "times 3 doses." Write out "for 3 days."

⊖ **CLINICAL ALERT**

"Once" means eleven in Spanish! The word for one is "uno" in Spanish or "una vez," one time. In the United Kingdom, qds means four times a day.

WORKSHEET 3F (page 61)

1. Yes. Care must be taken in distinguishing this patient from other patients with the same or a similar name to avoid giving a medication to the wrong patient.

2. Yes. The patient is allergic to the intravenous iodine used in some contrast media tests and to products that contain aspirin. There are many.

3. One 24-hour day

4. Digoxin was withheld as denoted by a circle and the code "R."

5. Topical

6. Promethazine, a stat order

7. Morphine sulfate; left arm denoted by "C."

8. 05/09/12 at 0700

9. 05/07/12 at 2000; 8 pm

10. Having both the initials and the nurse's signature identifies the nurse who administered the medication more clearly. More than one staff member may have the same initials or some initials may be illegible.

WORKSHEET 3G (page 62)

1. The route is not specified.

2. The dose is not specified. Aspirin is supplied in more than one dose (e.g., 325 mg per tablet, 650 mg per tablet). The number of tablets should *not* be mentioned in the order.

3. The route is not specified. Ampicillin can be administered by more than one route (PO, IM, IV).

4. The time or frequency is not specified—for example, stat, one time only, or more than one time.

5. The dose and form are not specified. Tylenol is supplied in tablet, liquid suspension, intravenous, and suppository forms and in a variety of doses targeted to infants, children, and adults. Teaspoons should not be mentioned in the order

WORKSHEET 3H (page 64)

1. b. Correct identification of patient is always the first priority. Answers a, c, and d would all be appropriate after the patient is identified.

2. a. Answers b, c, and d would all be appropriate after the patient was assessed.

3. a. Answer b is the total amount of drug in the container. Answer c is the total volume in mL. Answer d is the usual ordered adult dosage on the first day.

4. **d.** Answers a, b, and c are inappropriate actions.

5. **b.** Refer to the international/military time clock on page 55.

6. **a.** Answers b, c, and d are false statements.

7. **d.** Refer to the legend below the TJC "Do Not Use" list on page 44.

8. **d.** The right route is usually the one that is ordered but not in this case. There is a conflict, and common sense dictates that the nurse must clarify. The patient is NPO and there must be a written order to be able to give a medication by mouth. Some medications are totally unsuitable for nasogastric tube administration, and some just obstruct the tube. Some orders may specify to crush the tablet, dilute with water, and give via the tube.

9. **a.** Be very aware that there are many drugs with similar names but different uses.

10. **b.** Giving a medication after the expiration date, whether automatically established by the agency or written by the physician, is illegal. All other actions are appropriate.

CHAPTER 3 FINAL: SAFE MEDICATION ADMINISTRATION (page 68)

1. **a.** Right patient
   b. Right drug
   c. Right dose
   d. Right time
   e. Right route
   f. Right documentation
   g. Right to refuse

2.

Term/Abbreviation	Meaning	Term/Abbreviation	Meaning
c̄	with	s̄	without
po	by mouth	NPO	nothing by mouth
IV	intravenous	IM	intramuscular
supp	suppository	bid	twice a day
tid	three times daily	q6h	every 6 hours
prn	whenever necessary	ad lib*	freely, as desired
ac	before meals	pc	after meals
subcut	subcutaneous	ID	intradermal
SL	sublingual	NG	nasogastric
stat	immediately	top	topical

*ad lib is used for fluids and activity but not for medications.

3.

Term	Abbreviation
milligram	mg
microgram	mcg
gram	g
kilogram	kg
liter	L
milliliter	mL

4.

Traditional Time	24-Hour Clock	24-Hour Clock	Traditional Time
12 Noon (12 pm)	1200 hours	2100 hours	9 pm
Midnight (12 am)	2400 hours	1400 hours	2 pm
1 pm	1300 hours	0145 hours	1:45 am
9 am	0900 hours	0030 hours	12:30 am
5 pm	1700 hours	1645 hours	4:45 pm

5. **a.** Generic name: acyclovir

   b. Drug form: capsule

   c. Unit dose per capsule: 200 mg

   d. Unit dose or multidose container: multidose

6. Generic name, proprietary, trade, or brand name, unit dose, form, total amount in container, recommended routes, preparation directions, storage directions, and expiration date.

7. Aspirin tablet 325 milligrams by mouth every 4 hours as needed for headache.

8. The Joint Commission's Do Not Use list contains the prohibited abbreviations that have been misinterpreted and led to medication errors.

9. If an order is unclear it should be clarified with the prescriber.

10. Decimals can be missed altogether or mistaken for the number 1.

4 Drug Measurements and Dose Calculations

WORKSHEET 4A (page 73)

1. 1000 mg	**2.** 2000 mg	**3.** 500 mg	**4.** 1500 mg
5. 250 mg	**6.** 50 mcg	**7.** 50 mg	**8.** 100 mg
9. 300 mg	**10.** 1100 mg	**11.** 0.025 g	**12.** 5000 mcg
13. 3 g	**14.** 1.5 g	**15.** 15 g	**16.** 0.010 g
17. 0.1 mg	**18.** 0.0005 g	**19.** 0.0075 g	**20.** 2500 mcg

WORKSHEET 4B (page 77)

1. KNOW   WANT TO KNOW

1000 mg : 1 g :: 4 mg : x g

$$\frac{\cancel{1000}}{\cancel{1000}} x = \frac{4}{1000}$$

$$x = 0.004 \text{ g}$$

PROOF

$1000 \times 0.004 = 4$

$1 \times 4 = 4$

2. KNOW   WANT TO KNOW

1000 mg : 1 g :: 200 mg : x g

$$\frac{\cancel{1000}}{\cancel{1000}} x = \frac{200}{1000}$$

$$x = 0.2 \text{ g}$$

PROOF

$1000 \times 0.2 = 200$

$1 \times 200 = 200$

3. KNOW   WANT TO KNOW

1000 mg : 1 g :: 350 mg : x g

$$\frac{\cancel{1000}}{\cancel{1000}} x = \frac{350}{1000}$$

$$x = 0.35 \text{ g}$$

PROOF

$1000 \times 0.35 = 350$

$1 \times 350 = 350$

4. KNOW   WANT TO KNOW

1000 mg : 1 g :: 25 mg : x g

$$\frac{\cancel{1000}}{\cancel{1000}} x = \frac{25}{1000}$$

$$x = 0.025 \text{ g}$$

PROOF

$1000 \times 0.025 = 25$

$1 \times 25 = 25$

5. KNOW   WANT TO KNOW

1000 mg : 1 g :: 15 mg : x g

$\dfrac{\cancel{1000}}{\cancel{1000}} x = \dfrac{15}{1000}$

$\qquad\qquad x = 0.015$ g

PROOF

$1000 \times 0.015 = 15$

$1 \times 15 = 15$

6. KNOW   WANT TO KNOW

1 g : 1000 mg :: 2.5 g : x mg

$x = 1000 \times 2.5$

$x = 2500$ mg

PROOF

$1 \times 2500 = 2500$

$1000 \times 2.5 = 2500$

7. KNOW   WANT TO KNOW

1 g : 1000 mg :: 4.6 g : x mg

$x = 1000 \times 4.6$

$x = 4600$ mg

PROOF

$1 \times 4600 = 4600$

$1000 \times 4.6 = 4600$

8. KNOW   WANT TO KNOW

1 g : 1000 mg :: 0.03 g : x mg

$x = 1000 \times 0.03$

$x = 30$ mg

PROOF

$1 \times 30 = 30$

$1000 \times 0.03 = 30$

9. KNOW   WANT TO KNOW

1 g : 1000 mg :: 0.5 g : x mg

$x = 1000 \times 0.5$

$x = 500$ mg

PROOF

$1 \times 500 = 500$

$1000 \times 0.5 = 500$

10. KNOW   WANT TO KNOW

1 g : 1000 mg :: 0.01 g : x mg

$x = 1000 \times 0.01$

$x = 10$ mg

PROOF

$1 \times 10 = 10$

$1000 \times 0.01 = 10$

11. KNOW   WANT TO KNOW

1000 mcg : 1 mg :: 150 mcg : x mg

$\dfrac{\cancel{1000}}{\cancel{1000}} x = \dfrac{15\cancel{0}}{100\cancel{0}}$

$\qquad\qquad x = 0.15$ mg

PROOF

$1000 \times 0.15 = 150$

$1 \times 150 = 150$

12. KNOW   WANT TO KNOW

1000 mcg : 1 mg :: 500 mcg : x mg

$\dfrac{\cancel{1000}}{\cancel{1000}} x = \dfrac{50\cancel{0}}{100\cancel{0}}$

$\qquad\qquad x = 0.5$ mg

PROOF

1000×0.5 mg $= 500$

$1 \times 500 = 500$

13. KNOW   WANT TO KNOW

1000 mcg : 1 mg :: 50 mcg : x mg

$\dfrac{\cancel{1000}}{\cancel{1000}} x = \dfrac{5\cancel{0}}{100\cancel{0}}$

$\qquad\qquad x = 0.05$ mg

PROOF

$1000 \times 0.05 = 50$

$1 \times 50 = 50$

14. KNOW   WANT TO KNOW

1000 mcg : 1 mg :: 2500 mcg : x mg

$\dfrac{\cancel{1000}}{\cancel{1000}} x = \dfrac{250\cancel{0}}{100\cancel{0}}$

$\qquad\qquad x = 2.5$ mg

PROOF

$1000 \times 2.5 = 2500$

$1 \times 2500 = 2500$

15. KNOW   WANT TO KNOW

1000 mcg : 1 mg :: 3000 mcg : x mg

$\dfrac{\cancel{1000}}{\cancel{1000}} x = \dfrac{300\cancel{0}}{100\cancel{0}}$

$\qquad\qquad x = 3$ mg

PROOF

$1000 \times 3 = 3000$

$1 \times 3000 = 3000$

16. KNOW   WANT TO KNOW

1 mg : 1000 mcg :: 20 mg : x mcg

$x = 1000 \times 20$

$x = 20,000$ mcg

PROOF

$1 \times 20,000 = 20,000$

$1000 \times 20 = 20,000$

356   Answer Key

4.

Traditional Time	24-Hour Clock	24-Hour Clock	Traditional Time
12 Noon (12 pm)	1200 hours	2100 hours	9 pm
Midnight (12 am)	2400 hours	1400 hours	2 pm
1 pm	1300 hours	0145 hours	1:45 am
9 am	0900 hours	0030 hours	12:30 am
5 pm	1700 hours	1645 hours	4:45 pm

5. **a.** Generic name: acyclovir
   b. Drug form: capsule
   c. Unit dose per capsule: 200 mg
   d. Unit dose or multidose container: multidose

6. Generic name, proprietary, trade, or brand name, unit dose, form, total amount in container, recommended routes, preparation directions, storage directions, and expiration date.

7. Aspirin tablet 325 milligrams by mouth every 4 hours as needed for headache.

8. The Joint Commission's Do Not Use list contains the prohibited abbreviations that have been misinterpreted and led to medication errors.

9. If an order is unclear it should be clarified with the prescriber.

10. Decimals can be missed altogether or mistaken for the number 1.

4 Drug Measurements and Dose Calculations

WORKSHEET **4A** (page 73)

1.	1000 mg	**2.**	2000 mg	**3.**	500 mg	**4.**	1500 mg
5.	250 mg	**6.**	50 mcg	**7.**	50 mg	**8.**	100 mg
9.	300 mg	**10.**	1100 mg	**11.**	0.025 g	**12.**	5000 mcg
13.	3 g	**14.**	1.5 g	**15.**	15 g	**16.**	0.010 g
17.	0.1 mg	**18.**	0.0005 g	**19.**	0.0075 g	**20.**	2500 mcg

WORKSHEET **4B** (page 77)

1. KNOW   WANT TO KNOW

$1000 \text{ mg} : 1 \text{ g} :: 4 \text{ mg} : x \text{ g}$

$\frac{\cancel{1000}}{\cancel{1000}} x = \frac{4}{1000}$

$x = 0.004 \text{ g}$

PROOF

$1000 \times 0.004 = 4$

$1 \times 4 = 4$

2. KNOW   WANT TO KNOW

$1000 \text{ mg} : 1 \text{ g} :: 200 \text{ mg} : x \text{ g}$

$\frac{\cancel{1000}}{\cancel{1000}} x = \frac{200}{1000}$

$x = 0.2 \text{ g}$

PROOF

$1000 \times 0.2 = 200$

$1 \times 200 = 200$

3. KNOW   WANT TO KNOW

$1000 \text{ mg} : 1 \text{ g} :: 350 \text{ mg} : x \text{ g}$

$\frac{\cancel{1000}}{\cancel{1000}} x = \frac{350}{1000}$

$x = 0.35 \text{ g}$

PROOF

$1000 \times 0.35 = 350$

$1 \times 350 = 350$

4. KNOW   WANT TO KNOW

$1000 \text{ mg} : 1 \text{ g} :: 25 \text{ mg} : x \text{ g}$

$\frac{\cancel{1000}}{\cancel{1000}} x = \frac{25}{1000}$

$x = 0.025 \text{ g}$

PROOF

$1000 \times 0.025 = 25$

$1 \times 25 = 25$

5. KNOW   WANT TO KNOW

1000 mg : 1 g :: 15 mg : x g

$\dfrac{\cancel{1000}}{\cancel{1000}}x = \dfrac{15}{1000}$

$\qquad x = 0.015$ g

PROOF

$1000 \times 0.015 = 15$

$1 \times 15 = 15$

6. KNOW   WANT TO KNOW

1 g : 1000 mg :: 2.5 g : x mg

$x = 1000 \times 2.5$

$x = 2500$ mg

PROOF

$1 \times 2500 = 2500$

$1000 \times 2.5 = 2500$

7. KNOW   WANT TO KNOW

1 g : 1000 mg :: 4.6 g : x mg

$x = 1000 \times 4.6$

$x = 4600$ mg

PROOF

$1 \times 4600 = 4600$

$1000 \times 4.6 = 4600$

8. KNOW   WANT TO KNOW

1 g : 1000 mg :: 0.03 g : x mg

$x = 1000 \times 0.03$

$x = 30$ mg

PROOF

$1 \times 30 = 30$

$1000 \times 0.03 = 30$

9. KNOW   WANT TO KNOW

1 g : 1000 mg :: 0.5 g : x mg

$x = 1000 \times 0.5$

$x = 500$ mg

PROOF

$1 \times 500 = 500$

$1000 \times 0.5 = 500$

10. KNOW   WANT TO KNOW

1 g : 1000 mg :: 0.01 g : x mg

$x = 1000 \times 0.01$

$x = 10$ mg

PROOF

$1 \times 10 = 10$

$1000 \times 0.01 = 10$

11. KNOW   WANT TO KNOW

1000 mcg : 1 mg :: 150 mcg : x mg

$\dfrac{\cancel{1000}}{\cancel{1000}}x = \dfrac{15\cancel{0}}{100\cancel{0}}$

$\qquad x = 0.15$ mg

PROOF

$1000 \times 0.15 = 150$

$1 \times 150 = 150$

12. KNOW   WANT TO KNOW

1000 mcg : 1 mg :: 500 mcg : x mg

$\dfrac{\cancel{1000}}{\cancel{1000}}x = \dfrac{5\cancel{00}}{10\cancel{00}}$

$\qquad x = 0.5$ mg

PROOF

1000×0.5 mg $= 500$

$1 \times 500 = 500$

13. KNOW   WANT TO KNOW

1000 mcg : 1 mg :: 50 mcg : x mg

$\dfrac{\cancel{1000}}{\cancel{1000}}x = \dfrac{5\cancel{0}}{100\cancel{0}}$

$\qquad x = 0.05$ mg

PROOF

$1000 \times 0.05 = 50$

$1 \times 50 = 50$

14. KNOW   WANT TO KNOW

1000 mcg : 1 mg :: 2500 mcg : x mg

$\dfrac{\cancel{1000}}{\cancel{1000}}x = \dfrac{25\cancel{00}}{10\cancel{00}}$

$\qquad x = 2.5$ mg

PROOF

$1000 \times 2.5 = 2500$

$1 \times 2500 = 2500$

15. KNOW   WANT TO KNOW

1000 mcg : 1 mg :: 3000 mcg : x mg

$\dfrac{\cancel{1000}}{\cancel{1000}}x = \dfrac{3\cancel{000}}{1\cancel{000}}$

$\qquad x = 3$ mg

PROOF

$1000 \times 3 = 3000$

$1 \times 3000 = 3000$

16. KNOW   WANT TO KNOW

1 mg : 1000 mcg :: 20 mg : x mcg

$x = 1000 \times 20$

$x = 20,000$ mcg

PROOF

$1 \times 20,000 = 20,000$

$1000 \times 20 = 20,000$

17. KNOW WANT TO KNOW
1 mg : 1000 mcg :: 200 mg : x mcg
$x = 1000 \times 200$
$x = 200,000$ mcg
PROOF
$1 \times 200,000 = 200,000$
$1000 \times 200 = 200,000$

18. KNOW WANT TO KNOW
1 mg : 1000 mcg :: 5 mg : x mcg
$x = 1000 \times 5$
$x = 5000$ mcg
PROOF
$1 \times 5000 = 5000$
$1000 \times 5 = 5000$

19. KNOW WANT TO KNOW
1 mg : 1000 mcg :: 0.1 mg : x mcg
$x = 1000 \times 0.1$
$x = 100$ mcg
PROOF
$1 \times 100 = 100$
$1000 \times 0.1 = 100$

20. KNOW WANT TO KNOW
1 mg : 1000 mcg :: 0.04 mg : x mcg
$x = 1000 \times 0.04$
$x = 40$ mcg
PROOF
$1 \times 40 = 40$
$1000 \times 0.04 = 40$

21. KNOW WANT TO KNOW
1 kg : 1000 g :: 5.5 kg : x g
$x = 1000 \times 5.5$
$x = 5500$ g
PROOF
$1 \times 5500 = 5500$
$1000 \times 5.5 = 5500$

22. KNOW WANT TO KNOW
1 kg : 1000 g :: 12 kg : x g
$x = 1000 \times 12$
$x = 12,000$ g
PROOF
$1 \times 12,000 = 12,000$
$1000 \times 12 = 12,000$

23. KNOW WANT TO KNOW
1 kg : 1000 g :: 3 kg : x g
$x = 1000 \times 3$
$x = 3000$ g
PROOF
$1 \times 3000 = 3000$
$1000 \times 3 = 3000$

24. KNOW WANT TO KNOW
1 kg : 1000 g :: 1.3 kg : x g
$x = 1000 \times 1.3$
$x = 1300$ g
PROOF
$1 \times 1300 = 1300$
$1000 \times 1.3 = 1300$

25. KNOW WANT TO KNOW
1 kg : 1000 g :: 0.5 kg : x g
$x = 1000 \times 0.5$
$x = 500$ g
PROOF
$1 \times 500 = 500$
$1000 \times 0.5 = 500$

26. KNOW WANT TO KNOW
1 L : 1000 mL :: 0.5 L : x mL
$x = 1000 \times 0.5$
$x = 500$ mL
PROOF
$1 \times 500 = 500$
$1000 \times 0.5 = 500$

27. KNOW WANT TO KNOW
1 L : 1000 mL :: 1.3 L : x mL
$x = 1000 \times 1.3$
$x = 1300$ mL
PROOF
$1 \times 1300 = 1300$
$1000 \times 1.3 = 1300$

28. KNOW WANT TO KNOW
1 L : 1000 mL :: 1.5 L : x mL
$x = 1000 \times 1.5$
$x = 1500$ mL
PROOF
$1 \times 1500 = 1500$
$1000 \times 1.5 = 1500$

29.
KNOW   WANT TO KNOW
1 L : 1000 mL :: 3 L : x mL
$x = 1000 \times 3$
$x = 3000$ mL
PROOF
$1 \times 3000 = 3000$
$1000 \times 3 = 3000$

30.
KNOW   WANT TO KNOW
1 L : 1000 mL :: 2.8 L : x mL
$x = 1000 \times 2.8$
$x = 2800$ mL
PROOF
$1 \times 2800 = 2800$
$1000 \times 2.8 = 2800$

WORKSHEET 4C (page 79)

1. more
2. more
3. same (one serving)
4. more
5. less
6. less
7. more
8. less
9. same (one serving)
10. more

---

*USP refers to the *United States Pharmacopoeia,* a national listing of drugs.
**It is critical to distinguish mg from mEq on medication orders and labels. This means that the fine print must be scrutinized for critical information.

WORKSHEET 4D (page 80)

1.
KNOW   WANT TO KNOW
250 mg : 1 cap :: 500 mg : x cap
$\dfrac{\cancel{250}}{\cancel{250}} x = \dfrac{500}{250}$
$x = 2$ caps
PROOF
$250 \times 2 = 500$
$1 \times 500 = 500$

2.
KNOW   WANT TO KNOW
175 mcg : 1 tab :: 350 mcg : x tab
$\dfrac{\cancel{175}}{\cancel{175}} x = \dfrac{350}{175}$
$x = 2$ tabs
PROOF
$175 \times 2 = 350$
$1 \times 350 = 350$

3.
KNOW   WANT TO KNOW
0.125 mg : 1 tab :: 0.0625 mg : x tab
$\dfrac{\cancel{0.125}}{\cancel{0.125}} x = \dfrac{0.0625}{0.125}$
$x = 0.5$ or $\dfrac{1}{2}$ tab
PROOF
$0.125 \times 0.5 = 0.0625$
$1 \times 0.0625 = 0.0625$

4.
KNOW   WANT TO KNOW
200 mg : 5 mL :: 300 mg : x mL
$\dfrac{\cancel{200}}{\cancel{200}} x = \dfrac{5 \times \cancel{300}}{\cancel{200}}$ or $\dfrac{\cancel{1500}}{\cancel{200}}$
$x = 7.5$ mL
PROOF
$200 \times 7.5 = 1500$
$5 \times 300 = 1500$

5.
KNOW   WANT TO KNOW
80 mg : 0.8 mL :: 40 mg : x mL
$\dfrac{\cancel{80}}{\cancel{80}} x = \dfrac{32}{80}$
$x = 0.4$ mL
PROOF
$80 \times 0.4 = 32$
$0.8 \times 40 = 32$

1. KNOW   WANT TO KNOW

50 mg : 1 tab :: 75 mg : x tab

$\dfrac{\cancel{50}}{\cancel{50}}x = \dfrac{75}{50}$

$x = 1.5$ tabs

PROOF

$50 \times 1.5 = 75$

$1 \times 75 = 75$

2. KNOW   WANT TO KNOW

15 mg : 1 tab :: 30 mg : x tab

$\dfrac{\cancel{15}}{\cancel{15}}x = \dfrac{30}{15}$

$x = 2$ tabs

PROOF

$15 \times 2 = 30$

$1 \times 30 = 30$

3. KNOW   WANT TO KNOW

300 mg : 1 tab :: 450 mg : x tab

$\dfrac{\cancel{300}}{\cancel{300}}x = \dfrac{45\cancel{0}}{30\cancel{0}}$

$x = 1.5$ tabs

PROOF

$300 \times 1.5 = 450$

$1 \times 450 = 450$

4. KNOW   WANT TO KNOW

0.125 mg : 1 tab :: 0.25 mg : x tab

$\dfrac{\cancel{0.125}}{\cancel{0.125}}x = \dfrac{0.25}{0.125}$

$x = 2$ tabs

PROOF

$0.125 \times 2 = 0.25$

$1 \times 0.25 = 0.25$

5. KNOW   WANT TO KNOW

0.1 mg : 1 tab :: 0.2 mg : x tab

$\dfrac{\cancel{0.1}}{\cancel{0.1}}x = \dfrac{0.2}{0.1}$

$x = 2$ tabs

PROOF

$0.1 \times 2 = 0.2$

$1 \times 0.2 = 0.2$

6. KNOW   WANT TO KNOW

8 mEq : 5 mL :: 20 mEq : x mL

$\dfrac{\cancel{8}}{\cancel{8}}x = \dfrac{100}{8}$

$x = 12.5$ mL

PROOF

$8 \times 12.5 = 100$

$5 \times 20 = 100$

mEq and mL are not interchangeable.

7. KNOW   WANT TO KNOW

0.01 mg : 1 tab :: 0.02 mg : x tab

$\dfrac{\cancel{0.01}}{\cancel{0.01}}x = \dfrac{0.02}{0.01}$

$x = 2$ tabs

PROOF

$0.01 \times 2 = 0.02$

$1 \times 0.02 = 0.02$

8. KNOW   WANT TO KNOW

10 mg : 1 tab :: 5 mg : x tab

$\dfrac{\cancel{10}}{\cancel{10}}x = \dfrac{5}{10}$

$x = 0.5$ tab

PROOF

$10 \times 0.5 = 5$

$1 \times 5 = 5$

9. KNOW   WANT TO KNOW

400 mg : 1 tab :: 800 mg : x tab

$400 x = 800$

$x = 2$ tabs

PROOF

$400 \times 2 = 800$

$1 \times 800 = 800$

10. KNOW   WANT TO KNOW

150 mg : 1 tab :: 450 mg : x tab

$\dfrac{\cancel{150}}{\cancel{150}}x = \dfrac{45\cancel{0}}{15\cancel{0}}$

$x = 3$ tabs

PROOF

$150 \times 3 = 450$

$1 \times 450 = 450$

1. **Step 1:**

   KNOW WANT TO KNOW

   1000 mg : 1 g :: x mg : 0.5 g

   $x = 1000 \times 0.5$

   $x = 500$ mg

   PROOF

   $1000 \times 0.5 = 500$

   $1 \times 500 = 500$

   Step 2:

   KNOW WANT TO KNOW

   500 mg : 1 tab :: 500 mg : x tab

   $\dfrac{\cancel{500}}{\cancel{500}} x = \dfrac{\cancel{500}}{\cancel{500}}$

   $x = 1$ tab

   PROOF

   $500 \times 1 = 500$

   $1 \times 500 = 500$

2. **Step 1:**

   KNOW WANT TO KNOW

   1000 mg : 1 g :: x mg : 0.3 g

   $x = 1000 \times 0.3$

   $x = 300$ mg

   PROOF

   $1000 \times 0.3 = 300$

   $1 \times 300 = 300$

   Step 2:

   KNOW WANT TO KNOW

   100 mg : 1 cap :: 300 mg : x cap

   $\dfrac{\cancel{100}}{\cancel{100}} x = \dfrac{\cancel{300}}{\cancel{100}}$

   $x = 3$ caps*

   PROOF

   $100 \times 3 = 300$

   $1 \times 300 = 300$

3. **Step 1:**

   KNOW WANT TO KNOW

   1000 mg : 1 g :: x mg : 1 g

   $x = 1000$ mg

   PROOF

   $1000 \times 1 = 1000$

   $1 \times 1000 = 1000$

   Step 2:

   KNOW WANT TO KNOW

   500 mg : 1 tab :: 1000 mg : x tab

   $\dfrac{\cancel{500}}{\cancel{500}} x = \dfrac{\cancel{1000}}{\cancel{500}}$

   $x = 2$ tabs

   PROOF

   $500 \times 2 = 1000$

   $1 \times 1000 = 1000$

4. **Step 1:**

   KNOW WANT TO KNOW

   1000 mg : 1 g :: x mg : 0.3 g

   $x = 1000 \times 0.3$

   $x = 300$ mg

   PROOF

   $1000 \times 0.3 = 300$

   $1 \times 300 = 300$

   Step 2:

   KNOW WANT TO KNOW

   300 mg : 1 cap :: 300 mg : x cap

   $\dfrac{\cancel{300}}{\cancel{300}} x = \dfrac{\cancel{300}}{\cancel{300}}$

   $x = 1$ cap

   PROOF

   $300 \times 1 = 300$

   $1 \times 300 = 300$

---

*When giving more than 1 or 2 times the unit dose (more than 1 or 2 capsules), recheck the order and the math. Consult a current drug guide for the recommended dose.

5. **Step 1:**

KNOW   WANT TO KNOW

1000 mg : 1 g :: x mg : 0.6 g

$x = 1000 \times 0.6$

$x = 600$ mg

PROOF

$1000 \times 0.6 = 600$

$1 \times 600 = 600$

Step 2:

KNOW   WANT TO KNOW

600 mg : 1 tab :: 600 mg : x tab

$\dfrac{\cancel{600}}{\cancel{600}} x = \dfrac{\cancel{600}}{\cancel{600}}$

$\qquad x = 1$ tab

PROOF

$600 \times 1 = 600$

$1 \times 600 = 600$

WORKSHEET **4G** (page 86)

1. KNOW   WANT TO KNOW

0.25 mg : 1 tab :: 0.5 mg : x tab

$\dfrac{\cancel{0.25}}{\cancel{0.25}} x = \dfrac{0.5}{0.25}$

$\qquad x = 2$ tabs

PROOF

$0.25 \times 2 = 0.5$

$1 \times 0.5 = 0.5$

2. **Step 1:**

KNOW   WANT TO KNOW

1000 mg : 1 g :: x mg : 0.2 g

$x = 1000 \times 0.2$

$x = 200$ mg

Step 2:

HAVE   WANT TO HAVE

100 mg : 1 cap :: 200 mg : x cap

$\dfrac{\cancel{100}}{\cancel{100}} x = \dfrac{\cancel{200}}{\cancel{100}}$

$\qquad x = 2$ caps

PROOF

$100 \times 2 = 200$

$1 \times 200 = 200$

3. KNOW   WANT TO KNOW

4 mg : 5 mL :: 6 mg : x mL

$\dfrac{\cancel{4}}{\cancel{4}} x = \dfrac{30}{4}$

$\quad x = 7.5$ mL

PROOF

$4 \times 7.5 = 30$

$5 \times 6 = 30$

4. **Step 1:**

KNOW   WANT TO KNOW

1000 mg : 1 g :: x mg : 0.5 g

$x = 1000 \times 0.5$

$x = 500$ mg

PROOF

$1000 \times 0.5 = 500$

$1 \times 500 = 500$

Step 2:

HAVE   WANT TO HAVE

250 mg : 1 tab :: 500 mg : x tab

$\dfrac{\cancel{250}}{\cancel{250}} x = \dfrac{\cancel{500}}{\cancel{250}}$

$\qquad x = 2$ tabs

PROOF

$250 \times 2 = 500$

$1 \times 500 = 500$

5.

KNOW   WANT TO KNOW

$20 \text{ mg} : 5 \text{ mL} :: 25 \text{ mg} : x \text{ mL}$

$\dfrac{\cancel{20}}{\cancel{20}} x = \dfrac{125}{20}$

$x = 6.25 \text{ mL, rounded to } 6.3 \text{ mL}$

PROOF

$20 \times 6.25 = 125$

$5 \times 25 = 125$

WORKSHEET **4H** (page 88)

1. **Step 1:**

KNOW   WANT TO KNOW

$1000 \text{ mcg} : 1 \text{ mg} :: 125 \text{ mcg} : x \text{ mg}$

$\dfrac{\cancel{1000}}{\cancel{1000}} x = \dfrac{125}{1000}$

$x = 0.125 \text{ mg}$

PROOF

$1000 \times 0.125 = 125$

$1 \times 125 = 125$

Step 2:

HAVE   WANT TO HAVE

$0.125 \text{ mg} : 1 \text{ tab} :: 0.125 \text{ mg} : x \text{ tab}$

$\dfrac{\cancel{0.125}}{\cancel{0.125}} x = \dfrac{0.125}{0.125}$

$x = 1 \text{ tab}$

PROOF

$0.125 \times 1 = 0.125$

$1 \times 0.125 = 0.125$

2. **Step 1:**

KNOW   WANT TO KNOW

$1000 \text{ mg} : 1 \text{ g} :: x \text{ mg} : 0.01 \text{ g}$

$x = 1000 \times 0.01$

$x = 10 \text{ mg}$

PROOF

$1000 \times 0.01 \text{ g} = 10$

$1 \times 10 = 10$

Step 2:

HAVE   WANT TO HAVE

$5 \text{ mg} : 1 \text{ tab} :: 10 \text{ mg} : x \text{ tab}$

$\dfrac{\cancel{5}}{\cancel{5}} x = \dfrac{10}{5}$

$x = 1 \text{ tab}$

PROOF

$5 \times 2 = 10$

$1 \times 10 = 10$

3. **Step 1:**

KNOW   WANT TO KNOW

$1000 \text{ mg} : 1 \text{ g} :: x \text{ mg} : 0.2 \text{ g}$

$x = 1000 \times 0.2$

$x = 200 \text{ mg}$

PROOF

$1000 \times 0.2 = 200$

$1 \times 200 = 200$

Step 2:

HAVE   WANT TO HAVE

$100 \text{ mg} : 1 \text{ cap} :: 200 \text{ mg} : x \text{ cap}$

$\dfrac{\cancel{100}}{\cancel{100}} x = \dfrac{\cancel{200}}{\cancel{100}}$

$x = 2 \text{ caps}$

PROOF

$100 \times 2 = 200$

$1 \times 200 = 200$

4. **Step 1:**

KNOW   WANT TO KNOW

$1000 \text{ mg} : 1 \text{ g} :: x \text{ mg} : 0.05 \text{ g}$

$x = 1000 \times 0.05$

$x = 50 \text{ mg}$

PROOF

$1000 \times 0.05 = 50$

$1 \times 50 = 50$

Step 2:

HAVE   WANT TO HAVE

$25 \text{ mg} : 1 \text{ tab} :: 50 \text{ mg} : x \text{ tab}$

$\dfrac{\cancel{25}}{\cancel{25}} x = \dfrac{50}{25}$

$x = 2 \text{ tabs}$

PROOF

$25 \times 2 = 50$

$1 \times 50 = 50$

5. Step 1:

KNOW WANT TO KNOW

1000 mcg : 1 mg :: x mcg : 0.25 mg

$x = 1000 \times 0.25$

$x = 250$ mcg

PROOF

$1000 \times 0.25 = 250$

$1 \times 250 = 250$

Step 2:

HAVE WANT TO HAVE

125 mcg : 1 tab :: 250 mcg : x tab

$\dfrac{\cancel{125}}{\cancel{125}} x = \dfrac{250}{125}$

$x = 2$ tabs

PROOF

$125 \times 2 = 250$

$1 \times 250 = 250$

WORKSHEET 4I (page 89)

1. KNOW WANT TO KNOW

1000 mg : 1 g :: x mg : 0.5 g

$x = 1000 \times 0.5$

$x = 500$ mg

PROOF

$1000 \times 0.5 = 500$

$1 \times 500 = 500$

HAVE WANT TO HAVE

250 mg : 1 tab :: 500 mg : x tab

$\dfrac{\cancel{250}}{\cancel{250}} x = \dfrac{50\cancel{0}}{25\cancel{0}}$

$x = 2$ tabs

PROOF

$250 \times 2 = 500$

$1 \times 500 = 500$

2. KNOW WANT TO KNOW

1000 mg : 1 g :: x mg : 0.5 g

$x = 1000 \times 0.5$

$x = 500$ mg

PROOF

$1000 \times 0.5 = 500$

$1 \times 500 = 500$

HAVE WANT TO HAVE

250 mg : 1 cap :: 500 mg : x cap

$\dfrac{\cancel{250}}{\cancel{250}} x = \dfrac{50\cancel{0}}{25\cancel{0}}$

$x = 2$ caps

PROOF

$250 \times 2 = 500$

$1 \times 500 = 500$

3. KNOW WANT TO KNOW

1000 mg : 1 g :: x mg : 0.3 g

$x = 1000 \times 0.3$

$x = 300$ mg

PROOF

$1000 \times 0.3 = 300$

$1 \times 300 = 300$

HAVE WANT TO HAVE

250 mg : 5 mL :: 300 mg : x mL

$\dfrac{\cancel{250}}{\cancel{250}} x = \dfrac{150\cancel{0}}{25\cancel{0}}$

$x = 6$ mL

PROOF

$250 \times 6 = 1500$

$5 \times 300 = 1500$

4. KNOW WANT TO KNOW

1000 mg : 1 g :: x mg : 1 g

$x = 1000 \times 1$

$x = 1000$ mg

PROOF

$1000 \times 1 = 1000$

$1 \times 1000 = 1000$

HAVE WANT TO HAVE

500 mg : 1 cap :: 1000 mg : x cap

$\dfrac{\cancel{500}}{\cancel{500}} x = \dfrac{100\cancel{0}}{50\cancel{0}}$

$x = 2$ caps

PROOF

$500 \times 2 = 1000$

$1 \times 1000 = 1000$

5.

KNOW   WANT TO KNOW

$1000 \text{ mcg} : 1 \text{ mg} :: x \text{ mcg} : 0.2 \text{ mg}$

$x = 1000 \times 0.2$

$x = 200 \text{ mcg}$

PROOF

$1000 \times 0.2 = 200$

$1 \times 200 = 200$

HAVE   WANT TO HAVE

$100 \text{ mcg} : 1 \text{ tab} :: 200 \text{ mcg} : x \text{ tab}$

$\frac{\cancel{100}}{\cancel{100}} x = \frac{200}{100}$

    $x = 2 \text{ tabs}$

PROOF

$100 \times 2 = 200$

$1 \times 200 = 200$

WORKSHEET 4J (page 92)

1. **a.** (one-step)

HAVE   WANT TO HAVE

$8 \text{ mEq} : 5 \text{ mL} :: 20 \text{ mEq} : x \text{ mL}$

$8x = 100 \quad x = 12.5 \text{ mL}$

PROOF

$8 \times 12.5 = 100$

$5 \times 20 = 100$

2. **c.** KNOW   WANT TO KNOW

$1000 \text{ mg} : 1 \text{ g} :: x \text{ mg} : 0.3 \text{ g}$

$x = 1000 \times 0.3 = 300 \text{ mg}$

PROOF

$1000 \times 0.3 = 300$

$1 \times 300 = 300$

HAVE   WANT TO HAVE

$150 \text{ mg} : 1 \text{ tab} :: 300 \text{ mg} : x \text{ tabs}$

$150x = 300$

$\frac{\cancel{150}}{\cancel{150}} x = \frac{30\cancel{0}}{15\cancel{0}}$

    $x = 2 \text{ tabs}$

PROOF

$150 \times 2 = 300$

$1 \times 300 = 300$

3. **c.** (two-step)

KNOW   WANT TO KNOW

$1000 \text{ mg} : 1 \text{ g} :: x \text{ mg} : 2 \text{ g}$

$x = 2000 \text{ mg}$

PROOF

$1000 \times 2 = 2000$

$1 \times 2000 = 2000$

HAVE   WANT TO HAVE

$500 \text{ mg} : 1 \text{ tab} :: 2000 \text{ mg} : x \text{ tabs}$

$\frac{\cancel{500}}{\cancel{500}} x = \frac{20\cancel{00}}{5\cancel{00}}$

    $x = 4 \text{ tabs}$

PROOF

$500 \times 4 = 2000$

$1 \times 2000 = 2000$

4. **d.** (two-step)

KNOW   WANT TO KNOW

$1000 \text{ mg} : 1 \text{ g} :: x \text{ mg} : 0.2 \text{ g}$

$x = 1000 \times 0.2 \quad x = 200 \text{ mg}$

PROOF

$1000 \times 0.2 = 200$

$1 \times 200 = 200$

HAVE   WANT TO HAVE

$100 \text{ mg} : 1 \text{ tab} :: 200 \text{ mg} : x \text{ tabs}$

$\frac{\cancel{100}}{\cancel{100}} x = \frac{2\cancel{00}}{1\cancel{00}}$

    $x = 2 \text{ tabs}$

PROOF

$100 \times 2 = 200$

$1 \times 200 = 200$

*When more than 1 or 2 tablets or capsules are ordered, more than 1 or 2 unit dose servings, recheck the order, consult a current drug reference , and or instructor, and/or prescriber to verify the order.

5. b. (one-step)

HAVE   WANT TO HAVE

0.125 mg : 1 tab :: 0.25 mg : x mg

$\dfrac{\cancel{0.125}}{\cancel{0.125}} x = \dfrac{0.25}{0.125}$

$x = 2$ tabs

PROOF

$0.125 \times 2 = 0.250$

$1 \times 0.25 = 0.25$

6. b. (two-step)

KNOW   WANT TO KNOW

1000 mg : 1 g :: x mg : 0.5 g

$x = 1000 \times 0.5\, x = 500$ mg

PROOF

$1000 \times 0.5 = 500$

$1 \times 500 = 500$

HAVE   WANT TO HAVE

500 mg : 1 tab :: $250 : x$ tabs

$\dfrac{\cancel{500}}{\cancel{500}} x = \dfrac{25\cancel{0}}{50\cancel{0}}$

$x = \dfrac{1}{2}$ tab

PROOF

$500 \times \dfrac{1}{2} = 250$

$1 \times 250 = 250$

7. c. (one-step)

HAVE   WANT TO HAVE

0.125 mg : 1 tab :: 0.25 mg : x tab

$\dfrac{\cancel{0.125}}{\cancel{0.125}} x = \dfrac{0.25}{0.125}$

$x = 2$ tabs

PROOF

$0.125 \times 2 = 0.25$

$1 \times 0.25 = 0.25$

8. b. (two-step)

KNOW   WANT TO KNOW

1000 mg : 1 g :: x mg : 1 g

$x = 1000$ mg

PROOF

$1000 \times 1 = 1000$

$1 \times 1000 = 1000$

HAVE   WANT TO HAVE

500 mg : 1 tab :: 1000 mg : x tab

$\dfrac{\cancel{500}}{\cancel{500}} x = \dfrac{100\cancel{0}}{50\cancel{0}}$

$x = 2$ tabs

PROOF

$500 \times 2 = 1000$

$1 \times 1000 = 1000$

9. c. (two-step)

KNOW   WANT TO KNOW

1000 mg : 1 g :: x mg : 0.75 g

$x = 1000 \times 0.75$

$x = 750$ mg

PROOF

$1000 \times 0.75 = 750$

$1 \times 750 = 750$

HAVE   WANT TO HAVE

250 mg : 1 tab :: 750 mg : x tabs

$250x = 750$

$\dfrac{25\cancel{0}}{25\cancel{0}} x = \dfrac{75\cancel{0}}{25\cancel{0}}$

$x = 3$ tabs

PROOF

$250 \times 3 = 750$

$1 \times 750 = 750$

10. a. (two-step)

KNOW   WANT TO KNOW

1000 mg : 1 g :: x mg : 0.12 g

$x = 1000 \times 0.12 \quad x = 120$ mg

PROOF

$1000 \times 0.12 = 120$

$1 \times 120 = 120$

HAVE   WANT TO HAVE

120 mg : 1 cap :: 120 mg : x caps

$\dfrac{\cancel{120}}{\cancel{120}} x = \dfrac{\cancel{120}}{\cancel{120}}$

$x = 1$ cap

PROOF

$120 \times 1 = 120$

$1 \times 120 = 120$

· When more than 1 or 2 tablets or capsules are ordered, more than 1 or 2 unit dose servings, recheck the order, consult a current drug reference, and or instructor, and/ or prescriber to verify the order.

1. 2 caps
2. 2 tabs
3. 3 tabs
4. 2 tabs
5. 1 tab
6. 12.5 mL
7. 20 mL
8. 3 tabs. Clarify the order before giving because this amount exceeds the 1 to 2 tablets usually given to patients.
9. 2 tabs
10. Give 4 tabs. Clarify the order before giving because this amount exceeds the 1- to 2-unit doses usually given to patients. If the order is correct, check with the pharmacy for a different strength so that the patient will not have to take so many tablets.

5 Injectable Medications

WORKSHEET **5A** (page 101)

1. a. 3 mL
   b. 0.1 mL
   c. 1.2 mL

2. a. 5 mL
   b. 0.2 mL
   c. 4.4 mL

3. a. 1 mL
   b. 0.01 mL
   c. 0.25 mL

4. a. 10 mL
   b. 0.2 mL
   c. 6.8 mL

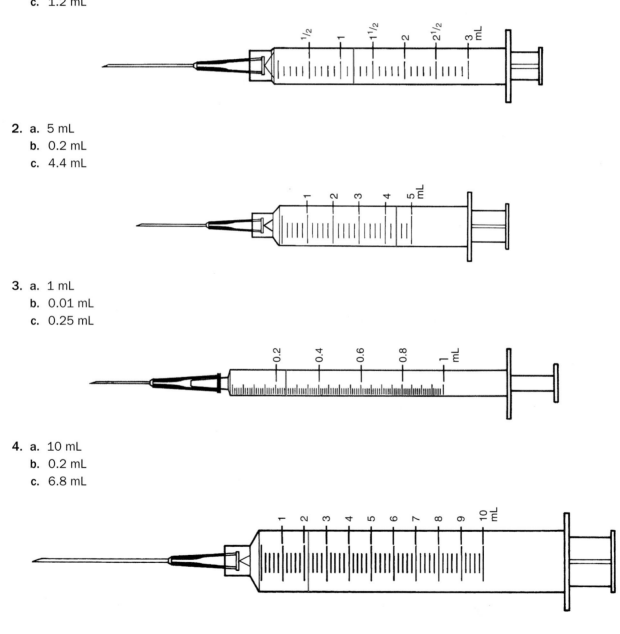

5. a. 20 mL
 b. 1 mL
 c. 13 mL

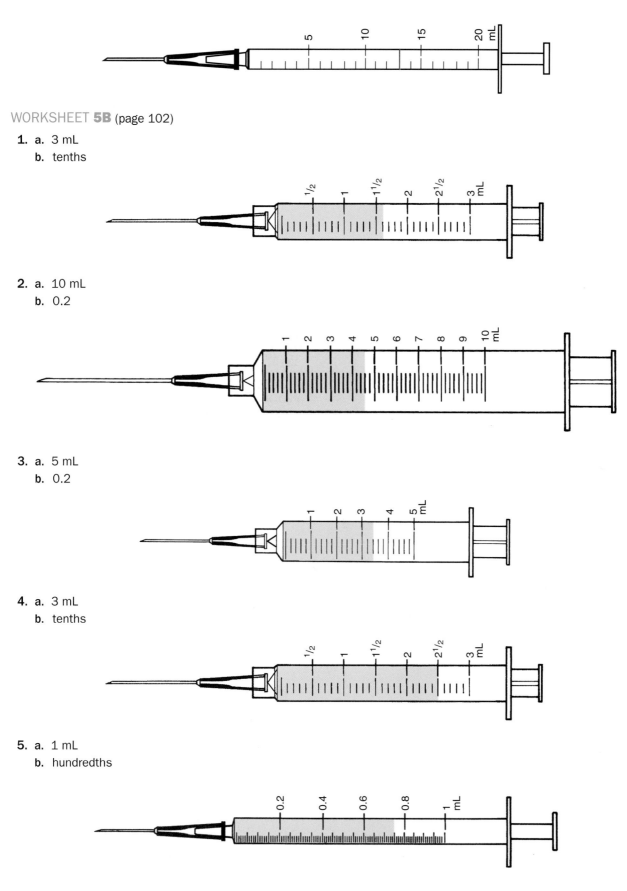

WORKSHEET **5B** (page 102)

1. a. 3 mL
 b. tenths

2. a. 10 mL
 b. 0.2

3. a. 5 mL
 b. 0.2

4. a. 3 mL
 b. tenths

5. a. 1 mL
 b. hundredths

1. two-step

KNOW	WANT TO KNOW

Step 1: 1000 mg : 1 g :: x mg : 0.2 g

$x = 1000 \times 0.2$ or 200 mg

PROOF

$1000 \times 0.2 = 200$

$1 \times 200 = 200$

(more)

HAVE	WANT TO HAVE

Step 2: 150 mg : 1 mL :: 200 mg : x mL

$\frac{\cancel{150}}{\cancel{150}} x = \frac{\cancel{200}}{\cancel{150}}$

$x = 1.3$ mL

PROOF

$150 \times 1.3 = 195$

$1 \times 200 = 200$

(rounding to 1.3 affects answer)

2. one-step; less

HAVE	WANT TO HAVE

4 mg : 1 mL :: 3 mg : x mL

$4x = 3$

$\frac{\cancel{4}x}{\cancel{4}} \times \frac{3}{4} = 0.75$ mL $\quad x = 0.75$ mL

PROOF

$4 \times 0.75 = 3$

$1 \times 3 = 3$

3. two-step

KNOW	WANT TO KNOW

Step 1: 1000 mg : 1 g :: x mg : 0.2 g

$x = 1000 \times 0.2$ or 200 mg

PROOF

$1000 \times 0.2 = 200$

$1 \times 200 = 200$

(less)

HAVE	WANT TO HAVE

Step 2: 250 mg : 2 mL :: 200 mg : x mL

$\frac{\cancel{250}}{\cancel{250}} x = \frac{\cancel{400}}{\cancel{250}}$

$x = 1.6$ mL

PROOF

250 3 1.6 5 400

$2 \times 200 = 400$

4. one-step

HAVE	WANT TO HAVE

125 mg : 2 mL :: 75 mg : x mL

$\frac{\cancel{125}}{\cancel{125}} x = \frac{150}{125}$

$x = 1.2$ mL

PROOF

$125 \times 1.2 = 150$

$2 \times 75 = 150$

(less)

5. two-step; less

KNOW	WANT TO KNOW

1000 mcg : 1 mg :: 500 mcg : x mg

$1000x = 500$

$\frac{\cancel{1000}x}{\cancel{1000}} \times \frac{\cancel{500}}{\cancel{1000}}$

$x = 0.5$ mg

PROOF

$1000 \times 0.5 = 500$

$1 \times 500 = 500$

HAVE	WANT TO HAVE

1 mg : 1 mL :: 0.5 mg : x mL

$x = 1 \times 0.5$

$x = 0.5$ mL

PROOF

$1 \times 0.5 = 0.5$

$1 \times 0.5 = 0.5$

6. one-step; less

HAVE	WANT TO HAVE

5000 units : 1 mL :: 4000 units : x mL

$5000x = 4000$

$\frac{\cancel{5000}x}{\cancel{5000}} \times \frac{\cancel{4000}}{\cancel{5000}}$

$x = 0.8$ mL

PROOF

$5000 \times 0.8 = 4000$

$1 \times 4000 = 4000$

7. one-step

HAVE	WANT TO HAVE
300 mg : 1 mL :: 250 mg : x mL	

$$\frac{3\cancel{00}}{3\cancel{00}}x = \frac{25\cancel{0}}{30\cancel{0}}$$

$x = 0.83$ or 0.8 mL

PROOF

$300 \times 0.8 = 240$

$1 \times 250 = 250$

(rounding 0.83 to 0.8 affects answer)

(less)

8. two-step

KNOW	WANT TO KNOW

Step 1: 1000 mg : 1 g :: x mg : 0.3 g

$x = 1000 \times 0.3 = 300$ mg

PROOF

$1000 \times 0.3 = 300$

$1 \times 300 = 300$

(less)

HAVE	WANT TO HAVE

Step 2: 400 mg : 1 mL :: 300 mg : x mL

$$\frac{4\cancel{00}}{4\cancel{00}}x = \frac{3\cancel{00}}{4\cancel{00}}$$

$x = 0.75$ or 0.8 mL

PROOF

$400 \times 0.8 = 320$

$1 \times 300 = 300$

(rounding 0.75 to 0.8 affects answer)

9. one-step; less

HAVE	WANT TO HAVE
500,000 units : 2.5 mL :: 400,000 units : x mL	

$500,000x = 1,000,000$

$x = 2$ mL

PROOF

$500,000 \times 2 = 1,000,000$

$2.5 \times 400,000 = 1,000,000$

10. one-step; less

HAVE	WANT TO HAVE
2.5 g : 5 mL :: 1 g : x mL	

$2.5x = 5$

$x = 2$ mL

PROOF

$2.5 \times 2 = 5$

$1 \times 5 = 5$

WORKSHEET **5D** (page 109)

1. a. 4 mg per mL

b. 0.75 mL hydromorphone

HAVE	WANT TO HAVE
4 mg : 1 mL :: 3 mg : x mL	

$$\frac{\cancel{4}}{\cancel{4}}x = \frac{3}{4}$$

$x = 0.75$ mL

PROOF

$4 \times 0.75 = 3$

$1 \times 3 = 3$

c. 5 mg per mL Compazine (prochlorperazine)

d.

HAVE	WANT TO HAVE
5 mg : 1 mL :: 2.5 mg : x mL	

$$\frac{\cancel{5}}{\cancel{5}}x = \frac{2.5}{5}$$

$x = 0.5$ mL

PROOF

$5 \times 0.5 = 2.5$

$1 \times 2.5 = 2.5$

e. $0.75 + 0.5 = 1.25$ mL*

(total amount in syringe)

*Hundredths of a mL can be drawn up in a 1 mL syringe and added to the 3mL syringe when needed. They do not need to be rounded. The total volume is 1.25 mL which can't be shaded exactly on the 3 mL syringe.

2. a. 10 mg/mL

b. 0.6 mL morphine

    HAVE   WANT TO HAVE

    10 mg : 1 mL :: 6 mg : x mL

$$\frac{\cancel{10}}{\cancel{10}}\,x = \frac{6}{10}$$

       $x = 0.6$ mL

    PROOF

    $10 \times 0.6 = 6$

    $1 \times 6 = 6$

c. 25 mg/mL

d. 1 mL promethazine

    HAVE   WANT TO HAVE

    25 mg : 1 mL :: 25 mg : x mL

$$\frac{\cancel{25}}{\cancel{25}}\,x = \frac{\cancel{25}}{\cancel{25}}$$

       $x = 1$ mL

    PROOF

    $25 \times 1 = 25$

    $1 \times 25 = 25$

e. $0.6 + 1 = 1.6$ mL
(total amount in syringe)

3. a. 75 mg/mL

b. 0.4 mL Duramorph

    KNOW   WANT TO KNOW

    10 mg : 1 mL :: 4 mg : x mL

    $10x = 4$

       $x = 0.4$ mL

    PROOF

    $10 \times 0.4 = 4$

    $1 \times 4 = 4$

c. 0.4 mg/mL

d. 1.5 mL atropine sulfate

    KNOW   WANT TO KNOW

    0.4 mg : 1 mL :: 0.6 mg : x mL

    $0.4x = 0.6$

       $x = 1.5$ mL

    PROOF

    $0.4 \times 1.5 = 0.6$

    $1 \times 0.6 = 0.6$

e. $0.4 + 1.5 = 1.9$ mL
(total amount in syringe)

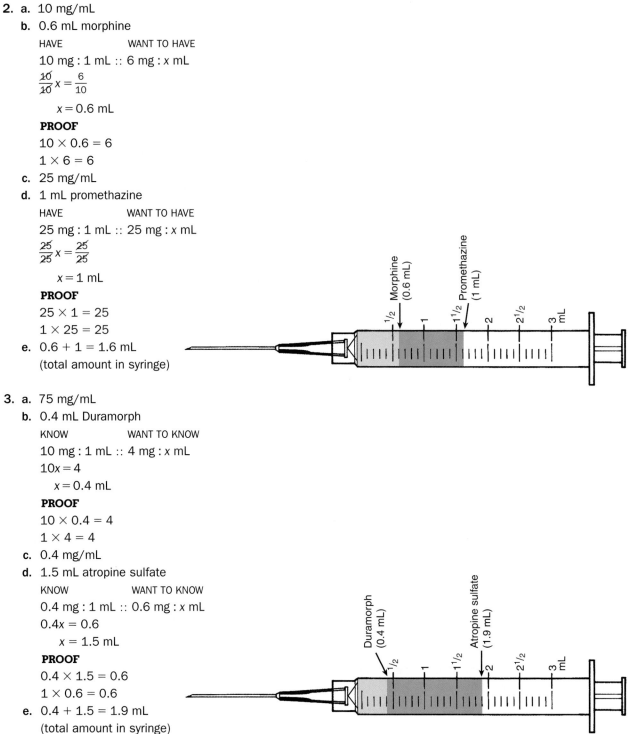

4. a. 0.7 mL morphine sulfate

KNOW   WANT TO KNOW

15 mg : 1 mL :: 10 mg : x mL

$$\frac{\cancel{15}}{\cancel{15}}\,x = \frac{\overset{2}{\cancel{10}}}{\underset{3}{\cancel{15}}} = 0.67\,\text{mL}$$

PROOF

15 × 0.67 = 10.05

1 × 10 = 10

b. 0.7 mL hydroxyzine

KNOW   WANT TO KNOW

50 mg : 1 mL :: 35 mg : x mL

$$\frac{\cancel{50}}{\cancel{50}}\,x = \frac{35}{50}$$

$x = 0.7$ mL

PROOF

50 × 0.7 = 35

1 × 35 = 35

c. 0.7 + 0.67 = 1.37 mL

(total amount in syringe)

5. a. 0.8 mL morphine sulfate

HAVE   WANT TO HAVE

10 mg : 1 mL :: 8 mg : x mL

$$\frac{\cancel{10}}{\cancel{10}}\,x = \frac{8}{10}$$

$x = 0.8$ mL

b. 0.5 mL Vistaril

HAVE   WANT TO HAVE

50 mg : 1 mL :: 25 mg : x mL

$$\frac{\cancel{50}}{\cancel{50}}\,x = \frac{25}{50}$$

$x = 0.5$ mL

c. 0.8 + 0.5 = 1.3 mL

(total amount in syringe)

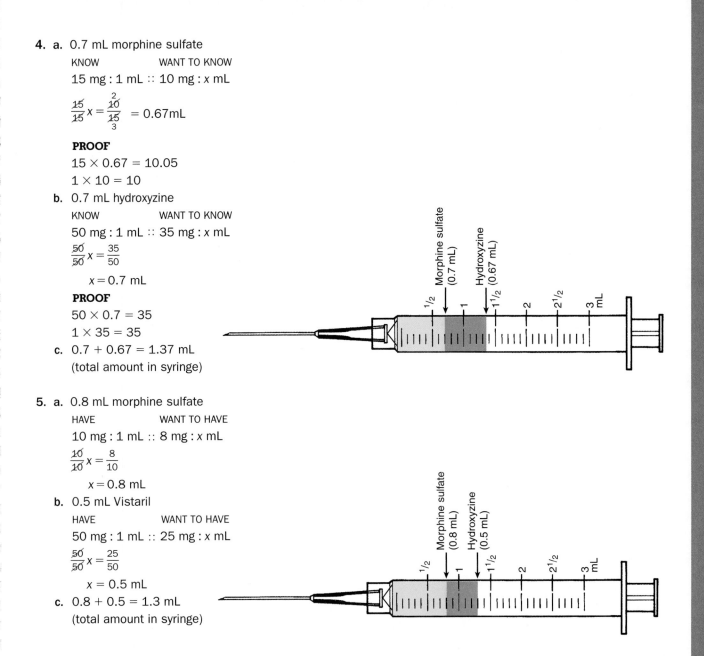

WORKSHEET **5E** (Multiple Choice) (page 112)

1. d.

HAVE   WANT TO HAVE

2 mg : 1 mL :: 1.8 mg : x mL

$$\frac{\cancel{2}}{\cancel{2}}\,x = \frac{1.8}{2}$$

$x = 0.9$ mL

PROOF

2 × 0.9 = 1.8

1 × 1.8 = 1.8

2. b.

HAVE   WANT TO HAVE

10 mg : 1 mL :: 25 mg : x mL

$$\frac{\cancel{8}}{\cancel{8}}\,x = \frac{100}{8}$$

$x = 2.5$ mL

PROOF

10 × 2.5 = 25

1 × 25 = 25

3. a.

HAVE	WANT TO HAVE

8 mEq : 5 mL :: 20 mEq : x mL

$\dfrac{\cancel{8}}{\cancel{8}}x = \dfrac{100}{8}$

$x = 12.5$ mL

PROOF

$8 \times 12.5 = 100$

$1 \times 100 = 100$

4. d.

HAVE	WANT TO HAVE

0.3 mg : 0.5 mL :: 0.4 mg : x mL

$\dfrac{\cancel{0.3}}{\cancel{0.3}}x = \dfrac{0.2}{0.3}$

$x = 0.666$ rounded to 0.67 mL

PROOF

$0.3 \times 0.67 = 0.21$

$0.5 \times 0.4 = 0.2$ (the difference is due to rounding)

5. c.

KNOW	WANT TO KNOW

1000 mcg : 1 mg :: x mcg : 0.5 mg

$x = 1000 \times 0.5$

$x = 500$ mcg

PROOF

$1000 \times 0.5 = 500$

$1 \times 500 = 500$

HAVE	WANT TO HAVE

500 mcg : 1 mL :: 1000 mcg : x mL

$x = 2$ mL

PROOF

$500 \times 2 = 1000$

$1 \times 1000 = 1000$

6. a.

2 mg : 2 mL :: 0.5 mg : x mL

$\dfrac{\cancel{2}}{\cancel{2}}x = \dfrac{1}{2}$

$x = 0.5$ mL

PROOF

$2 \times 0.5 = 1$

$2 \times 0.5 = 1$

7. c.

KNOW	WANT TO KNOW

1000 mg : 1 g :: x mg : 0.05 g

$x = 1000 \times 0.05$

$x = 50$ mg

PROOF

$1000 \times 0.05 = 50$

$1 \times 50 = 50$

8. d.

KNOW	WANT TO KNOW

1000 mcg : 1 mg :: x mcg : 0.1 mg

$x = 1000 \times 0.1$

$x = 100$ mcg

PROOF

$1000 \times 0.1 = 100$

$1 \times 100 = 100$

HAVE	WANT TO HAVE

50 mcg : 1 mL :: 100 mcg : x mL

$\dfrac{\cancel{50}}{\cancel{50}}x = \dfrac{100}{50}$

$x = 2$ mL

PROOF

$50 \times 2 = 100$

$1 \times 100 = 100$

9. b.

HAVE	WANT TO HAVE

5 mg : 1 mL :: 4 mg : x mL

$\dfrac{\cancel{5}}{\cancel{5}}x = \dfrac{4}{5}$

$x = 0.8$ mL

PROOF

$5 \times 0.8 = 4$

$1 \times 0.8 = 4$

10. b.

$10 \times 0.5 = 5$

1. 0.66 rounded to 0.7 mL

2. 1.2 mL

3. 0.5 mL

4. 0.7 mL; 0.75 mL; 1.45 mL total
5. a. safe dose   b. 0.5 mL
6. a. more   b. 2.5 mL

7. a. 300 mg per 2 mL   b. more (045 g = 450 mg, more than 300 mg)   c. 3 mL

8. 4.4 mL

9. 2.6 mL

10. 7 mL

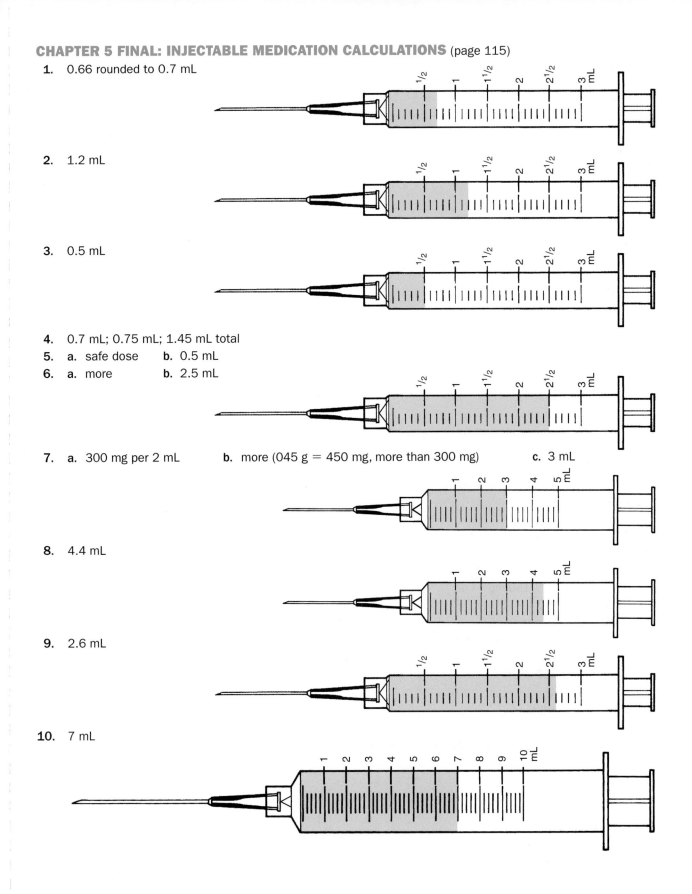

6 Medications from Powders and Crystals: Oral and Intramuscular

WORKSHEET **6A** (page 122)

1. **a.** 30 mL of water in two portions.

   b. KNOW   WANT TO KNOW

   100 mg : 5 mL :: x mg : 50 mL

   $5x = 100 \times 50 = 5000$

   $5x = 5000$

   $x = 1000$ mg in bottle

   PROOF

   $100 \times 50 = 5000$

   $5 \times 1000 = 5000$

   c. 7.5 mL of Lorabid.

   KNOW   WANT TO KNOW

   100 mg : 5 mL :: 150 mg : x mL

   $10\cancel{0}\,x = 5 \times 150 = 75\cancel{0}$

   $x = 7.5$ mL yields 150 mg

   PROOF

   $100 \times 7.5 = 750$

   $5 \times 150 = 750$

   d. 6.6 doses per bottle

   KNOW   WANT TO KNOW

   7.5 mL : 1 dose :: 50 mL : x dose

   $7.5x = 1 \times 50 = 50$

   $x = 6.6$

   PROOF

   $1 \times 50 = 50$

   $7.5 \times 6.6 = 49.5 = 50$

2. **a.** Add 112 mL water, half at a time

   b. KNOW   WANT TO KNOW

   62.5 mg : 5 mL :: 150 mg : x mL

   $62.5x = 5 \times 150 = 750$

   $62.5 = 750$

   $x = 12$ mL for the first dose

   PROOF

   $62.5 \times 12 = 750$

   $150 \times 5 = 750$

   c. 200 mL = 1 bottle

   <u>− 12 mL</u> first dose

   = 188 mL left in bottle divided by 5 mL per dose = 37.6 doses left in the bottle.

   OR

   KNOW   WANT TO KNOW

   5 mL : 1 dose :: 188 mL : x doses

   $5x = 188$

   $x = 37.6$ doses left in the bottle

   PROOF

   $1 \times 188 = 188$

   $37.6 \times 5 = 188$

3. a. 1000 mg

   b. KNOW   WANT TO KNOW

   250 mg : 5 mL :: 500 mg : x mL

   $25x = 5 \times 50 = 250$

   $x = 10$ mL

   PROOF

   $5 \times 500 = 2500$

   $250 \times 10 = 2500$

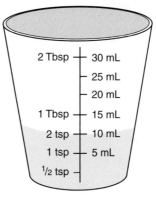

4. a. Add 90 mL of water.

   b. Amount in bottle 100 mL.

   c. Administer 8 mL.

   KNOW   WANT TO KNOW

   125 mg : 5 mL :: 200 mg : x mL

   $125x = 5 \times 200 = 1000$

   $x = 8$ mL

   PROOF

   $5 \times 200 = 1000$

   $125 \times 8 = 1000$

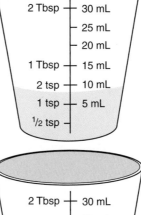

5. a. 60 mL of water in two portions.

   b. 200 mg: 5 mL :: x mg : 100 mL

   $5x = 200 \times 100 = 20,000$

   $5x = 20,000$

   $x = 4000$ mg in bottle

   PROOF

   $200 \times 100 = 20,000$

   $5x \times 4000 = 20,000$

   c. 10 mL.

   KNOW   WANT TO KNOW

   200 mg : 5 mL :: 400 mg : x mL

   $200x = 5 \times 400 = 2000$

   $x = 10$ mL

   PROOF

   $5 \times 400 = 2000$

   $200 \times 10 = 2000$

   d. 10 doses in the bottle.

   KNOW   WANT TO KNOW

   10 mL : 1 dose :: 100 mL : x dose

   $10x = 1 \times 100 = 100$

   $x = 10$

   PROOF

   $1 \times 100 = 100$

   $10 \times 10 = 100$

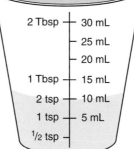

6. **a.** Add 46 mL of purified sterile water
   b. 50 mL total
   c. KNOW   WANT TO KNOW
   400 mg : 50 mL :: 40 mg : x mL
   400x = 50 × 40 = 2000
         x = 5 mL/dose
   PROOF
   400 × 5 = 2000
   50 × 40 = 2000
   d. KNOW   WANT TO KNOW
   5 mL : 1 dose :: 50 mL : x dose
   5x = 1 × 50 = 50
         x = 10 doses in the bottle
   PROOF
   5 × 10 = 50
   1 × 50 = 50

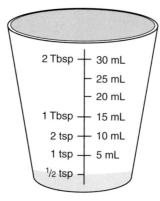

7. **a.** Add 20 mL of distilled water.
   b. 1000 mg Vancocin in the bottle.
   c. 6 mL of Vancocin.
        KNOW   WANT TO KNOW
   250 mg : 5 mL :: 300 mg : x mL
   25Ø x = 5 × 300 = 150Ø
         x = 6 mL
   PROOF
   5 × 300 = 1500
   250 × 6 = 1500

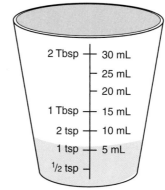

8. **a.** Add 78 mL of diluent.
   b. Amount in bottle: 2500 mg.
        KNOW   WANT TO KNOW
   125 mg : 5 mL :: x mg : 100 mL
   5x = 125 × 100 = 12,500
   5x = 12,500
         x = 2500 mg in bottle
   PROOF
   5 × 2500 = 12,500
   125 × 100 = 12,500
   c. Amount of fluid to be given per dose:
   20 mL/dose.
        KNOW   WANT TO KNOW
   125 mg : 5 mL :: 500 mg : x mL
   125x = 5 × 500 = 2500
         x = 20 mL/dose
   PROOF
   5 × 500 = 2500
   125 × 20 = 2500

   d. Doses in bottle: 5 doses.
        KNOW   WANT TO KNOW
   20 mL : 1 dose :: 100 mL : x doses
   20x = 100
         x = 5 doses in bottle
   PROOF
   1 × 100 = 100
   20 × 5 = 100

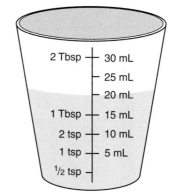

9. **a.** Add 24 mL of sterile water.

   b. KNOW   WANT TO KNOW

   10 mg : 1 mL :: 50 mg : x mL

   $10x = 1 \times 50 = 50$

   $x = 5$ mL to administer

   PROOF

   $1 \times 50 = 50$

   $10 \times 50 = 500$

   c. KNOW   WANT TO KNOW

   50 mg : 1 dose :: 350 mg : x dose

   $50x = 1 \times 350 = 350$

   $x = 7$ doses in the bottle

   PROOF

   $1 \times 350 = 350$

   $50 \times 7 = 350$

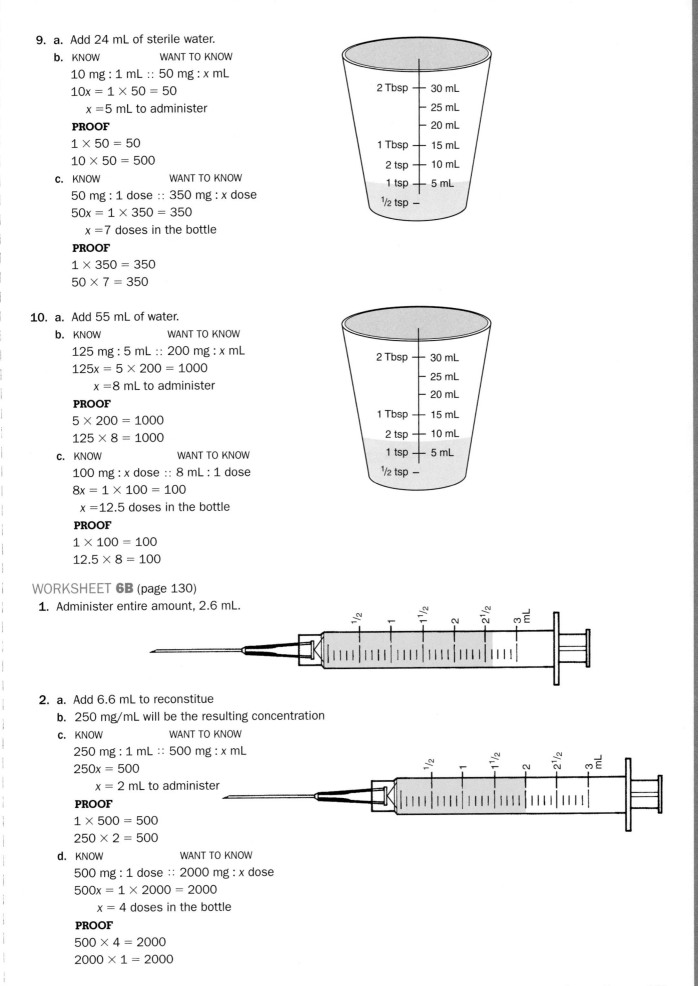

10. **a.** Add 55 mL of water.

   b. KNOW   WANT TO KNOW

   125 mg : 5 mL :: 200 mg : x mL

   $125x = 5 \times 200 = 1000$

   $x = 8$ mL to administer

   PROOF

   $5 \times 200 = 1000$

   $125 \times 8 = 1000$

   c. KNOW   WANT TO KNOW

   100 mg : x dose :: 8 mL : 1 dose

   $8x = 1 \times 100 = 100$

   $x = 12.5$ doses in the bottle

   PROOF

   $1 \times 100 = 100$

   $12.5 \times 8 = 100$

WORKSHEET **6B** (page 130)

1. Administer entire amount, 2.6 mL.

2. **a.** Add 6.6 mL to reconstitue

   b. 250 mg/mL will be the resulting concentration

   c. KNOW   WANT TO KNOW

   250 mg : 1 mL :: 500 mg : x mL

   $250x = 500$

   $x = 2$ mL to administer

   PROOF

   $1 \times 500 = 500$

   $250 \times 2 = 500$

   d. KNOW   WANT TO KNOW

   500 mg : 1 dose :: 2000 mg : x dose

   $500x = 1 \times 2000 = 2000$

   $x = 4$ doses in the bottle

   PROOF

   $500 \times 4 = 2000$

   $2000 \times 1 = 2000$

3. a. Administer 4 mL.

KNOW   WANT TO KNOW

250 mg : 1 mL :: 1000 mg : x mL

$250x = 1000$

$x = 4$ mL

PROOF

$1 \times 1000 = 1000$

$250 \times 4 = 1000$

b. Give 2 mL in each site = 500 mg per injection.

4. a. Add 2.7 mL of diluent

Administer: 3 mL.

b. KNOW   WANT TO KNOW

250 mg : 1.5 mL :: 500 mg : x mL

$250x = 1.5 \times 500 = 750$

$x = 3$ mL

This can be given in divided doses.

PROOF

$1.5 \times 0.5 = 0.75$

$0.25 \times 3 = 0.75$

5. a. Add 4.0 mL of diluent to yield 250,000 units/mL.

b. KNOW   WANT TO KNOW

250,000 units : 1 mL :: 300,000 units : x mL

$250,000x = 300,000$

$25x = 30$

$x = 1.2$ mL

PROOF

$250,000 \times 1.2 = 300,000$

$1 \times 300,000 = 300,000$

c. KNOW   WANT TO KNOW

300,000 units : 1 dose :: 1,000,000 units : x dose

$300,000x = 1,000,000$

$3x = 10$

$x = 3.3 = 3$ full doses in the vial

PROOF

$1 \times 1,000,000 = 1,000,000$

$3.3 \times 300,000 = 990,000$

If the 1.8 mL diluent were used, the resulting dosage would be 0.6 mL, which is concentrated and may create tissue inflammation.

6. a. Make the 500,000 units/mL

   b. Administer 0.6 mL.

      KNOW   WANT TO KNOW

      500,000 units : 1 mL :: 300,000 units : x mL

      $5x = 1 \times 3 = 3$

      $x = 0.6$ mL

      PROOF

      $1 \times 300,000 = 300,000$

      $500,000 \times 0.6 = 300,000$

      Or, you may give another concentration, depending on the assessment of body mass.

   a. Make the 200,000 units/mL.

   b. Administer 1.5 mL.

      KNOW   WANT TO KNOW

      200,000 units : 1 mL :: 300,000 units : x mL

      $2x = 1 \times 3 = 3$

      $x = 1.5$ mL

      PROOF

      $1 \times 300,000 = 300,000$

      $200,000 \times 1.5 = 300,000$

      Or, you may give another concentration, depending on the assessment of body mass.

   a. Make the 100,000 units/mL.

   b. Administer 3 mL.

      KNOW   WANT TO KNOW

      100,000 units : 1 mL :: 300,000 units : x mL

      $1x = 1 \times 3 = 3$

      $x = 3$ mL

      PROOF

      $1 \times 300,000 = 300,000$

      $100,000 \times 3 = 300,000$

7. a. Add 3 mL of sterile water for injection as the diluent.

   b. 280 mg/mL is the concentration.

   c. KNOW   WANT TO KNOW

      280 mg : 1 mL :: 250 mg : x mL

      $280x = 250$

      $x = 0.892 = 0.9$ mL

      PROOF

      $1 \times 250 = 250$

      $0.892 \times 280 = 250$

8. a. Add 1.2 mL of diluent.

   b. 1 hour

   c. 125 mg/mL

   d. KNOW   WANT TO KNOW

      125 mg : 1 mL :: 100 mg : x mL

      $125x = 100$

      $x = 0.8$ mL

      PROOF

      $125 \times 0.8 = 100$

      $100 \times 1 = 100$

9. a. Administer 1.7 mL.

KNOW WANT TO KNOW

500 mg : 1.2 mL :: 700 mg : x mL

5x = 1.2 × 7

5x = 8.4

x = 1.68 or 1.7 mL

PROOF

5 × 1.68 = 8.4

1.2 × 7 = 8.4

b. Patient will receive 2800 mg/day.

KNOW WANT TO KNOW

700 mg : 1 dose :: x mg : 4 doses

x = 4 × 700

x = 2800 mg/day

PROOF

700 × 4 = 2800

1 × 2800 = 2800

c. Need 2.8 or 3 vials per day.

KNOW WANT TO KNOW

1000 mg : 1 vial :: 2800 mg : x vials

10x = 280 = 2.8 or 3 vials needed for a 24-hr period

PROOF

1 × 2800 = 2800

1000 × 2.8 = 2800

10. a. Administer 4 mL in first dose.
   b. Divide into two equal injections.
   c. Give deep intramuscularly in the right or left ventrogluteal area.

WORKSHEET 6C (page 134)

1. KNOW WANT TO KNOW

250 mg : 1 mL :: 500 mg : x mL

250x = 500

x = 2 mL = 500 mg

PROOF

500 × 1 = 500

250 × 2 = 500

OR

KNOW WANT TO KNOW

350 mg : 1 mL :: 500 mg : x mL

350x = 1 × 500 = 500

x = 1.428 = 1.4 mL = 500 mg

PROOF

1 × 500 = 500

350 × 1.428 = 500

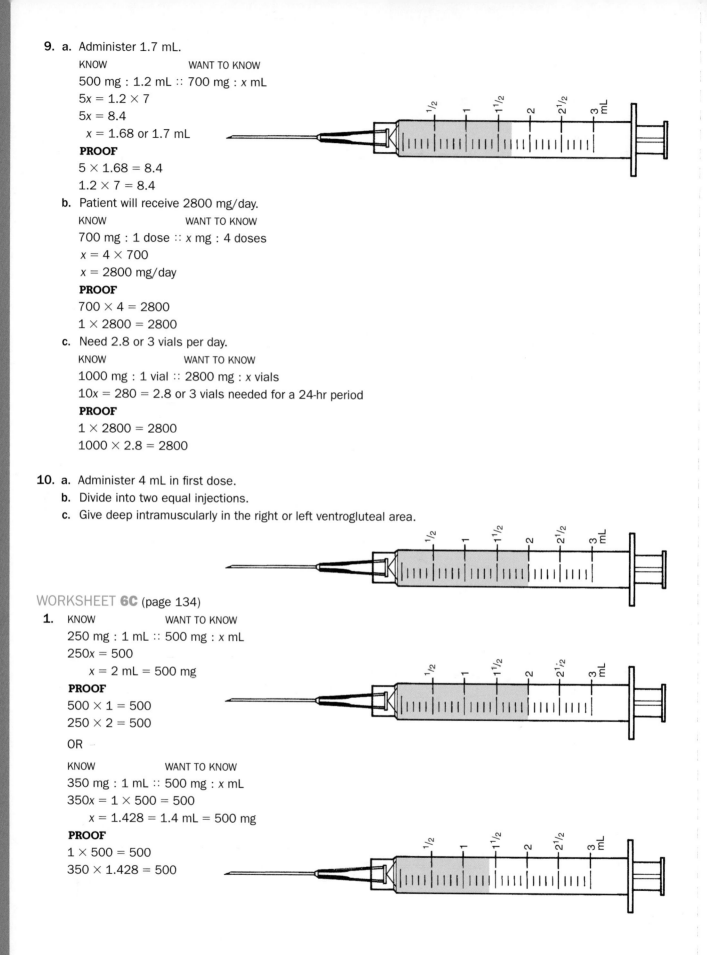

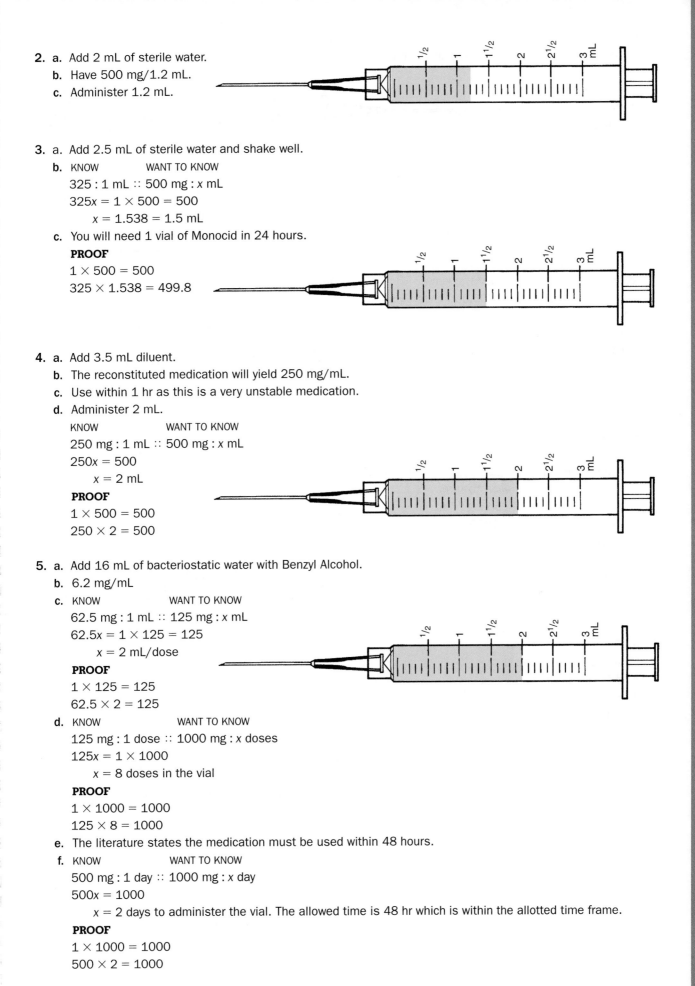

2. **a.** Add 2 mL of sterile water.
   b. Have 500 mg/1.2 mL.
   c. Administer 1.2 mL.

3. **a.** Add 2.5 mL of sterile water and shake well.
   b. KNOW   WANT TO KNOW
   325 : 1 mL :: 500 mg : x mL
   325x = 1 × 500 = 500
       x = 1.538 = 1.5 mL
   c. You will need 1 vial of Monocid in 24 hours.
   PROOF
   1 × 500 = 500
   325 × 1.538 = 499.8

4. **a.** Add 3.5 mL diluent.
   b. The reconstituted medication will yield 250 mg/mL.
   c. Use within 1 hr as this is a very unstable medication.
   d. Administer 2 mL.
   KNOW   WANT TO KNOW
   250 mg : 1 mL :: 500 mg : x mL
   250x = 500
       x = 2 mL
   PROOF
   1 × 500 = 500
   250 × 2 = 500

5. **a.** Add 16 mL of bacteriostatic water with Benzyl Alcohol.
   b. 6.2 mg/mL
   c. KNOW   WANT TO KNOW
   62.5 mg : 1 mL :: 125 mg : x mL
   62.5x = 1 × 125 = 125
       x = 2 mL/dose
   PROOF
   1 × 125 = 125
   62.5 × 2 = 125
   d. KNOW   WANT TO KNOW
   125 mg : 1 dose :: 1000 mg : x doses
   125x = 1 × 1000
       x = 8 doses in the vial
   PROOF
   1 × 1000 = 1000
   125 × 8 = 1000
   e. The literature states the medication must be used within 48 hours.
   f. KNOW   WANT TO KNOW
   500 mg : 1 day :: 1000 mg : x day
   500x = 1000
       x = 2 days to administer the vial. The allowed time is 48 hr which is within the allotted time frame.
   PROOF
   1 × 1000 = 1000
   500 × 2 = 1000

6. KNOW   WANT TO KNOW   **Option #1**

250,000 units : 1 mL :: 400,000 units : x mL

$25x = 40$

  $x = 1.6$ mL

PROOF

$1 \times 40 = 40$

$25 \times 1.6 = 40$

KNOW   WANT TO KNOW   **Option #2**

500,000 units : 1 mL :: 400,000 units : x mL

$5x = 1 \times 4 = 4$

  $x = 0.8$ mL

PROOF

$1 \times 4 = 4$

$5 \times 0.8 = 4$

KNOW   WANT TO KNOW   **Option #3**

1,000,000 units : 1 mL :: 400,000 units : x mL

$10x = 4$

    $x = 0.4$ mL

PROOF

$10 \times 0.4 = 4$

$1 \times 4 = 4$

7. a. Add 2 mL of sterile water for injection.

    b. The reconstituted medication will yield 1 g/2.6 mL.

    c. Use medication promptly.

    d. 1000 mg or 1 g.

    e. Administer 2 mL.

KNOW   WANT TO KNOW

1000 mg : 2.6 mL :: 750 mg : x mL

$1000x = 2.6 \times 750 = 1950$

$1000x = 1950$

     $x = 1.95 = 2$ mL

PROOF

$1000 \times 1.95 = 1950$

$2.6 \times 750 = 1950$

8. a. 500,000 units/mL.

    b. Add 1.6 mL diluent.

    c. Administer 1.5 mL.

    d. Refrigerated, 7 days.

KNOW   WANT TO KNOW

500,000 units : 1 mL :: 750,000 units : x mL

$50x = 1 \times 75$

$50x = 75$

   $x = 1.5$ mL

PROOF

$50 \times 1.5 = 75$

$1 \times 75 = 75$

9. If you add 4 mL of diluent

   KNOW   WANT TO KNOW

   250,000 units : 1 mL :: 400,000 units : x mL

   $25x = 40$

      $x = 1.6$ mL

   PROOF

   $25 \times 1.6 = 40$

   $1 \times 40 = 40$

   If you add 1.5 mL of diluent

   KNOW   WANT TO KNOW

   500,000 units : 1 mL :: 400,000 units : x mL

   $5x = 4$

      $x = 0.8$ mL

   PROOF

   $5 \times 0.8 = 4$

   $1 \times 4 = 4$

10. a. Add 2.7 mL of sterile water for injection.

   b. 1.5 mL/250 mg.

   c. Refrigerated, 7 days; room temperature, 3 days.

   d. 500 mg.

   e. Administer 2.7 mL.

      KNOW   WANT TO KNOW

      250 mg : 1.5 mL :: 450 mg : x mL

      $250x = 1.5 \times 450$

      $250x = 675$

         $x = 2.7$ mL

      PROOF

      $250 \times 2.7 = 675$

      $1.5 \times 450 = 675$

WORKSHEET **6D** (page 139)

1. c. KNOW   WANT TO KNOW

   4 mL : 2000 mg :: x mL :: 1000 mg

   $2000x = 4 \times 1000 = 4000$

   $2x = 4$

     $x = 2$ mL

   PROOF

   $2000 \times 2 = 4000$

   $4 \times 1000 = 4000$

2. b. Directions read: Add 1.2 mL of diluent to yield 125 mg/mL.

   d. KNOW   WANT TO KNOW

   250 mg : 1 dose :: x mg : 2 doses

   $x = 250 \times 2 = 500$

   $x = 500$ mg for 2 doses

   PROOF

   $1 \times 500 = 500$

   $500 \times 1 = 500$

   KNOW   WANT TO KNOW

   125 mg : 1 vial :: 500 mg : x vials

   $125x = 1 \times 500 = 500$

      $x = 4$ vials for 24 hr

   PROOF

   $1 \times 500 = 500$

   $125 \times 4 = 500$

3. d. The directions read: Add 5.7 mL sterile water for injection.

   b. KNOW   WANT TO KNOW

       250 mg : 1.5 mL :: 500 mg : x mL

       $250x = 1.5 \times 500$ mg $= 750$

          $x = 3$ mL

       PROOF

       $1.5 \times 500 = 750$

       $250 \times 3 = 750$

5. b. KNOW   WANT TO KNOW

       40 mcg : 1 mL :: 60 mcg : x mL

       $40x = 1 \times 60 = 60$

         $x = 1.5$ mL

       PROOF

       $1 \times 60 = 60$

       $40 \times 1.5 = 60$

7. c. KNOW   WANT TO KNOW

       500 mg : 1 dose :: x mg : 3 doses

       $x = 500 \times 3 = 1500$

       $x = 1500$ mg/24 hr

       PROOF

       $500 \times 3 = 1500$

       $1500 \times 1 = 1500$

       KNOW   WANT TO KNOW

       1000 mg : 1 vial :: 1500 mg : x vials

       $1000x = 1500$

          $x = 1.5$ vials

       PROOF

       $1 \times 1500 = 1500$

       $1000 \times 1.5 = 1500$

       You will need to have 2 vials on hand for 24 hr.

9. c. Add 9 mL of diluent $= 400$ mg/mL

   a. KNOW   WANT TO KNOW

       400,000 mg : 1 mL :: 500,000 mg : x mL

       $400,000 x = 1 \times 500,000 = 500,000$

       $4x = 5$

         $x = 1.25 = 1.3$ mL

       PROOF

       $1 \times 500,000 = 500,000$

       $400,000 \times 1.25 = 500,000$

4. b. KNOW   WANT TO KNOW

       2 mL : 1 g :: x mL : 1.5 g

       $x = 2 \times 1.5 = 3$

       $x = 3$ mL divided into 2 doses

       PROOF

       $1 \times 3 = 3$

       $2 \times 1.5 = 3$

   d. KNOW   WANT TO KNOW

       1000 mg : 1 vial :: 3000 mg : x vials

       $1000x = 3000$

           $x = 3$ vials needed

       PROOF

       $1000 \times 3 = 3000$

       $1 \times 3000 = 3000$

6. c. KNOW   WANT TO KNOW

       2.6 mL : 1000 mg :: x mL : 500 mg

       $10x = 2.6 \times 5 = 13$

         $x = 1.3$ mL

       PROOF

       $2.6 \times 500 = 1300$

       $1000 \times 1.3 = 1300$

8. c. Directions read: Add 1.5 mL of diluent $= 500,000$ units/mL

   d. KNOW   WANT TO KNOW

       500,000 units : 1 mL :: 400,000 units :

          x mL

       $500,000 x = 1 \times 400,000 = 400,000$

       $5x = 4$

         $x = 0.8$ mL

       PROOF

       $0.8 \times 500,000 = 400,000$

       $1 \times 400,000 = 400,000$

10. c. 330 mg : 1 mL :: 250 mg : x mL

       $330x = 250$

          $x = 0.757 = 0.8$ mL

       PROOF

       $1 \times 250 = 250$

       $0.757 \times 330 = 249.8$

1. a. Add 55 mL of water
   b. 125 mg per 5 mL
   c. Give 6 mL

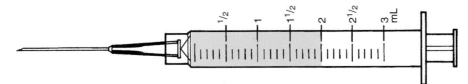

2. Administer 2 mL.

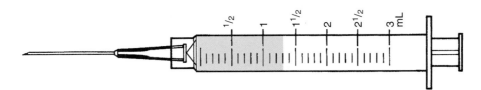

3. a. Add 3.5 mL diluent.
   b. Administer 1 mL.

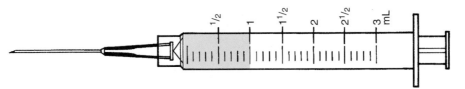

4. a. Add 2 mL of sterile water for injection.
   b. Administer 1.3 mL.

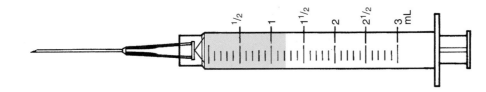

5. a. 250,000 units/mL
   b. 1.2 mL
   c. 16.6 doses in the vial

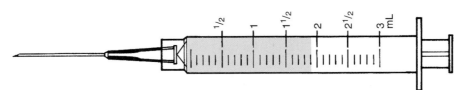

6. a. Add 9.5 mL of diluent.
   b. Give 1.9 mL IM.

7. a. Add 2.5 mL of sterile water for injection.
   b. Give 1.5 mL IM.

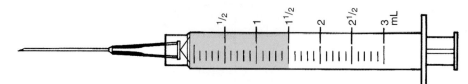

8. a. Add 9.6 mL of diluent to make
   100,000 units/mL. A more concentrated
   solution may be caustic to the tissue.
   b. Administer 1 mL.

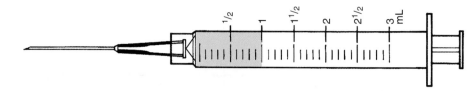

9. a. Add 2.7 mL sterile water for injection.
   b. Administer 1.5 mL.

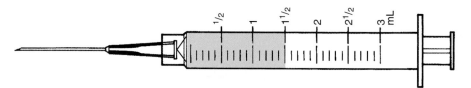

10. Administer 0.7 mL.

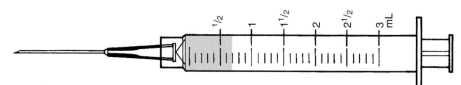

7 Basic Intravenous Calculations

WORKSHEET **7A** (page 156)

remember $1 \dfrac{TV}{TT \text{ in hr}} = \text{mL per hr}$

$2 \dfrac{Df}{\text{Time in min}} \times V \text{ per hr} = \text{drops per min}$

1.   Step 1: $\dfrac{1500}{12} = 125$ mL per hr

   Step 2: $\dfrac{15}{60} \times \dfrac{125}{1} = \dfrac{1}{4} \times \dfrac{125}{1} = 31.25$ or 31 drops per min

2.   Step 2: $\dfrac{60}{60} \times \dfrac{50}{1} = \dfrac{1}{1} \times \dfrac{50}{1} = \dfrac{50}{1} = 50$ drops per min

3.   Step 2: $\dfrac{10}{30} \times \dfrac{100}{1} = \dfrac{1}{3} \times \dfrac{100}{1} = \dfrac{100}{3} = 33.3$ or 33 drops per min

4.   Step 1: $\dfrac{TV}{TT} = \dfrac{1000}{8} = 125$ mL per hr

   Step 2: $\dfrac{10}{60} \times \dfrac{125 \text{ mL}}{1} = \dfrac{1}{6} \times \dfrac{125}{1} = \dfrac{125}{6} = 20.8$ or 21 drops per min

5. Step 2: $\frac{15}{60} \times \frac{200}{1} = \frac{1}{4} \times \frac{200}{1} = \frac{200}{4} = 50$ drops per min

6. Step 2: $\frac{20}{\overset{1}{\underset{3}{60}}} \times 150 = \frac{11}{33} \times \frac{150}{1} = \frac{150}{3} = 50$ drops per min

7. Step 2: $\frac{10}{45} \times \frac{75}{1} = \frac{750}{45} = 16.6$ or 17 drops per min

8. Step 2: $\frac{\overset{2}{60}}{\underset{3}{90}} \times \frac{150}{1} = \frac{300}{3} = 100$ drops per min

9. Step 2: $\frac{\overset{3}{15}}{\underset{8}{40}} \times 150 = \frac{3}{8} \times \frac{150}{1} = \frac{450}{8} = 56.25$ or 56 drops per min

10. Step 1: $\frac{1500}{8} = 188$ mL per hr

    Step 2: a. $\frac{10}{60} \times \frac{188}{1} = \frac{1}{6} \times \frac{188}{1} = \frac{188}{6} = 31.3$ or 31 drops per min

    b. $\frac{15}{60} = \frac{1}{4} \times \frac{188}{1} = 47$ drops per min

WORKSHEET 7B (page 157)

remember
$$1 \frac{TV}{TT \text{ in hr}} = \text{mL per hr}$$
$$2 \frac{Df}{\text{Time in min}} \times V \text{ per hr} = \text{drops per min}$$

1. Step 1: $\frac{TV}{TT} = \frac{2000}{24} = 83.3$ or 83 mL per hr

   Step 2: $\frac{\overset{1}{15}}{\underset{4}{60}} \times \frac{83}{1} = \frac{83}{4} = 20.75$ or 21 drops per min

2. Step 1: $\frac{TV}{TT} = \frac{500}{4} = 125$ mL per hr

   Step 2: $\frac{\overset{1}{15}}{\underset{4}{60}} \times \frac{125}{1} = \frac{125}{4} = 31.2$ or 31 drops per min

3. Step 1: $\frac{TV}{TT} = \frac{3000}{24} = 125$ mL per hr

   Step 2: $\frac{\overset{1}{15}}{\underset{4}{60}} \times \frac{125}{1} = \frac{125}{4} = 31$ drops per min

4. Step 1: $\frac{TV}{TT} = \frac{1500}{8} = 187.5$ or 188 mL per hr

   Step 2: $\frac{\overset{1}{15}}{\underset{4}{60}} \times \frac{188}{1} = 47$ drops per min

5. Step 1: $\frac{TV}{TT} = \frac{1000}{12} = 83.3$ or 83 mL per hr

   Step 2: $\frac{\overset{1}{60}}{\underset{1}{60}} \times \frac{83}{1} = \frac{83}{1} = 83$ drops per min

6. Start with Step 2 because we already know how many milliliters per 30 minutes.

   Step 2: $\frac{\overset{2}{20}}{\underset{3}{30}} \times \frac{100}{1} = \frac{200}{3} = 67$ drops per min

7. Step 1: $\frac{TV}{TT} = \frac{2000}{24} = 83.3$ or 83 mL per hr

8. **Step 1:** $\dfrac{TV}{TT} = \dfrac{250}{10} = 25$ mL per hr

   Step 2: $\dfrac{\overset{1}{\cancel{60}}}{\underset{1}{\cancel{60}}} \times \dfrac{25}{1} = 25$ drops per min

9. **Step 1:** $\dfrac{TV}{TT} = \dfrac{1500}{12} = 125$ mL per hr

   Step 2: $\dfrac{\overset{1}{\cancel{15}}}{\underset{4}{\cancel{60}}} \times \dfrac{125}{1} = \dfrac{125}{4} = 31.25$ or 31 drops per min

10. **MEMORIZE**   *   **Step 1:** $\dfrac{TV}{TT\ in\ hr} =$ mL per hr

   Step 2: $\dfrac{Df}{Time\ in\ min} \times V$ per hr = drops per min

WORKSHEET **7C** (page 157)

remember $1\ \dfrac{TV}{TT\ in\ hr} =$ mL per hr

  $2\ \dfrac{Df}{Time\ in\ min} \times V$ per hr = drops per min

1. **Step 2:** $\dfrac{15}{30} \times \dfrac{100}{1} = \dfrac{1}{2} \times \dfrac{100}{1} = \dfrac{100}{2} = 50$ drops per min

2. **Step 2:** $\dfrac{\cancel{10}}{\cancel{30}} \times \dfrac{50}{1} = \dfrac{50}{3} = 16.6$ or 17 drops per min

3. **Step 1:** $\dfrac{TV}{TT} = \dfrac{1000}{6} = 166.6$ or 167 mL per hr

   Step 2: $\dfrac{\overset{1}{\cancel{15}}}{\underset{4}{\cancel{60}}} \times \dfrac{167}{1} = \dfrac{167}{4} = 41.75$ or 42 drops per min

4. **Step 2:** $\dfrac{\overset{1}{\cancel{60}}}{\underset{1}{\cancel{60}}} \times \dfrac{100}{1} = 100$ drops per min   Yes, the mL per hr is the same as the drops per min rate.

5. **Step 2:** $\dfrac{20}{60} \times 85 = \dfrac{1}{3} \times \dfrac{85}{1} = \dfrac{85}{3} = 28.3$ or 28 drops per min

6. **Step 2:** $\dfrac{\cancel{10}}{\cancel{60}} \times 100 = \dfrac{100}{6} = 16.6$ or 17 drops per min

7. **Step 1:** $\dfrac{TV}{TT} = \dfrac{1500}{24} = 62.5$ or 63 mL per hr

   Step 2: $\dfrac{\overset{1}{\cancel{10}}}{\underset{6}{\cancel{60}}} \times \dfrac{63}{1} = \dfrac{63}{6} \times 10.5 = 11$ drops per min

8. **Step 1:** $\dfrac{TV}{TT} = \dfrac{500}{8} = 62.5$ or 63 mL per hr

   Step 2: $\dfrac{\overset{1}{\cancel{60}}}{\underset{1}{\cancel{60}}} \times \dfrac{63}{1} = 63$ drops per min

9. **Step 2:** $\dfrac{\overset{1}{\cancel{15}}}{\underset{4}{\cancel{60}}} \times \dfrac{75}{1} = \dfrac{75}{4} = 18.7$ or 19 drops per min

10. **Step 1:** $\dfrac{TV}{TT} = \dfrac{2000}{12} = 166.6$ or 167 mL per hr

   Step 2: $\dfrac{\overset{1}{\cancel{20}}}{\underset{3}{\cancel{60}}} \times \dfrac{167}{1} = \dfrac{167}{3} = 55.6 = 56$ drops per min

1. KNOW   WANT TO KNOW

5 g : 100 mL :: x g : 1000 mL

$x = 5 \times 10 = 50$

$x = 50$ g or mL dextrose

PROOF

$5 \times 1000 = 5000$

$100 \times 50 = 5000$

KNOW   WANT TO KNOW

0.9 g : 100 mL :: x g : 1000 mL

$x = 0.9 \times 10 = 9$

$x = 9$ g of sodium chloride

PROOF

$0.9 \times 1000 = 900$

$100 \times 9 = 900$

OSMO: HYPER

2. KNOW   WANT TO KNOW

5 g : 100 mL :: x g : 500 mL

$x = 5 \times 5 = 25$

$x = 25$ g or mL of dextrose

PROOF

$5 \times 500 = 2500$

$100 \times 25 = 2500$

KNOW   WANT TO KNOW

0.45 g : 100 mL :: x g : 500 mL

$x = 0.45 \times 5 = 2.25$

$x = 2.25$ g of sodium chloride

PROOF

$0.45 \times 500 = 2.25$

$100 \times 2.25 = 225$

OSMO: HYPER

3. KNOW   WANT TO KNOW

10 g : 100 mL :: x g : 500 mL

$x = 10 \times 5 = 50$

$x = 50$ g or mL of dextrose

PROOF

$10 \times 500 = 5000$

$100 \times 50 = 5000$

KNOW   WANT TO KNOW

0.9 g : 100 mL :: x g : 500 mL

$x = 0.9 \times 5$

$x = 4.5$ g or mL of sodium chloride

PROOF

$0.9 \times 500 = 450$

$4.5 \times 100 = 450$

OSMO: HYPER

4. KNOW   WANT TO KNOW

0.9 g : 100 mL :: x g : 1000 mL

$x = 0.9 \times 10 = 9$

$x = 9$ g or mL of sodium chloride

PROOF

$0.9 \times 1000 = 900$

$9 \times 100 = 900$

OSMO: ISO

5. KNOW   WANT TO KNOW

0.45 g : 100 mL :: x g : 500 mL

$x = 0.45 \times 5 = 2.25$

$x = 2.25$ g or mL of sodium chloride

PROOF

$0.45 \times 500 = 225$

$100 \times 2.25 = 225$

OSMO: HYPO

6. KNOW   WANT TO KNOW

5 g : 100 mL :: x g : 1000 mL

$x = 5 \times 10 = 50$

$x = 50$ g or mL of dextrose

PROOF

$5 \times 1000 = 500$

$100 \times 50 = 5000$

OSMO: ISO

7.

KNOW	WANT TO KNOW

5 g : 100 mL :: x g : 500 mL

$x = 5 \times 5 = 25$

$x = 25$ g or mL of dextrose

PROOF

$100 \times 25 = 2500$

$5 \times 500 = 2500$

OSMO: HYPER

8.

KNOW	WANT TO KNOW

600 mg : 100 mL :: x mg : 1000 mL

$x = 10 \times 600 = 6000$

$x = 6000$ mg of sodium chloride in 1000 mL

PROOF

$600 \times 1000 = 600,000$

$100 \times 6000 = 600,000$

KNOW	WANT TO KNOW

1 g : 1000 mg :: x g : 6000 mg

$x = 6 \times 1 = 6$

$x = 6$ g of sodium chloride in 1000 mL

PROOF

$1 \times 6000 = 6000$

$6 \times 1000 = 6000$

OSMO: ISO

9.

KNOW	WANT TO KNOW

5 g : 100 mL :: x g : 1000 mL

$x = 5 \times 10 = 50$

$x = 50$ g or mL of dextrose

PROOF

$5 \times 1000 = 5000$

$100 \times 50 = 5000$

KNOW	WANT TO KNOW

0.9 g : 100 mL :: x g : 1000 mL

$x = 0.9 \times 10 = 9$

$x = 9$ g or mL of sodium chloride

PROOF

$100 \times 9 = 900$

$0.9 \times 1000 = 900$

OSMO: HYPER

10.

KNOW	WANT TO KNOW

5 g : 100 mL :: x g : 500 mL

$x = 5 \times 5 = 25$

$x = 25$ g or mL of dextrose

PROOF

$5 \times 500 = 2500$

$100 \times 25 = 2500$

KNOW	WANT TO KNOW

0.45 g : 100 mL :: x g : 500 mL

$x = 0.45 \times 5 = 2.25$

$x = 2.25$ g or mL of sodium chloride

PROOF

$0.45 \times 500 = 225$

$100 \times 2.25 = 225$

OSMO: HYPER

WORKSHEET 7E (page 167)

1.

$$\frac{\text{Total volume}}{\text{Total time}} = \text{mL per hr}$$

$$\frac{1500 \text{ mL}}{4 \text{ hr}} = 375 \text{ mL per hr}$$

2.

KNOW	WANT TO KNOW

125 mL : 1 hr :: 1000 mL : x hr

$125x = 1000$

$x = 8$ hr

The IV will be completed by 1700 hours.

PROOF

$1 \times 1000 = 1000$

$125 \times 8 = 1000$

3.

HAVE	WANT TO HAVE

1000 mL : 6 hr :: x mL : 1 hr

$6x = 1000$

$x = 166.6 = 167$ mL per hr

PROOF

$1000 \times 1 = 1000$

$6 \times 166.6 = 999.96$

4.

$$\frac{\text{Total volume}}{\text{Total time}} = \text{mL per hr}$$

$$\frac{1000 \text{ mL}}{8 \text{ hr}} = 125 \text{ mL per hr}$$

The IV was started at $0715 + 8 = 1515$ for the hour of completion.

5. KNOW   WANT TO KNOW

$5 \text{ g} : 100 :: x \text{ g} : 125 \text{ mL}$

$100x = 5 \times 125 = 625$

$x = 6.25 \text{ g per hr}$

PROOF

$5 \times 125 = 625$

$100 \times 6.25 = 625$

6. HAVE   WANT TO HAVE

$30 \text{ mL} : 1 \text{ hr} :: 250 \text{ mL} : x \text{ hr}$

$30x = 250$

$x = 8.33 \text{ hr}$

Convert $0.33 \times 60 \text{ min} = 19.8 = 20 \text{ min}$

The IV will take 8 hr and 20 min to infuse.

The IVPB was started at 1330 hr + 8 hr

20 min = 2150 for the hour of completion.

PROOF

$1 \times 250 = 250$

$8.33 \times 30 = 249.9$

7. HAVE   WANT TO HAVE

$500 \text{ mL} : 4 \text{ hr} :: x \text{ mL} : 1 \text{ hr}$

$4x = 500 \times 1 = 500$

$x = 125 \text{ mL per hr}$

PROOF

$500 \times 1 = 500$

$4 \times 125 = 500$

8. HAVE   WANT TO HAVE

$40 \text{ mL} : 1 \text{ hr} :: 500 \text{ mL} : x \text{ hr}$

$40x = 500$

$x = 12.5 \text{ hr}$

IV started at 2100 hr + 12.5 hr (12 hr

30 min) = 0930 for the hour of completion.

PROOF

$1 \times 500 = 500$

$40 \times 12.5 = 500$

9. HAVE   WANT TO HAVE

$200 \text{ mL} : 3 \text{ hr} :: x \text{ mL} : 1 \text{ hr}$

$3x = 200$

$x = 66.66 = 67 \text{ mL per hr}$

OR

$\dfrac{\text{Total volume}}{\text{Total time}} = \text{mL per hr}$

$\dfrac{200 \text{ mL}}{3 \text{ hr}} = 66.66 = 67 \text{ mL per hr}$

PROOF

$200 \times 1 = 200$

$66.66 = 199.98$

10. $\dfrac{\text{Total volume}}{\text{Total time}} = \text{vol per hr}$

$\dfrac{500 \text{ mL}}{4 \text{ hr}} = 125 \text{ mL per hr}$

WORKSHEET **7F** (page 175)

1. a. $\dfrac{\overset{2}{\cancel{60}}}{\underset{1}{\cancel{30}}} \times 100 = 200 \text{ drops per min}$

b. The infusion device will be set at 200 mL per hr.

KNOW   WANT TO KNOW

$100 \text{ mL} : 30 \text{ min} :: x \text{ mL} : 60 \text{ min}$

$30x = 100 \times 60 = 6000$

$30x = 6000$

$x = 200 \text{ mL per hr}$

2. KNOW   WANT TO KNOW

$100 \text{ mL} : 60 \text{ min} :: x \text{ mL} : 60 \text{ min}$

$60x = 6000$

$x = 100 \text{ mL per hr}$

PROOF

$100 \times 60 = 6000$

$60 \times 100 = 6000$

3. KNOW   WANT TO KNOW

150 mL : 60 min :: 250 mL : x min

$150x = 250 \times 60 = 15{,}000$

$x = 100$ min $= 1.6$ hr $= 1$ hr 36 min

PROOF

$100 \times 150 = 15{,}000$

$250 \times 60 = 15{,}000$

4. a. KNOW   WANT TO KNOW

50 mL : 20 min :: x mL : 60 min

$20x = 50 \times 60 = 3000$

$x = 150$ mL per hr

PROOF

$20 \times 150 = 3000$

$50 \times 60 = 3000$

b. $\dfrac{15}{20} \times \dfrac{50}{1} = \dfrac{\overset{3}{\cancel{15}}}{\underset{4}{\cancel{20}}} \times \dfrac{50}{1} = \dfrac{150}{4}$

$= 37.5$ or 38 drops per min

5. a. $\dfrac{15}{60} \times \dfrac{100}{1} = \dfrac{1}{4} \times \dfrac{100}{1} = \dfrac{100}{4} = 25$ drops per min

b. 100 mL : 60 min :: x mL : 60 min

$60x = 100 \times 60 = 6000$

$60x = 6000$

$x = 100$ mL per hr

PROOF

$100 \times 60 = 6000$

$60 \times 100 = 6000$

6. a. KNOW   WANT TO KNOW

50 mL : 30 min :: x mL : 60 min

$30x = 50 \times 60 = 3000$

$x = 100$ mL per hr

PROOF

$30 \times 150 = 3000$

$50 \times 60 = 3000$

b. $\dfrac{60}{30} \times \dfrac{50}{1} = \dfrac{\overset{2}{\cancel{60}}}{\underset{1}{\cancel{30}}} \times \dfrac{50}{1} = 100$ drops per min

7. a. $\dfrac{\overset{2}{\cancel{60}}}{\underset{3}{\cancel{90}}} \times 200 = \dfrac{400}{3} = 133$ drops per min

OR

200 mL : 90 min :: x mL : 60 min

$90x = 200 \times 60 = 12{,}000$

$9\cancel{0}x = 12{,}00\cancel{0}$

$x = 133$ mL per hr

b. Set infusion device for 133 mL per hr.

8. Step 1: $\dfrac{1000}{12} = 83.3$ or 83 mL per hr

a. Step 2: $\dfrac{\overset{1}{\cancel{15}}}{\underset{4}{\cancel{60}}} \times 83 = \dfrac{83}{4}$

$= 20.8$ or 21 drops per min

b. The infusion device will be set at 83 mL per hr.

KNOW WANT TO KNOW

c. 0.9 g : 100 mL :: x g : 1000 mL

$x = 0.9 \times 10 = 9$

$x = 9$ g of sodium chloride (solute)

PROOF

$0.9 \times 1000 = 900$

$100 \times 9 = 900$

9. a. Step 1: $\dfrac{TV}{TT} = \dfrac{2000}{8} = 250$ mL per hr

b. Step 2: $\dfrac{\overset{1}{\cancel{15}}}{\underset{4}{\cancel{60}}} \times 250 = \dfrac{250}{4}$

$= 62.5$ or 63 drops per min

KNOW   WANT TO KNOW

c. 5 g : 100 mL :: x g : 2000 mL

$x = 5 \times 20 = 100$

$x = 100$ g of dextrose

PROOF

$5 \times 2000 = 10{,}000$

$100 \times 100 = 10{,}000$

10. a. $\dfrac{\overset{3}{\cancel{60}}}{\underset{2}{\cancel{40}}} \times 150 = \dfrac{450}{2}$

$= 225$ drops per min is the fastest rate or 225 mL per hr for the infusion device using the microdrip formula

b. $\dfrac{60}{60} \times 150 = 150$ drops per min is the slowest rate. Set infusion device for 150 mL per hr using the microdrip formula

WORKSHEET **7G** (page 176)

1. c. KNOW   WANT TO KNOW

2500 mL : 24 hr :: x mL : 1 hr

$24x = 2500$

$x = 104.16$ mL per hr

PROOF

$2500 \times 1 = 2500$

$24 \times 104.16 = 2500 = 104$ mL per hr

KNOW   WANT TO KNOW

15 gtt : 1 mL :: x gtt : 104.16 mL

OR

$\frac{15}{60} \times 104 = \frac{1560}{60} = 26$ drops per min

$x = 15 \times 104.16 = 1562$

$x = 1562$ divided by 60 min = 26 drops per min

PROOF

$15 \times 104.16 = 1562$

$1 \times 1562 = 1562$

3. d. $\frac{20 \text{ gtt}}{30 \text{ min}} \times 50 = \frac{100}{3} = 33$ drops per min

5. d. KNOW   WANT TO KNOW

12 mL : 1 hr :: 150 mL : x hr

$12x = 150$

$x = 12.5 = 12$ hr 30 min

PROOF

$1 \times 150 = 150$

$12.5 \times 12 = 150$

2. d. $\frac{15}{15} \times 50 = 50$ drops per min

4. b. KNOW   WANT TO KNOW

300 mL : 6 hr :: x mL : 1 hr

$6x = 300 \times 1 = 300$

$x = 50$ mL per hr. mL per hr and microdrip drops per min are the same, so 50 drops per min is correct

PROOF

$300 \times 1 = 300$

$6 \times 50 = 300$

OR

$\frac{\overset{1}{60} \text{ gtt}}{\underset{6}{360} \text{ min}} \times 300 \text{ mL} = \frac{300}{6} = 50$ drops per min and 50 mL per hr

6. d. KNOW   WANT TO KNOW

30 drops : 1 min :: 20 drops : x min

$30x = 20$

$x = 0.66$ min

PROOF

$1 \times 20 = 20$

$30 \times 0.66 = 20$

KNOW   WANT TO KNOW

1 mL : 0.66 min :: 500 mL : x min

$x = 0.66 \times 500 = 330$

$x = 330$ min ÷ 60 = 5.5 hr = 5 hr 30 min

PROOF

$1 \times 330 = 330$

$0.66 \times 500 = 330$

7. a.

KNOW	WANT TO KNOW

25 drops : 1 min :: 10 drops : x min

$25x = 10$

$\quad x = 0.4$ min = 1 mL

PROOF

$25 \times 0.4 = 10$

$1 \times 10 = 10$

KNOW	WANT TO KNOW

1 mL : 0.4 min :: 1000 mL : x min

$x = 0.4 \times 1000 = 400$

$x = 400$ min divided by 60

$\quad = 6.66$ hr = 6 hr 40 min

8. c.

KNOW	WANT TO KNOW

42 gtt : 1 min :: 10 drops : x min

$42x = 1 \times 10 = 10$

$\quad x = 0.238 = 0.24$ min per mL

PROOF

$1 \times 10 = 10$

$42 \times 0.24 = 10.08 = 10$

KNOW	WANT TO KNOW

1 mL : 0.24 min :: 500 mL : x min

$x = 0.24 \times 500 = 120$

$x = 120$ min divided by 60 = 2 hr

PROOF

$1 \times 120 = 120$

$0.24 \times 500 = 120$

The transfusion was started at 1100 hours.
The completion time will be 1300 hours.

9. c.

KNOW	WANT TO KNOW

30 mL : 1 hr :: 500 mL : x hr

$30x = 500$

$\quad x = 16.66$ hr = 16 hr 40 min

PROOF

$30 \times 16.6 = 499.8 = 500$

$1 \times 500 = 500$

10. d. $\frac{250}{2} = 125$ mL per hr

CHAPTER 7 FINAL: BASIC INTRAVENOUS CALCULATIONS (page 178)

1. 31 drops per min

2. 100 mL per hr
17 drops per min

3. 83 mL per hr
28 drops per min

4. 150 drops per min

5. 83 mL per hr
14 drops per min

6. 125 mL per hr
31 drops per min

7. 125 mL per hr
42 drops per min

8. Set infusion device at 267 mL per hr.

9. 83 drops per min

10. 42 drops per min or 167 mL per hr if infusion device is used

8 Advanced Intravenous Calculations

WORKSHEET 8A (page 186)

1. b. 9600 mcg/hr or 9.6 mg/hr
c. 9900 mcg or 9.9 mg/hr (121 lb = 55 kg)
d. 12,000 mcg/hr or 12 mg/hr
e. 72,000 mcg/hr or 72 mg/hr

3. b. $x = 30$ mL/hr (1 : 1 :: 30 : 30)
c. $x = 50$ mL/hr (1 : 10 :: 5 : 50)
d. $x = 6$ mL/hr (1 : 2 :: 3 : 6)
e. $x = 5$ mL/hr (2 : 1 :: 10 : 5)

5. b. (1 : 1 :: 9 : 9) 9 mL/hr
c. (2 : 1 :: 20 : 10) 10 mL/hr
d. (1 : 2 :: 15 : 30) 30 mL/hr
e. (8 : 5 :: 8 : 5) 5 mL/hr

2. b. 1 : 1
c. 1 : 10
d. 1 : 2
e. 1 : 2

4. b. (2 : 1 :: 12 : 6) 12 mg/hr
c. (1 : 2 :: 9 : 18) 9 mg/hr
d. (4 : 10 :: 4 : 10) 4 mg/hr
e. (2 : 1 :: 36 : 18) 36 mg/hr

		mg/hr	mcg/hr	mg/min	mcg/min
1.	**a.**	0.050	50	$0.050 \div 60 = 0.0008$	0.8
	b.	24	24,000	0.4	400
	c.	30	30,000	0.5	500
	d.	1.2	1200	0.02	20
	e.	7.5	7500	0.125	125

		kg	mg/hr	mg/kg/min	mcg/kg/min
2.	**a.**	85	25	$25 \div 85 \div 60 = 0.005$	5
	b.	70	$10 \times 70 \times 60 = 42{,}000$	10	10,000
	c.	62	0.37	0.0001	0.1
	d.	55	75	0.02	20
	e.	48	144	0.05	50

		IV Contents	TD : TV Reduced Ratio	HD (mg/hr)	HV (mL/hr)	mg/mL
3.	**a.**	500 mg/1000 mL	1 : 2	5	10	0.5
	b.	250 mg/500 mL	1 : 2	15	30	0.5
	c.	400 mg/250 mL	8 : 5	24	15	1.6
	d.	500 mg/500 mL	1 : 1	75	75	1
	e.	500 mg/250 mL	2 : 1	16	8	2

2. a. $1 : 2 :: x$ mg : 15 mL   ($x = 7.5$ mg/hr)
    PROOF
       $1 \times 15 = 15$
       $2 \times 7.5 = 15$
  b. 7.5 mg $\times$ 1000 = 7500 mcg/hr
  c. 7500 mcg $\div$ 60 = 125 mcg/min
  d. 125 mcg/min $\div$ 50 kg = 2.5 mcg/kg/min

3. a. $2 : 5 :: x$ mg : 5 mL   ($x = 2$ mg/hr)
    PROOF
       $2 \times 5 = 10$
       $5 \times 2 = 10$
  b. 2 mg/hr $\times$ 1000 = 2000 mcg/hr
  c. 2000 mcg/hr $\div$ 60 = 33.3 mcg/min
  d. 33.3 mcg/min $\div$ 55 kg = 0.605 or 0.6 mcg/kg/min

4. a. $4 : 1 :: x$ mg/hr : 10 mL/hr   ($x = 40$ mg)
    PROOF
       $4 \times 10 = 40$
       $10 \times 4 = 40$
  b. 40 $\times$ 1000 = 40,000 mcg/hr
  c. 40,000 mcg $\div$ 60 = 666.7 mcg/min
  d. 666.7 mcg/min $\div$ 60 kg = 11.1 mcg/kg/min

5. a. $2 : 1 :: x$ mg : 8 mL/hr   ($x = 16$ mL/hr)
    PROOF
       $2 \times 8 = 16$
       $1 \times 16 = 16$
  b. 16 mg $\times$ 1000 = 16,000 mcg/hr
  c. 16,000 mcg/hr $\div$ 60 = 266.7 mcg/min
  d. 266.7 mcg/min $\div$ 79.5 kg = 3.4 mcg/kg/min

2. a. 2 : 1 (500 mg : 250 mL)
  b. No. The nurse is incorrect. The nurse does not understand the mg to mL ratio.
  c. 250 mL per hr*

3. a. 20 mg per mL (1000 mg : 50 mL :: 20 mg : 1 mL
    PROOF: $1000 \times 1 = 1000$; $50 \times 20 = 1000$
  b. Yes. Safe.
  c. 100 mL per hr (50 mL : 30 min :: x mL : 60 min)
    PROOF: $50 \times 60 = 3000$
                 $30 \times 100 = 3000$

---

*Recheck the 250 mL per hr rate with current IV drug reference and pharmacist. It is very rapid but may be indicated for this patient.

4. a. 4 mg per mL (40 mg : 10 mL :: x mg : 1 mL)
   PROOF: $40 \times 1 = 40$; $10 \times 4 = 40$

   b. 0.4 mg per mL (40 mg : 100 mL :: x mg : 1 mL)
   PROOF: $40 \times 1 = 40$; $100 \times 0.4 = 40$

   c. Yes. (0.4 mg $\times$ 6.7 mL per min $\times$ 15 min = 40.2 mg total dose infused per label instructions

   d. 402 mL per hr (6.7 mg per min $\times$ 60 min) or approximately 100.5 mL in 15 minutes
   Recheck high rate calculations and check with Pharmacy if needed

WORKSHEET 8E (page 190)

2. a. 60 (132 ÷ 2.2)

   b. 300 mcg/min $\times$ 60 = 18,000 mcg/hr

   c. 18 mg/hr (decimal moved 3 places to left)

   d. 250 : 250 :: 1 : 1

   e. 18 mL/hr (1 : 1 :: 18 : x)
   PROOF
   $1 \times 18 = 18$
   $1 \times 18 = 18$

   f. Incorrect flow rate. Should be 18 mL/hr, not 36 mL/hr.

   g. Unsafe. Assess patient's vital signs, report per hospital policy, and contact physician for orders.

4. a. 1 mg : 250 mL

   b. 5 mcg $\times$ 60 = 300 mcg/hr or 0.3 mg/hr

   c. 1 : 250 mL :: 0.3 mg : x mL

   d. 0.3 $\times$ 250 = 75.Ø mL/hr
   PROOF
   $1 \times 75 = 75$
   $0.3 \times 250 = 75$

WORKSHEET 8F (page 192)

2. a. 10,000 milliunits : 1000 mL = 10 : 1

   b. 10 milliunits : 1 mL :: 1200 milliunits (hr) : x mL (120) (hr)
   PROOF
   $10 \times 120 = 1200$
   $1 \times 1200 = 1200$

   c. Rate should be 120 mL/hr; obtain order to increase.

5. a. 250 mg (5 mg $\times$ 50 kg)

   b. 1 : 1 (250 mg : 250 mL)

   c. 1.5 hr (60 min : 1 hr :: 90 min : 1.5 hr)
   PROOF: $60 \times 1.5 = 90$; $1 \times 90 = 90$

   d. 166.6 mL per hr (250 mL : 1.5 hr :: x mL : 1 hr)
   PROOF: $250 \times 1 = 250$; $166.6 \times 1.5 = 249.75$ rounded to approximately 250

   e. Current rate is too slow.

   f. Assess patient; contact prescriber promptly for appropriate rate change if any, report and document assessment, prescriber order and nurse action. Perform frequent followup assessments.

3. a. 1000 mg : 500 mL = 2 mg : 1 mL

   b. 4 mg $\times$ 60 = 240 mg/hr

   c. 2 : 1 :: 240 : x = 120 mL per hr
   PROOF
   $2 \times 120 = 240$
   $1 \times 240 = 240$

5. a. 1 mg : 250 mL :: x mg : 50 mL

   b. x = 0.2 mg/hr

   c. 200 mcg/hr

   d. 200 mcg ÷ 60 = 3.3 mcg/min
   PROOF
   $1 \times 50 = 50$
   $250 \times 0.2 = 50$

   e. 8 to 12 mcg/min

   f. Low; consult with provider

3. a. 5 : 500 = 1 mg : 100 mL

   b. 10 $\times$ 60 = 600 mcg/hr

   c. 0.6 mg/hr

   d. 1 : 100 :: 0.6 mg : x mL
   PROOF
   $1 \times 60 = 60$
   $100 \times 0.6 = 60$

   e. x = 60 mL/hr (for 30 min) will deliver 300 mcg total, as ordered.

4. a. 2Ø : 5ØØ = 1 : 25
   b. 1 g : 25 mL :: x g : 25 mL/hr
   PROOF
   1 × 25 = 25
   25 × 1 = 25
   c. x = 1 g/hr
   d. 2 hr

5. a. 10 units = 10,000 milliunits
   b. 10 milliunits : 1 mL
   c. 2 milliunits × 60 = 120 milliunits/hr
   d. 10 : 1 :: 120 : x
   PROOF
   10 × 12 = 120
   1 × 120 = 120
   e. x = 12 mL/hr

WORKSHEET 8G (page 193)

1. a. 65 kg
   b. 3250 to 13,000 mcg/min
   c. 195 to 780 mg/hr (mcg/min × 60 ÷ 1000)
   d. (5 g = 5000 mg) 10 : 1 :: x mg : 39 mL
   e. x = 390 mg/hr
   f. 390 ÷ 60 = 6.5 mg/min
   g. 6500 mcg/min
   h. 6500 mcg ÷ 65 kg = 100 mcg/kg/min
   i. Safe; continue

2. a. 5Ø mg : 5ØØ mL = 1 mg : 10 mL ::
      x mg/hr : 6 mL/hr
   b. x = 0.6 mg/hr (600 mcg/hr)
   PROOF
   1 × 6 = 6
   10 × 0.6 = 6
   c. 1 : 10 :: 0.6 : 6 mL/hr
   d. 0.6 ÷ 60 = 10 mcg/min
   e. Yes
   f. Safe; continue.

3. a. 1000 / : 500 / = 2 : 1 :: x mg : 50 mL
   b. x = 100 mg/hr
   c. 100 mg ÷ 60 = 1.66 or 1.7 mg
   d. Safe; continue.

4. a. 220 ÷ 2.2 = 100 kg
   b. 0.3 × 100 × 60 = 1800 mcg or 1.8 mg/hr
   c. 1 : 5 :: 1.8 mg : x mL   x = 9 mL/hr
   d. 15 mL/hr
   e. 3 mg/hr (1 : 5 :: x mg : 15)   (x = 3)
   f. Unsafe; assess patient; check vital signs;
      call for order to lower rate to 9 mL/hr.

5. a. 125 mg : 125 mL = 1 : 1 :: 15 : 15 mL
   b. Safe; continue infusion.

WORKSHEET 8H (page 197)

1. a. 5 × 60 = 300 sec
      300 ÷ 50 lines = 6 sec/line
   b. 10 mL : 5 min :: x mL : 1 min
      5x = 10
       x = 2 mL/min

2. a. 250 mcg : 1 mL :: 500 mcg : x mL
      (x = 2 mL)
   b. 10 × 60 = 600 sec
   c. 600 ÷ 10 lines = 60 sec/line
   d. 2 mL : 10 min :: x mL : 1 min
      x = 0.2 mL/min

3. a. 100 mg : 1 mL :: 900 mg : x mL
      (x = 9 mL)
   b. 50 mg : 1 min :: 900 mg : x min
      50x = 900
       x = 18 min
   c. 9 mL : 18 min :: x mL : 1 min
      18x = 9
       x = 0.5 mL/min

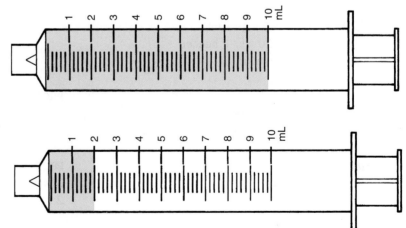

4. a. 10 mg : 1 mL :: 20 mg : x mL
   (x = 2 mL)

   b. 2 × 60 = 120 sec

   c. 120 ÷ 10 = 12 sec/line

   d. 2 mL : 2 min :: x mL : 1 min
   2x = 2
   x = 1 mL/min

5. a. 5 mL

   b. 5 minutes

   c. 5 mL : 5 min :: x mL : 1 min
   5x = 5
   x = 1 mL per minute

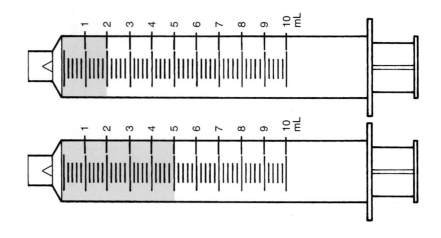

WORKSHEET 8I (page 199)

1. c
5 mcg : 1 min :: x mcg : 60 min or
5 × 60 = 300 mcg or 0.3 mg/hr

PROOF
5 × 60 = 300
1 × 300 = 300

2. a
250 mg : 1000 mL :: x mg : 1 mL
TD   TV
1 mg : 4 mL :: x mg : 1 mL
x = 0.25 mg/mL

PROOF
1 × 1 = 1
4 × 0.25 = 1

3. a
1 g = 1000 mg
TD   TV
1000 mg : 500 mL = 2 : 1

PROOF
1000 mg : 500 mL = 2 : 1 ratio

4. c
8 mcg × 60 min or 480 mcg/hr or
0.48 mg/hr = minimum drug
per hour
TD   TV   HD   HV
1 mg : 250 mL :: 0.48 mg : x mL
x = 250 × 0.48 or 120 mL/hr needed
to infuse 0.48 mg per hour

1 × 120 = 120
250 × 0.48 = 120

5. d
Step 1 total volume to be pushed
10 mg : 1 mL :: 30 mg : x ml
x = 3 mL
Step 2 mL/min
3 mL : 2 min :: x mL : 1 min
2x = 3 or x = 1.5 mL/min

PROOF
10 × 3 = 30
1 × 30 = 30

PROOF
3 × 1 = 3
2 × 1.5 = 3

6. b

Step 1 Convert milligrams to micrograms or micrograms to milligrams by moving decimals.

0.5 mg = 500 mcg OR

250 mcg = 0.25 mg

Step 2 Total mL

On Hand

250 mcg : 1 mL :: 500 mcg : x mL

OR

0.25 mg : 1 mL :: 0.5 mg : x mL

x = 2 mL total volume to be injected over 5 min

Step 3 mL/min

2 mL : 5 min :: x mL : 1 min

5x = 2 or 0.4 mL/1 min

PROOF

250 mcg : 1 mL :: 500 mcg : x mL

250x = 500 or 2 mL

OR

0.25x = 0.5 = 2 mL

PROOF

2 × 1 = 2

5 × 0.4 = 2

7. a

Step 1 Calculate SDR for maintenance for adult

1 mg : 1 min :: x mg : 60 min

x = 60 mg/hr is minimum SDR

6 mg : 1 min :: x mg : 60 min

x = 360 mg/hr is maximum SDR

SDR is 60 − 360 mg/hr.

Step 2 Calculate total drug/total volume ratio and ordered drug per hour and per minute.

1 g = 1000 mg

TD   TV   HD   HV

1000 mg : 500 mL :: x mg : 40 mL

2 mg : 1 mL :: x mg : 40 mL

x = 80 mg/hr being infused

80 mg ÷ 60 min = 1.3 mg/min

After reduction of TD : TV ratio, the answer is apparent.

PROOF

1 × 60 = 60

1 × 60 = 60

PROOF

6 × 60 = 360

1 × 360 = 360

PROOF

2 × 40 = 80

1 × 80 = 80

8. b

Step 1 Change total drug to milligrams to match hourly drug terms.

TD   TV   HD   HV

1 g : 1000 mL :: 60 mg : x mL

Need to change grams to milligrams by using memorized conversion

1000 mg = 1 g.

TD   TV

1000 mg :: 1000 mL :: 60 mg : x mL

Step 2 Calculate mL/hr infusing

Simplify: reduce the TD/TV ratio and math won't be needed to solve this question.

1 : 1 :: 60 : x mL/hr

1x = 60   x = 60 mL/hr

   x = 60 mL/hr

PROOF

1 × 60 = 60

1 × 60 = 60

9. c

TD   HD   HD HV

20 g :   500 mL $::$ x g : 30 mL

$500x = 600 = 1.2$ g/hr

PROOF

$20 \times 30 = 600$

$600 \times 1 = 600$

1.2 g : 1 hr $::$ 3 g : x hr

$1.2x = 3$

$x = 2.5$ hr or 2 hr 30 min

10. d

2.5 mcg $\times$ 70 kg $\times$ 60 min =

10,500 mcg/hr needed

500 mcg : 1 mL $::$ 10,500 mcg : x mL

$500x = 10,500$

$x = 21$ mL/hr flow rate to deliver 10,500 mcg/hr

PROOF

$500 \times 21 = 10{,}500$

$1 \times 500 = 500$

CHAPTER 8 FINAL: ADVANCED INTRAVENOUS CALCULATIONS (page 202)

1. a. 15,000 mcg (5 mcg $\times$ 50 kg $\times$ 60 min)

   b. 7.5 mL (2000 mcg : 1 mL $::$ 15,000 mcg : x mL)

2. a. 20 kg

   b. 60 mEq maximum per 24 hours

   c. 10 mEq

   d. Safe

   e. 5 mL

   f. $105 \div 4 = 26.25$ or 26 mL/hr (100 mL D5W plus 5 mL KCl)

3. a. 9.6 mg/hr (2 mcg $\times$ 80 kg $\times$ 60 min = 9600 mcg/hr)

   b. 12 mg/hr (400 mg : 500 mL $::$ x mg : 15 mL)

      $5x = 4 \times 15 = 60$

      $x = 12$ mg/hr

   c. 12 mL/hr (4 : 5 $::$ 9.6 : x mL)

      $4x = 48$ $x = 12$ mL/hr

   d. 15 mL/hr infusing

   e. Existing flow rate is too fast. Assess patient for side effects and contact physician for new order.

4. a. 50 kg

   b. 100-500 mcg/min   (2-10 mcg/kg/min)

   c. 200 mcg/min   (4 mcg/kg/min)

   d. Safe

   e. 4 : 5

   f. TD TV   HD HV

      4 : 5 $::$ x : 15 ($x = 12$ mg/hr)

   g. TD TV   HD HV

      4 : 5 $::$ 12 : x ($x = 15$ mL/hr)

   h. Correct

5. a. 0.75 mL

   b. 3 mL

   c. 3 min

   d. 1 mL per min

9 Parenteral Nutrition

WORKSHEET **9A** (page 211)

1. Total grams per bag:

   % × mL = g/L
   a. AA 0.055 × 400 = 22 g/L
   b. Dextrose 0.10 × 350 = 35 g/L
   c. Lipids 0.10 × 200 = 20 g/L

   g/L × TV/L = g/bag
   22 × 1.350 = 29.7 g/bag
   35 × 1.350 = 47.25 g/bag
   20 × 1.350 = 27 g/bag

2. Percentages of concentration per bag:

   g/bag ÷ TV = % of concentration
   a. AA 29.7 g ÷ 1350 = 2.2%
   b. Dextrose 47.25 ÷ 1350 = 3.5%
   c. Lipids 27 ÷ 1350 = 2%

3. **Percentages for additives per bag:**

   mEq/L × TV/L = mEq/bag
   a. Calcium gluconate 5 × 1.35 = 6.75 mEq/bag
   b. Magnesium sulfate 10 × 1.35 = 13.5 mEq/bag
   c. Potassium chloride 20 × 1.35 = 27 mEq/bag
   d. Sodium chloride 30 × 1.35 = 40.5 mEq/bag

   mEq/bag ÷ TV = % in bag
   6.75 ÷ 1350 = 0.5% Ca gluconate
   13.5 ÷ 1350 = 1% magnesium sulfate
   27 ÷ 1350 = 2% K chloride
   40.5 ÷ 1350 = 3% Na chloride

4. **kcal per bag:**   KNOW
   a. CHO 47.25 × 4 = 189
   b. PRO 29.7 × 4 = 118.8
   c. FAT 27 × 9 = 243
   d. Total kcal 550.8

   PRO = 4 kcal/g
   CHO = 4 kcal/g
   FAT = 9 kcal/g

5. **mL/hr to set infusion device**

   $\frac{TV}{TT}$ = mL/hr

   $\frac{1350}{12}$ = 112.5 = 113 mL/hr

WORKSHEET **9B** (page 214)

1. **% × mL = g/L**
   a. 0.085 × 500 = 42.5 g/L AA
   b. 0.50 × 500 = 250 g/L DEX
   c. 0.10 × 250 = 25 g/L LIP

   g/L × TV/L = g/bag
   42.5 × 1.5 = 63.75 g/bag
   250 × 1.5 = 375 g/bag
   25 × 1.5 = 37.5 g/bag

2. Percentage of concentration

   g/bag ÷ TV = % of concentration
   a. 63.75 ÷ 1500 = 4.25% AA
   b. 375 ÷ 1500 = 25% DEX
   c. 37.5 ÷ 1500 = 2.5% LIP

3. Percentage of additives

   mEq/L × TV/L = mEq/bag
   a. 5 × 1.5 = 7.5 Calcium gluconate
   b. 15 × 1.5 = 22.5 magnesium sulfate
   c. 8.3 × 1.5 = 12.45 potassium acetate
   d. 35 × 1.5 = 52.5 potassium phosphate
   e. 35 × 1.5 = 52.5 sodium chloride

   MmEq/bag × TV = % in bag
   7.5 ÷ 1500 = 0.5% Ca gluconate
   22.5 ÷ 1500 = 1.5% magnesium sulfate
   12.45 ÷ 1500 = 0.83% K acetate
   52.5 ÷ 1500 = 3.5% K phosphate
   52.5 ÷ 1500 = 3.5% Na chloride

4. **kcal per bag g/L 3**

   a. $63.75 \times 4 = 255$ kcal PRO   CHO = 4 kcal/g

   b. $375 \times 4 = 1500$ kcal CHO   PRO = 4 kcal/g

   c. $37.5 \times 9 = 337.5$ kcal FAT   FAT = 9 kcal/g

   d. Total kcal = 2092.5

5. **mL/hr to set infusion device**

   $\dfrac{TV}{TT} = mL/hr$ $\dfrac{1500}{12} = 125$ mL/hr

WORKSHEET 9C (page 216)

Total grams per bag

1. **Formula: 5 × mL = g/L**   **Formula: g/L × TV/L = g/bag**

   Shortcut method: % × mL = g/L × TV/L = g/bag

   AA $0.10 \times 900 = 90 \times 1.492 = 134.28$ g/bag

   Dex $0.70 \times 430 = 301 \times 1.492 = 449$ g/bag

   Percentage of concentrate per bag

2. **Formula: $\dfrac{g/bag}{TV}$ = %/bag**

   AA $\dfrac{134.28}{1492.74} = 0.0899 = 9\%$

   Dex $\dfrac{449}{1492.74} = 0.30 = 30\%$

   Percentage of additives

3. **Formula mEq/L × TV/L = mEq/bag**

   mEq/bag divided by TV = % in bag

   Shortcut method: mEq/L × TV/L divided by TV = % in bag

   a. Sodium chloride $140 \times 1.492 = 209$ divided by $1492 = 0.14 = 14\%$

   b. Potassium phosphate $41 \times 1.492 = 61$ divided by $1492 = 0.040 = 4\%$

   c. Potassium chloride $43 \times 1.492 = 64$ divided by $1492 = 0.042 = 4\%$

   d. Magnesium sulfate $7 \times 1.492 = 10$ divided by $1492 = 0.007 = 0.7\%$

   e. Calcium gluconate $7 \times 1.492 = 10$ divided by $1492 = 0.007 = 0.7\%$

   Total kcal per bag

4. a. Protein 134.28 g $\times 4 = 537$ kcal

   b. Carbohydrate 449 g $\times 4 = 1796$ kcal

   c. Total kcal = 2333

5. KNOW   WANT TO KNOW

   55 mL : 1 hr :: 1492 mL : x hr

   $55x = 1 \times 1492 = 1492$

   $x = 27.127 = 27$ hr

   PROOF

   55 mL $\times 27.127 = 1491.9 = 1492$

   $1 \times 1492 = 1492$

Total grams per bag

1. Formulas: % × mL = g/L
    g/L × TV/L = g/bag
    Shortcut method: % × mL = g/L × TV/L = g/bag
    AA 0.08 × 600 = 48 × 1.246 = 59.8 = 60 g/bag
    Dex 0.20 × 600 = 120 × 1.246 = 149.5 = 150 g/bag
    Percentage of concentrate per bag

2. Formula: $\frac{g/bag}{TV}$ = %/bag

    AA $\frac{60}{1246}$ = 0.048 = 4.8%/bag

    Dex $\frac{150}{1246}$ = 0.120 = 12%/bag
    Percentage of additives

3. Formula: mEq/L × TV/L = mEq/bag
    mEq/bag divided by TV = %/bag
    Shortcut method: mEq/L × TV/L divided by TV = %/bag
    Sodium chloride 42 × 1.246 = 52.3 divided by 1246 = 0.042 = 4.2%/bag
    Potassium phosphate 26 × 1.246 = 32.3 divided by 1246 = 0.026 = 2.6%/bag
    Potassium acetate 10 × 1.246 = 12.4 divided by 1246 = 0.01 = 1%/bag
    Calcium gluconate 6 × 1.246 = 7.4 divided by 1246 = 0.006 = 0.6%/bag
    Magnesium sulfate 6 × 1.246 = 7.4 divided by 1246 = 0.006 = 0.6%/bag
    kcal per bag

4. **Formula: 1 kcal of protein = 4 g; 1 kcal of dextrose = 4 g; 1 kcal of fat = 9 g**
    a. AA 60 × 4 = 240 kcal
    b. CHO 150 × 4 = 600 kcal
    c. Total kcal = 840

5. KNOW   WANT TO KNOW
    50 mL : 1 hr :: 1246 mL : x hr
    50x = 1 × 1246 = 1246
    x = 24.92   Convert .92 into minutes: 0.92 × 60 = 55 min
    x = 24 hr 55 min
    PROOF
    1 × 1246 = 1246
    50 × 24.92 = 1246

1. 14.3 : 100 :: x : 1400
    100x = 14.3 × 1400 = 20020
    100x = 20020
    x = 200.2 = 200 mL of 70% dextrose in 1400 mL
    PROOF
    100 × 200 = 20000
    14.3 × 1400 = 20020

2. 15 : 100 :: *x* : 1400

$100x = 15 \times 1400 = 21000$

$100x = 2100$

$x = 210$ mL of Aminosyn 15% in 1400 mL

PROOF

$100 \times 210 = 2100$

$15 \times 1400 = 2100$

3. 200 g of Dextrose × 4 Kcal = 800 Kcal

4. 210 g of Aminosyn × 4 Kcal = 840 Kcal

WORKSHEET 9F (page 218)

1. d. $0.085 \times 375 = 31.8 \times 1.500 = 47.8$ g/bag of AA

2. b. $\dfrac{47.8}{1500} = 0.03 = 3\%$ conc. of AA

3. a. $0.40 \times 400 = 160 \times 1.450 = 232$ g/bag of dextrose

4. b. $\dfrac{232}{1450} = 0.16 = 16\%$ conc. of dextrose

5. a. $0.20 \times 175 = 35 \times 1.200 = 42$ g lipids/bag

6. b. $\dfrac{42}{1200} = 0.035 = 3.5\%$ conc. of lipids

7. d. $6 \times 1.350 = 8.1 \div 1350 = 0.006 = 0.6\%$ calcium gluconate

8. a. $10 \times 1.258 = 12.5 \div 1258 = 0.01 = 1\%$ magnesium sulfate

9. c. $12 \times 1.385 = 16.62 \div 1385 = 0.012 = 1.2\%$ potassium

10. c. KNOW   WANT TO KNOW

110 mL : 1 hr :: 1275 mL : *x* hr

$110x = 1275$

$x = 11.59$ hr = 11 hr 35 min

PROOF

$1 \times 1275 = 1275$

$110 \times 11.59 = 1275$

IV started at 1800 hours plus 11 hr 35 min = 0535 hr

CHAPTER 9 FINAL: PARENTERAL NUTRITION (page 220)

1. a. 66.85 g/bag of AA
   b. 267.4 kcal of PRO

2. a. 73.62 g/bag of dextrose
   b. 294.52 kcal of CHO

3. a. 22.4 g/bag of AA
   b. 89.6 kcal of PRO

4. a. 212 g/bag of dextrose
   b. 848 kcal of dextrose

5. 0.4% potassium chloride

6. 2.5% sodium chloride

7. 1559 total kcal

8. a. 25 g/bag of lipids
   b. 225 kcal of fat

9. At 0709 hr the infusion will be completed

10. 11 hr to infuse

10 Insulin

WORKSHEET **10A** (page 233)

1. 27 units	**2.** 68 units	**3.** 16 units	**4.** 44 units
5. 32 units	**6.** 78 units	**7.** 42 units	**8.** 39 units
9. 23 units	**10.** 18 units		

WORKSHEET **10B** (page 234)

1. a	**2.** b	**3.** b	**4.** a
5. a			

WORKSHEET **10C** (page 239)

1. Total units: 48	**2.** Total units: 39	**3.** Total units: 23	**4.** Total units: 38
b is correct	**a** is correct	**a** is correct	**b** is correct

5. Total units: 68
   a is correct
   b insulins are reversed–drawn up incorrectly.

6. 15 units
   Peak: 1 to 3 hr

7. 10 units
   Onset: 15 min

8. 44 units
   Peak: 2 to 4 hr and 6 to 10 hr
   Duration: 3 to 4 hr and 10 to 16 hr

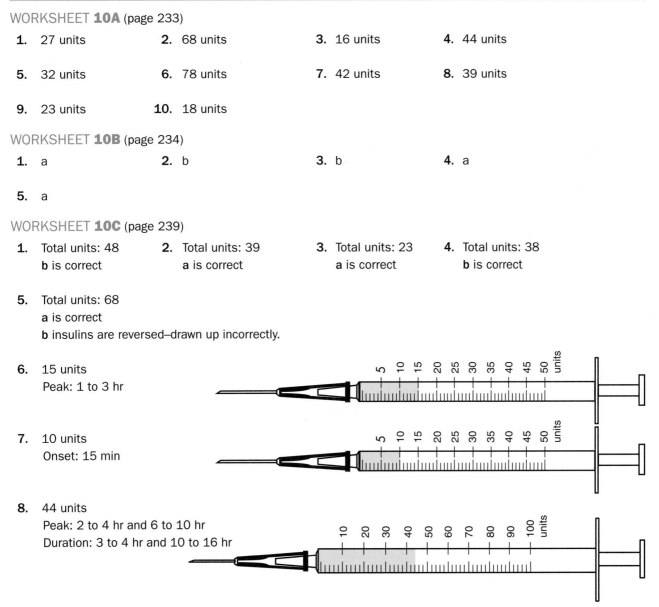

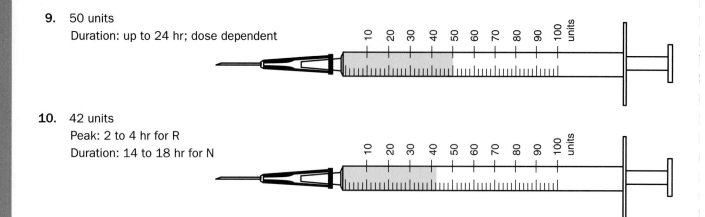

9. 50 units
   Duration: up to 24 hr; dose dependent

10. 42 units
   Peak: 2 to 4 hr for R
   Duration: 14 to 18 hr for N

WORKSHEET 10D (page 244)

1. BGL difference is 20 divided by 10 = 2 units of R
   CHO is 48 g divided by 8 = 6 units R

2. BGL difference is 5 divided by 10 = 0.5 = 1 unit R (rounded to nearest whole number)
   CHO is 71 g divided by 8 = 8.87 = 9 units R

3. BGL difference is 15 divided by 10 = 1.5 = 2 units R
   CHO is 34 g divided by 8 = 4.25 = 4 units R
   Snack: BGL difference is 15 divided by 10 = 1.5 = 2 units R
   CHO is 15 g divided by 8 = 1.87 = 2 units R
   Total insulin for the day = 28 units

4. BGL difference is −5 = 0 units R
   CHO is 43 g divided by 10 = 4.3 = 4 units R

5. BGL difference is 20 divided by 10 = 2 units
   CHO is 93 g divided by 10 = 9.3 = 9 units R

WORKSHEET 10E (page 245)

1. BGL difference is 30 divided by 20 = 1.5 = 2 units R
   CHO is 98 g divided by 6.5 = 7 units R
   Total = 9 units R

2. BGL difference is 50 divided by 20 = 2.5 = 3 units R
   CHO is 118 g divided by 15 = 7.8 = 8 units R
   Total = 11 units R

3. BGL difference is 20 divided by 20 = 2.5 = 1 unit R
   CHO is 40 g divided by 15 = 2.6 = 3 units R
   Total = 4 units R

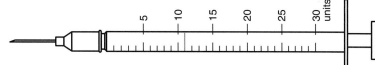

4. BGL difference is 90 divided by 3 = 3 units R
   CHO is 58 g divided by 10 = 5.8 = 6 units R
   Total = 9 units R

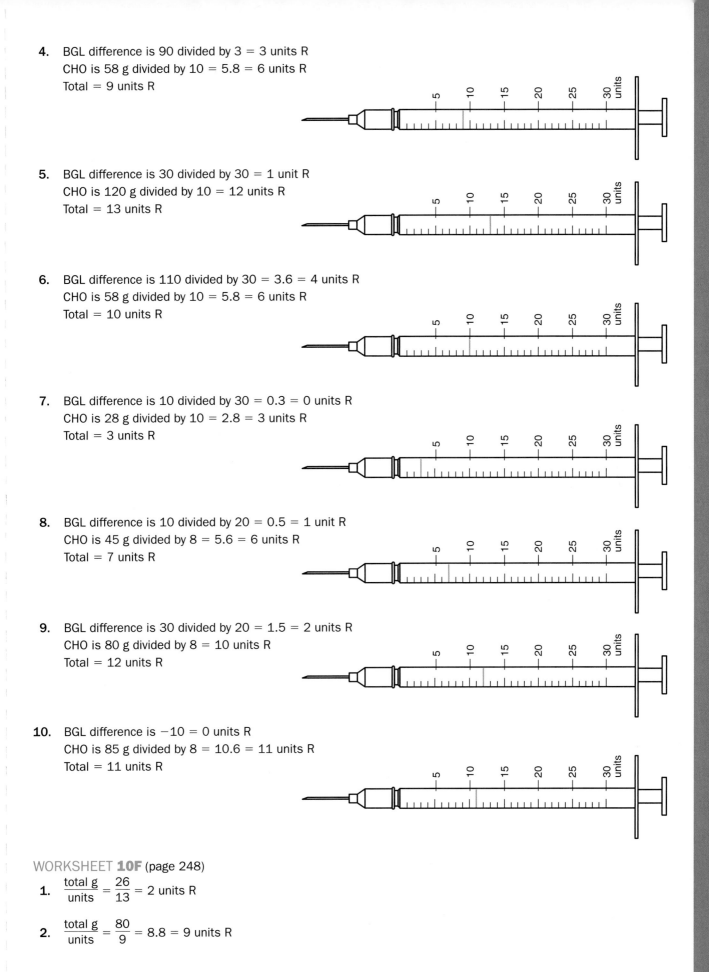

5. BGL difference is 30 divided by 30 = 1 unit R
   CHO is 120 g divided by 10 = 12 units R
   Total = 13 units R

6. BGL difference is 110 divided by 30 = 3.6 = 4 units R
   CHO is 58 g divided by 10 = 5.8 = 6 units R
   Total = 10 units R

7. BGL difference is 10 divided by 30 = 0.3 = 0 units R
   CHO is 28 g divided by 10 = 2.8 = 3 units R
   Total = 3 units R

8. BGL difference is 10 divided by 20 = 0.5 = 1 unit R
   CHO is 45 g divided by 8 = 5.6 = 6 units R
   Total = 7 units R

9. BGL difference is 30 divided by 20 = 1.5 = 2 units R
   CHO is 80 g divided by 8 = 10 units R
   Total = 12 units R

10. BGL difference is −10 = 0 units R
    CHO is 85 g divided by 8 = 10.6 = 11 units R
    Total = 11 units R

WORKSHEET **10F** (page 248)

1. $\dfrac{\text{total g}}{\text{units}} = \dfrac{26}{13} = 2$ units R

2. $\dfrac{\text{total g}}{\text{units}} = \dfrac{80}{9} = 8.8 = 9$ units R

3. $\dfrac{\text{total g}}{\text{units}} = \dfrac{18}{16} = 1.1 = 1$ unit R

4. $\dfrac{\text{total g}}{\text{units}} = \dfrac{90}{6} = 15$ units R

5. $\dfrac{\text{total g}}{\text{units}} = \dfrac{160}{11} = 14.5$ units $= 15$ units R for 24 hr

6. $\dfrac{\text{total g}}{\text{units}} = \dfrac{145}{7} = 20.7 = 21$ units R for 24 hr

7. $\dfrac{1}{2}$ of $45 = 22.5 + \dfrac{3}{4}$ of $75 = 56.25 = 78.75 = 9.8 = 10$ units R

8. 50 g divided by $2 = \dfrac{25 \text{ g}}{10} = 2.5 = 3$ units R

9. Total amount of CHO = 179 g
   $\dfrac{179}{12} = 14.9 = 15$ units for the day

10. $\dfrac{1}{2}$ of $38 = 19$ g; $\dfrac{1}{4}$ of $50 = 12.5$ g; 13 of $48 = 16$ g
    Total CHO grams $= 47.5 = 3$ units total for the 3 meals

WORKSHEET 10G (page 250)

1. **a.** 4 mL/hr
   b. 3 units/hr

2. **a.** KNOW   WANT TO KNOW
   100 units : 100 mL ∷ 2.5 units : x mL
   100x = 100 × 2.5 = 250
   $\quad x = 2.5$ mL/hr
   PROOF
   100 × 2.5 = 250
   100 × 2.5 = 250
   b. Change IV rate to 3 mL/hr
   c. 5.5 units

3. 19 total units
   Do not give inslin when BMBC is 120 mg per dL

4. **a.** KNOW   WANT TO KNOW
   50 mL : 100 units ∷ x mL : 5 units
   100x = 50 × 5 = 250
   $\quad x = 2.5$ mL/hr
   PROOF
   100 × 2.5 = 250
   50 × 5 = 250
   b. 5 units per hour × 16 hours = 80 units of insulin

5. a. KNOW   WANT TO KNOW

100 units : 50 mL :: x units : 3 mL

$50x = 100 \times 3 = 300$

$x = 6$ units/hr

PROOF

$100 \times 3 = 300$

$50 \times 6 = 300$

b. 8 hr $\times$ 6 units per hr = 48 units

6. KNOW   WANT TO KNOW

100 units : 150 mL :: 10 units : x mL

$100x = 150 \times 10 = 1500$

$100x = 1500$

$x = 15$ mL/hr = 10 units insulin

PROOF

$100 \times 15 = 1500$

$150 \times 10 = 1500$

KNOW   WANT TO KNOW

15 mL : 1 hr :: 150 mL : x hr

$15x = 150$

$x = 10$ hr to infuse 100 units insulin

PROOF

$15 \times 10 = 150$

$1 \times 150 = 150$

7. KNOW   WANT TO KNOW

50 mL : 50 units :: x mL : 8 units

$50x = 50 \times 8 = 400$

$50x = 400$

$x = 8$ mL/hr = 8 units of insulin

PROOF

$50 \times 8 = 400$

$50 \times 8 = 400$

KNOW   WANT TO KNOW

8 mL : 1 hr :: 50 mL : x hr

$8x = 50$

$x = 6.25$ hr to infuse 50 units insulin or

6 hr 15 min

PROOF

$8 \times 6.25 = 50$

$1 \times 50 = 50$

8. KNOW   WANT TO KNOW

50 mL : 75 units :: x mL : 15 units

$75x = 50 \times 15 = 750$

$75x = 750$

$x = 10$ mL/hr = 15 units

PROOF

$50 \times 15 = 750$

$75 \times 10 = 750$

KNOW   WANT TO KNOW

10 mL : 1 hr :: 50 mL : x hr

$10x = 50$

$x = 5$ hours to infuse

PROOF

$1 \times 50 = 50$

$10 \times 5 = 50$

9. KNOW   WANT TO KNOW

100 mL : 120 units :: x mL : 10 units

$120x = 100 \times 10 = 1000$

$120x = 1000$

$x = 8.33$ mL/hr to deliver 10 units of

insulin

PROOF

$120 \times 8.33 = 999.6$

$100 \times 10 = 1000$

KNOW   WANT TO KNOW

8 mL : 1 hr :: 100 mL : x hr

$8x = 1 \times 100 = 100$

$8x = 100$

$x = 12.5$ hr to infuse 120 units of regular insulin

PROOF

$8 \times 12.5 = 100$

$1 \times 100 = 100$

10. KNOW   WANT TO KNOW

150 mL : 150 units :: x mL : 12 units

$150x = 150 \times 12$

$150x = 1800$

$x = 12$ mL/hr to deliver 12 units

of insulin

PROOF

$150 \times 12 = 1800$

$12 \times 150 = 1800$

KNOW   WANT TO KNOW

12 mL : 1 hr :: 150 mL : x hr

$12x = 150$

$x = 12.5$ hr to infuse 150 units of regular

insulin, or 12 hr 30 min

$12 \times 12.5 = 150$

$1 \times 150 = 150$

1. d. 4 units

KNOW   WANT TO KNOW

250 mL : 100 units :: 10 mL : x units

$250x = 100 \times 10 = 1000$

$x = 4$ units/hr

PROOF

$250 \times 4 = 1000$

$100 \times 10 = 1000$

2. b. 25 hr

KNOW   WANT TO KNOW

4 units : 1 hr :: 100 units : x hr

$4x = 100$

$x = 25$ hr

PROOF

$1 \times 100 = 100$

$4 \times 25 = 100$

3. c. 3 mL/hr

KNOW   WANT TO KNOW

100 units : 100 mL :: 3 units : x mL

$100x = 100 \times 3 = 300$

$x = 3$ mL/hr

PROOF

$100 \times 3 = 300$

$100 \times 3 = 300$

4. b. 2.5 units/hr

KNOW   WANT TO KNOW

30 units : 12 hr :: x units : 1 hr

$12x = 30$

$x = 2.5$ units/hr

PROOF

$30 \times 1 = 30$

$12 \times 2.5 = 30$

a. 4 mL/hr

50 mL : 12 hr :: x mL : 1 hr

$12x = 50$

$x = 4.16 = 4$ mL/hr

PROOF

$50 \times 1 = 50$

$12 \times 4.16 = 4.9$

5. a. 50 mL/hr

KNOW   WANT TO KNOW

500 mL : 100 units :: x mL : 10 units

$100x = 500 \times 10 = 5000$

$x = 50$ mL/hr

PROOF

$100 \times 50 = 5000$

$500 \times 10 = 5000$

6. c. Humulin R

7. d. 24 hr

8. b. 4 to 10 hr

9. d. is peakless

10. b. anytime

CHAPTER 10 FINAL: INSULIN (page 255)

1. 15 units

    b

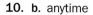

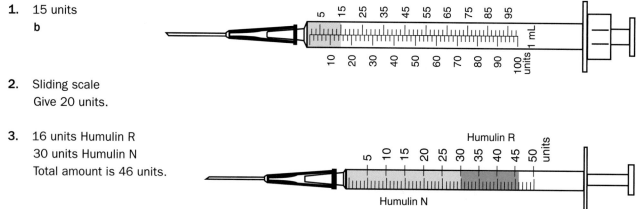

2. Sliding scale

    Give 20 units.

3. 16 units Humulin R

    30 units Humulin N

    Total amount is 46 units.

4. 18 units Humalog
   b is easier to read

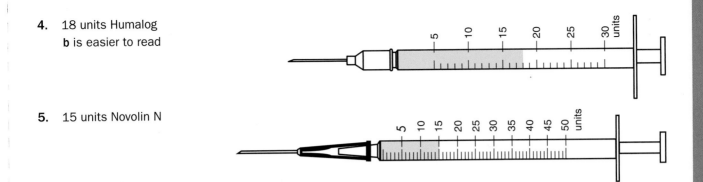

5. 15 units Novolin N

6. 20 mL per hr = 10 units
   25 hr to infuse. An IV solution can hang for only 24 hr (CDC guidelines).

7. 15 mL per hr to infuse 6 units insulin
   16.6 hr to infuse = 16 hr 36 min

8. 20 mL per hr to infuse 8 units insulin
   12.5 hr to infuse = 12 hr 30 min

9. 14 mL per hr to infuse 7 units insulin
   14.28 hr to infuse = 14 hr 17 min

10. 45 mL per hr to infuse 9 units insulin
   11.1 hr to infuse = 11 hr 6 min

11 Anticoagulants

WORKSHEET **11A** (page 262)

1. KNOW   WANT TO KNOW
   10,000 units : 1 mL :: 7000 units : x mL
   $10x = 7$
      $x = 0.7$ mL
   PROOF
   $1 \times 7000 = 7000$
   $10,000 \times 0.7 = 7000$

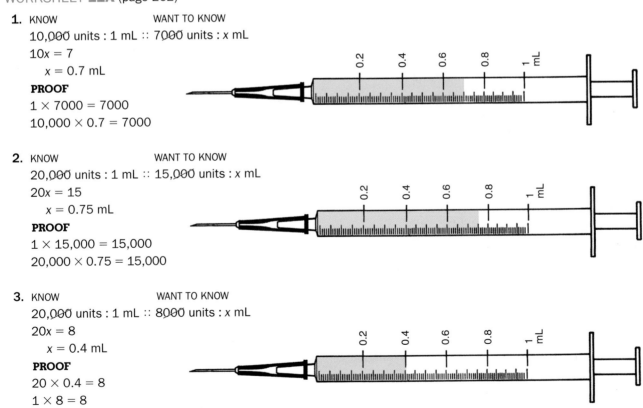

2. KNOW   WANT TO KNOW
   20,000 units : 1 mL :: 15,000 units : x mL
   $20x = 15$
      $x = 0.75$ mL
   PROOF
   $1 \times 15,000 = 15,000$
   $20,000 \times 0.75 = 15,000$

3. KNOW   WANT TO KNOW
   20,000 units : 1 mL :: 8000 units : x mL
   $20x = 8$
      $x = 0.4$ mL
   PROOF
   $20 \times 0.4 = 8$
   $1 \times 8 = 8$

4. KNOW   WANT TO KNOW   ⎫ use the 20,000

20,000 units : 1 mL :: 17,000 units : x mL ⎬ units per mL strength

20x = 17   ⎭

$\quad x = 0.85$ mL

PROOF

$1 \times 17 = 17$

$20 \times 0.85 = 17$

5. KNOW   WANT TO KNOW

10,000 international units : 1 mL :: 7500 international units : x mL

100x = 75

$\quad x = 0.75$ mL Fragmin

PROOF

$1 \times 75 = 75$

$100 \times 0.75 = 75$

6. KNOW   WANT TO KNOW

1000 units : 1 mL :: 750 units : x mL

1000x = 750

$\quad x = 0.75$ mL

PROOF

$1000 \times 0.75 = 750$

$1 \times 750 = 750$

7. KNOW   WANT TO KNOW

1000 units : 1 mL :: 800 units : x mL

10x = 8

$\quad x = 0.8$ mL

PROOF

$10 \times 0.8 = 8$

$1 \times 8 = 8$

8. KNOW   WANT TO KNOW

5000 units : 1 mL :: 3000 units : x mL

5x = 3

$\quad x = 0.6$ mL

PROOF

$1 \times 3 = 3$

$5 \times 0.6 = 3$

9. KNOW   WANT TO KNOW

10 units : 1 mL :: x units : 10 mL

$x = 10 \times 10 = 100$

$x = 100$ units in the vial

KNOW   WANT TO KNOW

10 units : 1 mL :: 5 units : x mL

10x = 5

$\quad x = 0.5$ mL

PROOF

$1 \times 5 = 5$

$10 \times 0.5 = 5$

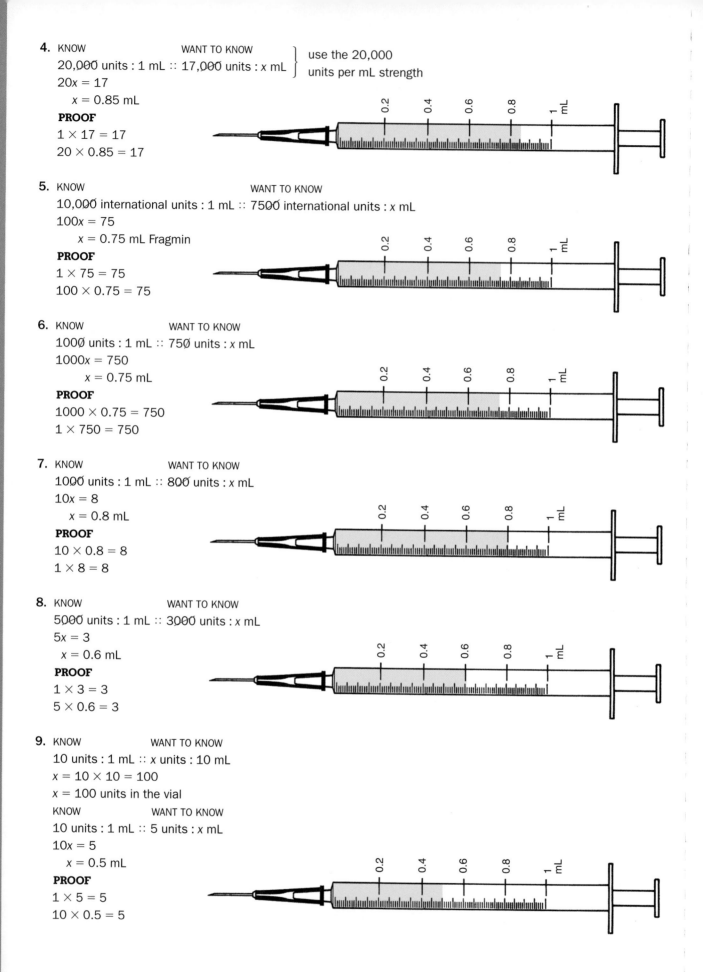

412   Answer Key

10. KNOW   WANT TO KNOW

100 units : 1 mL :: 50 units : x mL

10x = 5

    x = 0.5 mL

PROOF

1 × 5 = 5

10 × 0.5 = 5

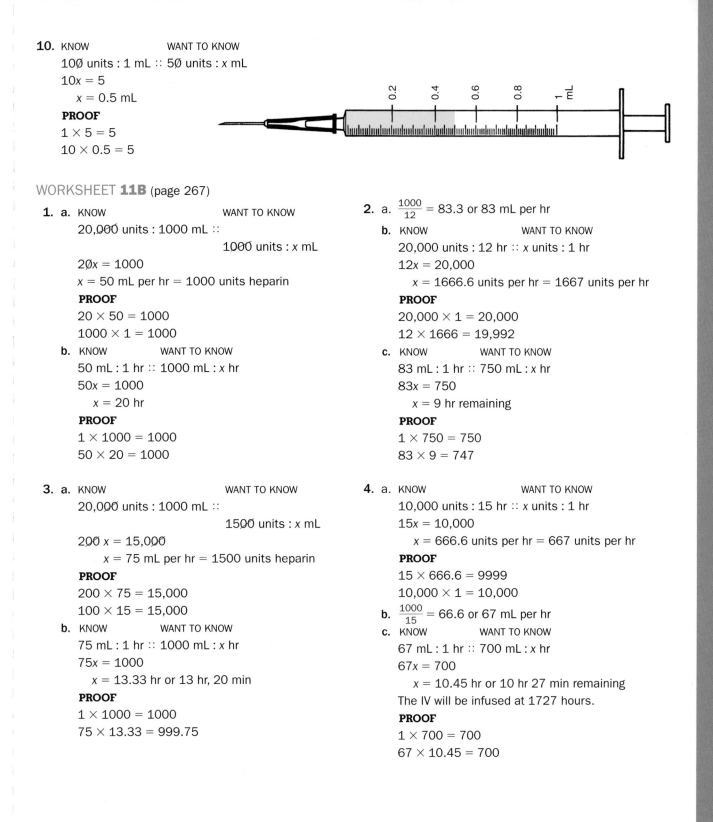

WORKSHEET **11B** (page 267)

1. a. KNOW   WANT TO KNOW

20,000 units : 1000 mL ::

                       1000 units : x mL

20x = 1000

x = 50 mL per hr = 1000 units heparin

PROOF

20 × 50 = 1000

1000 × 1 = 1000

b. KNOW   WANT TO KNOW

50 mL : 1 hr :: 1000 mL : x hr

50x = 1000

    x = 20 hr

PROOF

1 × 1000 = 1000

50 × 20 = 1000

3. a. KNOW   WANT TO KNOW

20,000 units : 1000 mL ::

                       1500 units : x mL

200 x = 15,000

    x = 75 mL per hr = 1500 units heparin

PROOF

200 × 75 = 15,000

100 × 15 = 15,000

b. KNOW   WANT TO KNOW

75 mL : 1 hr :: 1000 mL : x hr

75x = 1000

    x = 13.33 hr or 13 hr, 20 min

PROOF

1 × 1000 = 1000

75 × 13.33 = 999.75

2. a. $\frac{1000}{12}$ = 83.3 or 83 mL per hr

b. KNOW   WANT TO KNOW

20,000 units : 12 hr :: x units : 1 hr

12x = 20,000

    x = 1666.6 units per hr = 1667 units per hr

PROOF

20,000 × 1 = 20,000

12 × 1666 = 19,992

c. KNOW   WANT TO KNOW

83 mL : 1 hr :: 750 mL : x hr

83x = 750

    x = 9 hr remaining

PROOF

1 × 750 = 750

83 × 9 = 747

4. a. KNOW   WANT TO KNOW

10,000 units : 15 hr :: x units : 1 hr

15x = 10,000

    x = 666.6 units per hr = 667 units per hr

PROOF

15 × 666.6 = 9999

10,000 × 1 = 10,000

b. $\frac{1000}{15}$ = 66.6 or 67 mL per hr

c. KNOW   WANT TO KNOW

67 mL : 1 hr :: 700 mL : x hr

67x = 700

    x = 10.45 hr or 10 hr 27 min remaining

The IV will be infused at 1727 hours.

PROOF

1 × 700 = 700

67 × 10.45 = 700

5. a. KNOW   WANT TO KNOW

10,000 units : 500 mL ::

$\qquad\qquad\qquad$ 1200 units : x mL

$100x = 6000$

$x = 60$ mL per hr

PROOF

$500 \times 12 = 6000$

$100 \times 60 = 6000$

b. KNOW   WANT TO KNOW

60 mL : 1 hr :: 500 mL : x hr

$60x = 500$

$x = 8.33$ hr or 8 hr 20 min

PROOF

$60 \times 8.33 = 499.8$

$1 \times 500 = 500$

6. a. KNOW   WANT TO KNOW

50,000 units : 1000 mL ::

$\qquad\qquad\qquad$ 2500 units : x mL

$500x = 25 \times 1000 = 25,000$

$5x = 250$

$x = 50$ mL per hr

PROOF

$500 \times 50 = 25,000$

$1000 \times 25 = 25,000$

b. KNOW   WANT TO KNOW

50 mL : 1 hr :: 1000 mL : x hr

$50x = 1000$

$x = 20$ hr

PROOF

$50 \times 20 = 1000$

$1 \times 1000 = 1000$

7. a. KNOW   WANT TO KNOW

25,000 units : 500 mL ::

$\qquad\qquad\qquad$ 1500 units : x mL

$250x = 500 \times 15 = 7500$

$25x = 750$

$x = 30$ mL per hr

PROOF

$25 \times 750 = 7500$

$500 \times 15 = 7500$

b. KNOW   WANT TO KNOW

30 mL : 1 hr :: 500 mL : x hr

$30x = 500$

$3x = 50$

$x = 16.6$ hr = 16 hr 36 min

PROOF

$1 \times 500 = 500$

$30 \times 16.6 = 499.9$

8. a. KNOW   WANT TO KNOW

25,000 units : 500 mL ::

$\qquad\qquad\qquad$ 1300 units : x mL

$250x = 6500$

$x = 26$ mL per hr

PROOF

$26 \times 250 = 6500$

$500 \times 13 = 6500$

b. KNOW   WANT TO KNOW

26 mL : 1 hr :: 500 mL : x hr

$26x = 500$

$x = 19.23$ hr or 19 hr 14 min

PROOF

$1 \times 500 = 500$

$26 \times 19.23 = 499.98$

9. a. KNOW   WANT TO KNOW

25,000 units : 250 mL ::

$\qquad\qquad\qquad$ 1800 units : x mL

$250x = 4500$

$x = 18$ mL per hr

PROOF

$250 \times 18 = 4500$

$250 \times 18 = 4500$

b. KNOW   WANT TO KNOW

18 mL : 1 hr :: 250 mL : x hr

$18x = 250$

$x = 13.88$ hr or 13 hr 53 min

PROOF

$1 \times 250 = 250$

$18 \times 13.8 = 248.4$

10. a. KNOW   WANT TO KNOW

20,000 units : 250 mL ::

$\qquad\qquad\qquad$ 1000 units : x mL

$20x = 250$

$x = 12.5$ mL per hr or 13 mL per hr

PROOF

$20 \times 12.5 = 250$

$250 \times 1 = 250$

b. KNOW   WANT TO KNOW

13 mL : 1 hr :: 250 mL : x hr

$13x = 250$

$x = 19.23$ hr or 19 hr 14 min

PROOF

$1 \times 250 = 250$

$13 \times 19.2 = 249.8$

414   Answer Key

1. lb to kg = 172 ÷ 2.2 = 80 kg

   a. KNOW   WANT TO KNOW

   70 units : 1 kg :: x units : 80 kg

   x = 70 × 80 = 5600 units loading dose

   PROOF

   1 × 5600 = 5600

   70 × 80 = 5600

   b. KNOW   WANT TO KNOW

   20 units : 1 kg per hr :: x units : 80 kg per hr

   x = 20 × 80 = 1600

   x = 1600 units per hr

   PROOF

   1 × 1600 = 16,000

   20 × 80 = 16,000

   c. KNOW   WANT TO KNOW

   1000 mL : 25,000 units ::

                  x mL : 1600 units

   250x = 1000 × 16 = 16,000

   250x = 64 mL/hr

   PROOF

   64 × 250 = 16,000

   16 × 1000 = 16,000

2. lb to kg = 160 lb divided by 2.2 kg =
                            72.7 = 73 kg

   a. KNOW   WANT TO KNOW

   80 units : 1 kg :: x units : 73 kg

   x = 80 × 73 = 5840

   x = 5840 units loading dose

   PROOF

   1 × 5840 = 5840

   73 × 80 = 5840

   b. KNOW   WANT TO KNOW

   1000 mL : 30,000 units ::

                     x mL : 1500 units

   300x = 1000 × 15 = 15,000

   3x = 150

    x = 50 mL per hr

   PROOF

   50 × 300 = 15,000

   15 × 1000 = 15,000

3. lb to kg = 210 lb divided by 2.2 =
                            95.5 = 96 kg

   a. KNOW   WANT TO KNOW

   90 units : 1 kg :: x units : 96 kg

   x = 90 × 96 = 8640

   x = 8640 units loading dose

   PROOF

   1 × 8640 = 8640

   90 × 96 = 8640

   b. KNOW   WANT TO KNOW

   25 units : 1 kg :: x units : 96 kg/hr

   x = 25 × 96 = 2400

   x = 2400 units per hr

   PROOF

   25 × 96 = 2400

   c. KNOW   WANT TO KNOW

   1000 mL : 25,000 units ::

                     x mL : 2400 units

   250x = 1000 × 24 = 24,000

   25x = 2400 = 96

    x = 96 mL per hr

   PROOF

   96 × 25 = 24,000

   24 × 1000 = 24,000

4. lb to kg = 300 lb divided by 2.2 =
                            136.3 = 136 kg

   a. KNOW   WANT TO KNOW

   75 units : 1 kg :: x units : 136 kg

   x = 75 × 136 = 10,200

   x = 10,200 units bolus dose

   PROOF

   1 × 2720 = 10,200

   75 × 136 = 10,200

   b. KNOW   WANT TO KNOW

   20 units : 1 kg :: x units : 136 kg

   x = 20 × 136 = 2720

   x = 2720 units per hr

   PROOF

   1 × 2720 = 2720

   20 × 136 = 2720

   c. KNOW   WANT TO KNOW

   1000 mL : 50,000 units ::

                     x mL : 2720 units

   5000x = 1000 × 272 = 272,000

    5x = 272

     x = 54.4 = 54 mL per hr

   PROOF

   1000 × 272 = 272,000

   54.4 × 5000 = 272,000

5. lb to kg = 185 divided by 2.2 =

$$84.09 = 84 \text{ kg}$$

   a. KNOW   WANT TO KNOW

      75 units : 1 kg :: x units : 84 kg

      $x = 75 \times 84 = 6300$

      $x = 6300$ units bolus dose

      PROOF

      $1 \times 6300 = 6300$

      $75 \times 84 = 6300$

   b. KNOW   WANT TO KNOW

      17 units : 1 kg per hr :: x units : 84 kg per hr

      $x = 17 \times 84 = 1428$

      $x = 1428$ units per hr

      PROOF

      $1 \times 1428 = 1428$

      $17 \times 84 = 1428$

   c. KNOW   WANT TO KNOW

      1000 mL : 20,000 units ::

                     x mL : 1428 units

      $20{,}000x = 1000 \times 1428 = 1{,}428{,}000$

         $20x = 1428$

           $x = 71.4 = 71$ mL per hr

      PROOF

      $1000 \times 1428 = 1{,}428{,}000$

      $20{,}000 \times 71.4 = 1{,}428{,}000$

6. lb to kg = 145 divided by 2.2 =

$$65.9 = 66 \text{ kg}$$

   a. KNOW   WANT TO KNOW

      65 units : 1 kg :: x units : 66 kg

      $x = 65 \times 66 = 4290$

      $x = 4290$ units bolus dose

      PROOF

      $1 \times 4290 = 4290$

      $65 \times 66 = 4290$

   b. KNOW   WANT TO KNOW

      15 units : 1 kg per hr :: x units : 66 kg per hr

      $x = 15 \times 66 = 990$ units

      $x = 990$ units per hr

      PROOF

      $1 \times 990 = 990$

      $15 \times 66 = 990$

   c. KNOW   WANT TO KNOW

      500 mL : 30,000 units :: x mL : 990 units

      $30{,}000x = 500 \times 990 = 495{,}000$

         $30x = 495$

           $x = 16.5 = 17$ mL per hr

      PROOF

      $990 \times 500 = 495{,}000$

      $30{,}000 \times 16.5 = 495{,}000$

7. a. KNOW   WANT TO KNOW

      80 units : 1 kg :: x units : 120 kg

      $x = 80 \times 120 = 9600$

      $x = 9600$ units bolus dose

      PROOF

      $1 \times 9600 = 9600$

      $80 \times 120 = 9600$

   b. KNOW   WANT TO KNOW

      1000 mL : 25,000 units ::

                   x mL : 1000 units

      $25x = 1000$

        $x = 40$ mL per hr

      PROOF

      $25 \times 40 = 1000$

      $1 \times 1000 = 1000$

8. lb to kg = 194 divided by 2.2 = 88 kg

   a. KNOW   WANT TO KNOW

      70 units : 1 kg :: x units : 88 kg

      $x = 70 \times 88 = 6160$

      $x = 6160$ units bolus dose

      PROOF

      $1 \times 6160 = 6160$

      $70 \times 88 = 6160$

   b. KNOW   WANT TO KNOW

      18 units : 1 kg :: x units : 88 kg

      $x = 18 \times 88 = 1584$

      $x = 1584$ units per hr

      PROOF

      $1 \times 1584 = 1584$

      $18 \times 88 = 1584$

   c. KNOW   WANT TO KNOW

      1000 mL : 30,000 units ::

                   x mL : 1584 units

      $30{,}000x = 1584 \times 1000 = 1{,}584{,}000$

         $30x = 1584$

           $x = 52.8 = 53$ mL per hr

      PROOF

      $30 \times 52.8 = 1584$

      $1 \times 1584 = 1584$

9. a. KNOW   WANT TO KNOW

95 units : 1 kg :: x units : 136 kg

$x = 95 \times 136 = 12{,}920$

$x = 12{,}920$ units loading dose

PROOF

$1 \times 12{,}920 = 12{,}920$

$95 \times 136 = 12{,}920$

b. KNOW   WANT TO KNOW

20 units : 1 kg per hr :: x units : 136 kg per hr

$x = 20 \times 136 = 2720$

$x = 2720$ units per hr

PROOF

$1 \times 2720 = 2720$

$20 \times 136 = 22{,}720$

c. KNOW   WANT TO KNOW

1000 mL : 20,000 units ::

             x mL : 2720 units

$2000x = 1000 \times 272 = 272{,}000$

   $2x = 272 = 136$

     $x = 136$ mL per hr

PROOF

$2000 \times 136 = 272{,}000$

$1000 \times 272 = 272{,}000$

10. a. KNOW   WANT TO KNOW

1000 units : 1 kg :: x units : 108 kg

$x = 100 \times 108 = 10{,}800$

$x = 10{,}800$ units loading dose

PROOF

$1 \times 10{,}800 = 10{,}800$

$1000 \times 108 = 10{,}800$

b. KNOW   WANT TO KNOW

18 units : 1 kg :: x units : 108 kg

$x = 18 \times 108 = 1944$

$x = 1944$ units per hr

PROOF

$1 \times 1944 = 1944$

$18 \times 108 = 1944$

c. KNOW   WANT TO KNOW

1000 mL : 35,000 units ::

             x mL : 1944 units

$35x = 1944$

   $x = 55.54 = 56$ mL per hr

PROOF

$35 \times 55.54 = 1939$

$1944 \times 1 = 1944$

WORKSHEET **11D** (page 270)

1. Give initial bolus dose = 80 units/kg

KNOW   WANT TO KNOW   **PROOF**

80 units : 1 kg :: x units : 70 kg $80 \times 70 = 5600$

$x = 70 \times 80 = 5600$ $1 \times 5600 = 5600$

$x = 5600$ units initial bolus dose

2. Initial infusion rate: 18 units per kg per hr

KNOW   WANT TO KNOW   **PROOF**

18 units : 1 kg per hr :: x units : 70 kg $18 \times 70 = 1260$

$x = 70 \times 18 = 1260$ $1 \times 1260 = 1260$

$x = 1260$ units per hr round off units to nearest whole number = 1300 units per hr

3. KNOW   WANT TO KNOW   **PROOF**

250 mL : 25000 units :: x mL : 1300 units $250 \times 1300 = 325{,}000$

$x = 250 \times 1300 = 325000$ $13 \times 25000 = 325{,}000$

$x = 13$ mL per hr

After 6 hours the APTT is 30. Rebolus with 80 units/kg (5600 units). Increase the rate by 4 units per kg per hr.

4. a. KNOW   WANT TO KNOW   **PROOF**

4 units : 1 kg :: x units : 70 kg $4 \times 70 = 280$

$x = 4 \times 70 = 280$ units round to 300 units $1 \times 280 = 280$

b. 1300 units/hr increased by 300 units = 1600 units/hr

5. Reset infusion rate to:

KNOW   WANT TO KNOW   **PROOF**

250 mL : 25000 units :: x mL : 1600 units $250 \times 1600 = 400{,}000$

$25000x = 250 \times 1600 = 400{,}000$ $16 \times 25000 = 400{,}000$

     $25x = 400$

       $x = 16$ mL per hr is the new rate for the infusion

After 6 hours the APTT is 40. Increase IV rate by 2 units per kg per hr. Rebolus with 40 units per kg.

6. KNOW   WANT TO KNOW   **PROOF**

    40 units : 1 kg :: x units : 70 kg $40 \times 70 = 2800$

    $x = 40 \times 70 = 28{,}000$ $1 \times 2800 = 2800$

    $x = 2800$ units bolus dose

7. KNOW   WANT TO KNOW   **PROOF**

    a. 2 units : 1 kg :: x units : 70 kg $2 \times 70 = 140$

         $x = 2 \times 70 = 140$ $1 \times 140 = 140$

         $x = 140$ units per hr rounded to 100 units

    b. 1600 units per hr increased by 100 units = 1700 units per hr

    Reset infusion rate to:

8. KNOW   WANT TO KNOW   **PROOF**

    250 mL : 25000 units :: x mL : 1700 units $250 \times 1700 = 425{,}000$

    $25{,}000x = 250 \times 1700 = 425{,}000$ $17 \times 25{,}000 = 425{,}000$

               $x = 17$ mL per hr is the new rate for the infusion

    6 hour APTT is 55 = no change in the rate.

    6 hour APTT is 85. Decrease rate by 2 units per kg per hr.

9. KNOW   WANT TO KNOW   **PROOF**

    a. 2 units : 1 kg :: x units : 70 kg $2 \times 70 = 140$

         $x = 2 \times 70 = 140$ $1 \times 140 = 140$

         $x = 140$ rounded to 100 units per hr decrease

    b. 1700 units/hr decreased by 100 units/hr = 1600 units per hr new rate

    Reset infusion rate to:

10. KNOW   WANT TO KNOW   **PROOF**

    250 mL : 25,000 units :: x mL : 1600 units $250 \times 1600 = 400{,}000$

    $250{,}000x = 250 \times 1600 = 400{,}000$ $16 \times 25{,}000 = 400{,}000$

    $25x = 400$

      $x = 16$ mL per hr new rate to set the IV pump

    6 hr APTT is 95. Decrease rate by 3 units per kg per hr.

11. KNOW   WANT TO KNOW   **PROOF**

    a. 3 units : 1 kg :: x units : 70 kg $3 \times 70 = 210$

         $x = 3 \times 70 = 210$ $1 \times 210 = 210$

         $x = 210$ units = 200 units/hr decrease

    b 1600 units per hr decreased by 200 units per hr = 1400 units per hr new rate

    Reset infusion rate to:

12. KNOW   WANT TO KNOW   **PROOF**

    250 mL : 250 units :: x mL : 14 units $250 \times 1300 = 325{,}000$

    $250x = 250 \times 14 = 3500$ $13 \times 25{,}000 = 325{,}000$

        $250x = 3500$

    $x = 14$ mL per hr new IV rate. **Stop infusion for 1 hour before resuming IV rate. Next APTT in 6 hours.**

1. c. KNOW   WANT TO KNOW

120 international units : 1 kg ::

          x international units : 84 kg

$x = 120 \times 84 = 10{,}080$

$x = 10{,}080$ international units of

      Fragmin

PROOF

$120 \times 84 = 10{,}080$

$1 \times 10{,}080 = 10{,}080$

2. b. KNOW   WANT TO KNOW

25,000 international units : 1 mL ::

              10,080 : x mL

$25{,}000x = 10{,}080$

    $x = 0.4$ mL

PROOF

$1 \times 10{,}080 = 10{,}080$ (units can be

rounded up or down)

$0.4 \times 25{,}000 = 10{,}000$

3. c. KNOW   WANT TO KNOW

1 kg : 2.2 lb :: x kg : 132 lb

$2.2x = 132$

   $x = 60$ kg

PROOF

$1 \times 132 = 132$

$2.2 \times 60 = 132$

d. KNOW   WANT TO KNOW

120 international units : 1 kg ::

        x international units : 60 kg

$x = 60 \times 120$

$x = 7200$ international units q12h

PROOF

$1 \times 7200 = 7200$

$60 \times 120 = 7200$

4. a. KNOW   WANT TO KNOW

10,000 international units : 1 mL ::

      7200 international units : L : x mL

$10{,}000x = 7200$

    $x = 0.72 = 0.7$ mL

PROOF

$7200 \times 1 = 7200$

$10{,}000 \times 0.72 = 7200$

5. a. KNOW   WANT TO KNOW

80 units : 1 kg :: x units : 73 kg

$x = 80 \times 73 = 5840$

$x = 5840$ units of heparin

PROOF

$1 \times 5840 = 5840$

$80 \times 73 = 5840$

6. d. KNOW   WANT TO KNOW

18 units : 1 kg :: x units : 80 kg

$x = 18 \times 80 = 1440$

$x = 1440$ units/hr

PROOF

$1 \times 1440 = 1440$

$18 \times 80 = 1440$

d. KNOW   WANT TO KNOW

1000 mL : 20,000 units ::

             x mL : 1440 units

$20{,}000x = 1000 \times 1440 = 1{,}440{,}000$

    $x = 72$ mL per hr

PROOF

$1000 \times 1440 = 1{,}440{,}000$

$72 \times 20{,}000 = 1{,}440{,}000$

7. b. KNOW   WANT TO KNOW

1000 mL : 25,000 units ::

            x mL : 3000 units

$25{,}000x = 3{,}000{,}000$

   $25x = 120$ mL per hr

PROOF

$25 \times 120 = 3000$

$1000 \times 3 = 3000$

8. d. KNOW   WANT TO KNOW

10,000 units : 500 mL :: 500 units : x mL

$10{,}000x = 250{,}000$

   $x = 25$ mL per hr

PROOF

$25 \times 10{,}000 = 250{,}000$

$500 \times 500 = 250{,}000$

9. a. 220 divided by 2.2 = 100 kg

d. KNOW   WANT TO KNOW
120 international units : 1 kg ::
    x international units : 100 kg
$x = 120 \times 100 = 12,000$
$x = 12,000$ international units Fragmin

PROOF
$1 \times 12,000 = 12,000$
$100 \times 120 = 12,000$

10. c. KNOW   WANT TO KNOW
25,000 international units : 1 mL ::
    12,000 international units : x mL
$25,000x = 12,000$
    $x = 0.48$ mL

PROOF
$1 \times 12,000 = 12,000$
$25,000 \times 0.48 = 12,000$

CHAPTER 11 FINAL: ANTICOAGULANTS (page 275)

1. 0.8 mL

2. 0.25 mL

3. 0.2 mL using the 10,000 units per mL strength or 0.4 mL using the 5000 units per mL strength Give 0.2mL the smallest amount. Use the 1000 units per mL vial

4. 0.35 mL using the 20,000 units per mL strength or 0.7 mL using the 10,000 units per mL strength or 1.4 mL using the 5,000 units per mL strength Give the 2.5 mL the smallest amount

5. 0.8 mL

6. 17.5 mL/hr or 18 mL/hr
27 hr, 42 min

7. 30 mL per hr
16 hr, 40 min

8. 42 mL per hr
1041.6 units per hr

9. 42 mL per hr
1458 units per hr

10. 100 mL per hr via infusion device
10 hr to infuse

12 Children's Dosages

WORKSHEET 12A (page 279)

1. a. Estimate: 7 kg
  Actual: 6.4 kg
b. Estimate: 6 kg
  Actual: 12.1 lb (2 steps)
    5.5 kg
c. Estimate: 5 kg
  Actual: 4.5 kg
d. Estimate: 28 lb
  Actual: 30.8 lb
e. Estimate: 20 lb
  Actual: 22 lb

2. a. 150 mg $\times$ 3 = 450 mg
b. 200 mg $\times$ 4 = 800 mg
c. 400 mcg $\times$ 6 = 2400 mcg or 2.4 mg
d. 50 mg $\times$ 3 = 150 mg
e. 750 mcg $\times$ 2 = 1500 mcg or 1.5 mg

3. a. 1 g or 1000 mg ÷ 4 = 250 mg

   b. 750 mg ÷ 3 = 250 mg

   c. 2 g or 2000 mg ÷ 4 = 500 mg

      2 g or 2000 mg ÷ 6 = 333.3 mg

   d. 16 g a day ÷ 2 = 8 g

      16 g a day ÷ 4 = 4 g

   e. 500 mg/4 = 125 mg

4. a. 10 × 5 = 50 mg

   b. 5 × 7.3 = 36.5 mg (low dose)

      8 × 7.3 = 58.4 mg (high dose)

      SDR is 36.5 to 58.4 mg.

   c. 8 lb = approximately 4 kg estimated

      Step 1: 8 lb = 3.6 kg actual

      Step 2: *Low dose:* 6 × 3.6 = 21.6 mg

              High dose: 8 × 3.6 = 28.8 mg

      SDR is 21.6 to 28.8 mg.

   d. 5 lb, 8 oz = approximately 2.5 kg

      Step 1: *oz to lb:* 8 oz/16 = 0.5 lb

      Step 2: *lb to kg:* 5.5 lb ÷ 2.2 = 2.5 kg

      Step 3: *Low dose:* 3 × 2.5 = 7.5 mg

              High dose: 6 × 2.5 = 15 mg

      SDR is 7.5 to 15 mg.

   e. 4 lb, 6 oz = approximately 2 kg

      Step 1: *oz to lb:* 6 oz/16 = 0.37 rounded to 0.4 lb

      Step 2: *lb to kg:* 4.4 lb ÷ 2.2 = 2 kg

      Step 3: *Low dose:* 200 mcg × 2 = 400 mcg

              or 0.4 mg

              High dose: 400 mcg × 2 = 800 mcg

              or 0.8 mg

      SDR is 400 to 800 mcg or 0.4 to 0.8 mg.

5. a. 36 to 54 mg (2 × 18 = 36)

      (3 × 18 = 54)

   b. 12 to 18 mg (36 ÷ 3)

      (54 ÷ 3)

   c. 150 mg/day; 50 mg per dose

      (50 × 3)   (150 ÷ 3)

   d. Unsafe to give. Overdose ordered. Hold and clarify promptly with the physician.

WORKSHEET 12B (page 280)

1. a. Estimated wt in kg: 10 kg

   b. Actual wt in kg: 9.09 rounded to 9.1 kg

   c. SDR for this child: 18.2 to 36.4 mg per day

      2 × 9.1 = 18.2 mg

      4 × 9.1 = 36.4 mg

   d. Dose ordered: 50 mg daily

   e. Evaluation and decision: Hold and clarify promptly (overdose)

2. a. Estimated wt in kg: 16.5 kg

   b. Actual wt in kg: 15 kg

   c. SDR for this child: 1500 to 3000 mcg per day or 1.5 to 3 mg/day

      15 × 100 mcg = 1500 mcg or 1.5 mg

      15 × 200 mcg = 3000 mcg or 3 mg

   d. Dose ordered: 0.5 mg tid or 1.5 mg per day

   e. Evaluation and decision: Safe to give

3. a. Estimated wt in kg: 12.5 kg

   b. Actual wt in kg: 11.54 rounded to 11.5 kg

      (25.4/2.2)

   c. SDR for this child: 115 to 345 mg per day

      10 × 11.5 = 115 mg

      30 × 11.5 = 345 mg

   d. Dose ordered: 100 mg tid or 300 mg per day

   e. Evaluation and decision: Safe to give

4. a. Estimated wt in kg: 42.5 kg

   b. Actual wt in kg: 38.63 rounded to 38.6 kg

   c. SDR for this child: 386 mg to 579 mg per day in divided doses

   d. Dose ordered: 100 mg q6h or 100 × 4 = 400 mg per day

   e. Evaluation and decision: Safe to give

5. **a.** Estimated wt in kg: 2.5 kg

    b. Actual wt in kg: 2.27 rounded to 2.3 kg

    c. SDR for this child: 23-46 mcg per day

        $10 \times 2.3 = 23$ mcg

        $20 \times 2.3 = 46$ mcg

    d. Dose ordered: 0.03 mg $\times 4 = 0.12$ mg per day
or 120 mcg per day

    e. Evaluation and decision: Hold and clarify
promptly (overdose)

WORKSHEET **12C** (page 283)

1. 0.15 m²
$10 \times 0.15 = 1.5$ mg

2. 0.20 m²*
$15 \times 0.2 = 3$ mg

3. 0.27 m²
$5 \times 0.27 = 1.35$ mg

4. $4 \times 10 = 40$ mg

5. $15 \times 6 = 90$ mg

6. $5 \times 10 = 50$ mg

7. $10 \times 1.8 = 18$ mg

8. 2.72 kg
$2 \times 2.7 = 5.4$ mg

9. $\dfrac{60 \times 100}{3600} = 1.66$

    $\sqrt{1.66} = 1.29$ m²

10. $\dfrac{30 \times 35}{3131} = 0.335$

    $\sqrt{0.335} = 0.578$ rounded to 0.58 m²

---

*Note: Trailing zeros are seen in BSA square meters. Delete them for math calculations.

WORKSHEET **12D** (page 283)

1. **a.** Estimated wt in kg: 13 kg

    b. Actual wt in kg: 11.8 kg

    c. SDR: 1000 to 2000 mg in 4 divided doses

    d. Dose ordered: 500 mg $\times 4$ or 2000 mg

    e. Evaluation and decision: Safe to give

2. **a.** SDR for this child: 4.0 to 6.4 mg four times daily

        5×0.8 m² $= 4.0$ mg (low safe dose)

        8×0.8 m² $= 6.4$ mg (high safe dose)

    b. Dose ordered: 4 mg daily

    c. Evaluation and decision: Safe to give

3. **a.** Estimated wt in kg: 9.5 kg

    b. Actual wt in kg: 8.63 rounded to 8.6 kg

    c. SDR for this child: 0.9 to 2.6 mg in
2 divided doses or 860 to 2600 mcg in
2 divided doses
$0.1 \times 8.6 = 0.86$ mg rounded to 0.9 mg
(low safe dose)
$0.3 \times 8.6 = 2.58$ rounded to 2.6 mg
(high safe dose)

    d. Dose ordered: 2500 mcg bid or
2.5 mg $\times 2 = 5$ mg per day

    e. Evaluation and decision: Hold and
clarify promptly (overdose)

4. **a.** Estimated wt in kg: 4.5 kg

    b. Actual wt in kg: 4.09 rounded to 4.1 kg

    c. SDR for this child: 4.1 to 20.5 mcg/day

        $1 \times 4.1 = 4.1$ mcg

        $5 \times 4.1 = 20.54$ mcg

    d. Dose ordered: 0.01 mg or 10 mcg daily

    e. Evaluation and decision: Safe to give

5. **a.** Estimated wt in kg: 7 kg

    b. Actual wt in kg: 6.36 rounded to 6.4 kg

    c. SDR for this child: 0.13 to 0.32 mg/day
$0.02 \times 6.4 = 0.128$ mg (low safe dose)
$0.05 \times 6.4 = 0.32$ mg (high safe dose)

    d. Dose ordered: 150 mcg $\times 2 = 300$ mcg per day or 0.3 mg/day

    e. Evaluation and decision: Safe to give

1. **a.** Estimated wt in lb: 14 × 2 or 28 lb

b. Actual wt in lb: 30.8 lb

c. SDR for this child: For 24 to 35 lb, 1 tsp

d. Dose ordered: 160 mg

e. Evaluation and decision: Safe to give

f. Give: 1 tsp or 5 mL (80 mg per $\frac{1}{2}$ tsp)

2. **a.** Estimated wt in kg: 66 ÷ 2 = 33 kg

b. Actual wt in kg: 30 kg

c. SDR for this child: 300 to 900 mg per day in 3 to 4 doses

10 × 30 = 300 mg (low safe daily dose)

30 × 30 = 900 mg (maximum safe daily dose)

d. Dose ordered: 300 × 3 = 900 mg per day.

e. Evaluation and decision: Safe to give

f. Give

HAVE   WANT TO HAVE

75 mg : 5 mL :: 300 mg : x mL

$\frac{\cancel{75}}{\cancel{75}} x = \frac{1500}{75}$

$x = 20$ mL

PROOF

75 × 20 = 1500

1 × 1500 = 1500

3. **a.** SDR for this child: 400 to 800 mg/day in 3 to 4 doses

b. Dose ordered in mg:

0.25 g = 250 mg × 3 = 750 mg per day

HAVE   WANT TO HAVE

1 g : 1000 mg :: 0.25 g : x mg

$x = 1000 × 0.25$ or 250 mg

PROOF

1 × 250 = 250

1000 × 0.25 = 250

c. Evaluation and decision: Safe to give

d. Give 12.5 mL

HAVE   WANT TO HAVE

100 mg : 5 mL :: 250 mg : x mL

$\frac{\cancel{100}}{\cancel{100}} x = \frac{\cancel{1250}}{\cancel{100}}$ (5 × 250)

$x = 12.5$ mL

PROOF

100 × 12.5 = 1250

5 × 250 = 1250

4. **a.** SDR for this child:

10 × 0.5 × 4 = 20 mg per day

b. Dose ordered: 20 mg per day divided in 4 doses

c. Evaluation and decision: Safe to give

d. Give 1 tab

5. **a.** Estimated wt in kg: 13.5

b. Actual wt in kg: 12.27 rounded to 12.3 kg

c. SDR for this child: 492 mg per day

(40 mg × 12.3 kg) 164 mg tid

d. Dose ordered: 180 mg per dose or 540 mg per day

e. Evaluation and decision: Slight overdose. Hold and clarify promptly with prescriber.

f. Not applicable

1. a. 22 kg (44 ÷ 2)

   b. 20 kg (44 ÷ 2.2)

   c. SDR for this child: 10 mg (0.5 mg × 20 kg)

   d. Dose ordered: 10 mg

   e. Safe to give

   f. 0.33 mL

      HAVE   WANT TO HAVE

      30 mg : 1 mL :: 10 : x mL

$$\frac{\cancel{30}}{\cancel{30}}x = \frac{\cancel{10}}{\cancel{30}}$$

$$x = 0.33 \text{ mL}$$

      PROOF

      30 × 0.33 = 9.9

      1 × 10 = 10

2. a. Estimated wt: 27 kg

   b. Actual wt: 25.2 kg (2 steps)

      HAVE   WANT TO HAVE

      16 oz : 1 lb :: 8 oz : x lb

      16x = 8

      x = 0.5 lb   Child weighs 55.5 lb ÷ 2.2

                      or 25.2 kg

   c. SDR for this child: 2.52 to 5.04 mg q4h

      0.1 × 25.2 = 2.52 mg

      0.2 × 25.2 = 5.04 mg

   d. Dose ordered: 5 mg IM

   e. Evaluation and decision: Safe to give

   f. Give 0.5 mL

      HAVE   WANT TO HAVE

      10 mg : 1 mL :: 5 mg : x mL

$$\frac{\cancel{10}}{\cancel{10}}x = \frac{5}{10}$$

$$x = 0.5 \text{ mL}$$

      PROOF

      10 × 0.5 = 5

      1 × 5 = 5

3. a. Estimated wt: 8.5 kg

   b. Actual wt: 8 kg (2 steps)

      HAVE   WANT TO HAVE

      16 oz : 1 lb :: 9 oz : x lb

$$\frac{\cancel{16}}{\cancel{16}}x = \frac{9}{16}$$

$$x = 0.56 \text{ or } 0.6 \text{ lb}$$

      Child weighs 17.6 lb ÷ 2.2 or 8 kg

   c. SDR for a child between 7 and 9 kg: 0.2 mg

   d. Dose ordered: 0.2 mg

   e. Evaluation and decision: Safe to give

   f. Give 0.5 mL

      HAVE   WANT TO HAVE

      0.4 mg : 1 mL :: 0.2 mg : x mL

$$\frac{\cancel{0.4}}{\cancel{0.4}}x = \frac{0.2}{0.4}$$

$$x = 0.5 \text{ mL}$$

      PROOF

      0.4 × 0.5 = 0.2

      1 × 0.2 = 0.2

4. a. Estimated wt : 3.5 kg

   b. Actual wt 3.2 kg (1 step)

   c. SDR for this child: 320 to 640 mg per day (based on 3.2 kg wt)

   d. Dose ordered: 1000 mg/day

   e. Evaluation and decision: Overdose. Hold and clarify promptly. Also ask whether IV route is preferred.

   f. Not applicable.

5. a. 88 ÷ 2 = 44 lb

b. Actual wt in kg: 40 kg

KNOW   WANT TO KNOW

1 kg : 2.2 lb :: x kg : 88 lb

$$\frac{\cancel{2.2}}{\cancel{2.2}} x = \frac{8.8}{2.2}$$

$$x = 40 \text{ kg}$$

c. SDR: 0.004 × 40 kg = 0.16 mg

d. 0.16 mg

e. Safe to give

f.

HAVE   WANT TO HAVE

0.4 mg : 2 mL :: 0.16 mg : x mL

$$\frac{\cancel{0.4}}{\cancel{0.4}} x = \frac{0.32}{0.4}$$

$$x = 0.8 \text{ mL}$$

PROOF

0.4 × 0.8 = 0.32

2 × 0.16 = 0.32

WORKSHEET 12G (page 293)

1. a. Estimated wt in kg: 31 kg

b. Actual wt in kg: 28.18 rounded to 28.2 kg

c. SDR for this child: 28.2 to 84.6 mg q24h

d. Dose ordered: 65 mg IV stat

e. Evaluation and decision: Safe to give

f. Dose withdrawn from vial: 0.5 mL

130 mg : 1 mL :: 65 mg : x mL

130x = 195

$$x = 0.5 \text{ mL}$$

PROOF

130 × 1.5 = 195

3 × 65 = 195

2. a. Estimated wt in kg: 27.5 kg

b. Actual wt in kg: 25 kg

c. SDR for this child: 25 to 150 mg

(1 to 6 mg/kg)

1 × 25 = 25

6 × 25 = 150

d. Dose ordered: 25 mg IV stat

e. Evaluation and decision: Safe to give

(The initial dose for this drug must not exceed the lowest dose in the SDR.)

f. Give 2.5 mL

HAVE   WANT TO HAVE

40 mg : 4 mL :: 25 mg : x mL

$$\frac{\cancel{40}}{\cancel{40}} x = \frac{\cancel{100}}{\cancel{40}} (4 \times 25)$$

$$x = 2.5 \text{ mL}$$

PROOF

40 × 2.5 = 100

4 × 25 = 100

3. **a.** Estimated wt in kg: 6.5 kg

   b. Actual wt in kg: 6 kg

   c. SDR for this child: 12 to 15 mg q8h

      2 mg $\times$ 6 kg = 12 mg

      2.5 mg $\times$ 6 kg = 15 mg

   d. Dose ordered: 15 mg q8h

   e. Evaluation and decision: Safe to give

   f. Amount withdrawn from vial: Give 1.8 mL

     HAVE   WANT TO HAVE

     20 mg : 2 mg :: 15 mg : x mL

$$\frac{\cancel{20}}{\cancel{20}}x = \frac{30}{20}$$

$$x = 1.5 \text{ mL}$$

   g. Further dilute *to* 50 mL and administer at 50 mL/hr for 60 min.*

4. **a.** Estimated wt in kg: 12 kg (24 lb $\div$ 2)

   b. Actual wt in kg: 11.09 kg (two-step)

     KNOW   WANT TO KNOW

     1 lb : 16 oz :: x lb : 6 oz

$$\frac{\cancel{16}}{\cancel{16}}x = \frac{\cancel{6}^{\;3}}{\cancel{16}_{\,8}} \qquad x = 0.37 \text{ lb rounded to } 0.4 \text{ lb}$$

     24.4 lb $\div$ 2.2 = 11.09 kg rounded to 11.1 kg

   c. SDR IV for this child: 0.17 mg to 3.9 mg per day

     0.015 $\times$ 11.1 = 0.166 rounded to 0.17 mg per day

     0.35 $\times$ 11.1 = 3.88 rounded to 3.9 mg per day

   d. 0.5 mg IV

   e. Safe to give. 0.5 mg is within the SDR

   f. 2 mL (0.5 mg = 500 mcg)

     KNOW   WANT TO KNOW

     1 mg : 1000 mcg :: 0.5 mg : x mcg

     x = 500 mcg

     PROOF

     1 $\times$ 500 = 500

     1000 $\times$ 0.5 = 500

   g. Infuse at 40 mL per hr for 30 minutes

     HAVE   WANT TO HAVE

     20 mL : 30 min :: x mL : 60 min

     30x = 1200

        x = 40 mL per hr

     PROOF

     20 $\times$ 60 = 1200

     30 $\times$ 40 = 1200

5. **a.** Estimated wt in kg: 13 kg

   b. Actual wt in kg: 11.81 rounded to 11.8 kg

   c. SDR for this child: 590 to 5900 mg

     divided into 4 doses = 1475 mg

     maximum unit dose

     50 $\times$ 11.8 = 590

     500 $\times$ 11.8 = 5900

   d. Dose ordered: 2 g or 2000 mg q6h

   e. Evaluation and decision: Hold and clarify promptly (overdose)

   f. Not applicable

   g. Not applicable

---

*Dilute *"to"* is interpreted as, "Add diluent to the prepared medicine to make 50 mL total volume."

†Dilution *"with"* a substance adds to the volume. Dilution *"to"* an amount does not add to the volume.

1. a. Estimated wt in kg: 16.5 kg
   b. Actual wt in kg: $33 \div 2.2 = 15$
   c. SDR for this child: 300 mg $\div$ 3 or 100 mg tid
   d. Dose ordered: 100 mg $\times$ 3 or 300 mg/day
   e. Evaluation and decision: Safe to give
   f. Give 2 mL

HAVE	WANT TO HAVE
250 mg : 5 mL ::	100 mg : x mL

   $250x = 500$
   $x = 2$ mL

   PROOF
   $250 \times 2 = 500$
   $5 \times 100 = 500$

2. a. SDR for this child: $5 \times 30 = 150$ mg per day in 2 or 3 divided doses
   b. Dose ordered: 75 mg bid or 150 mg per day
   c. Evaluation and decision: Safe to give
   d. Give 11.3 mL

HAVE	WANT TO HAVE
100 mg : 15 mL ::	75 mg : x mL

   $100x = 1125$
   $x = 11.25$ rounded to 11.3 mL

   PROOF
   $100 \times 11.25 = 1125$
   $15 \times 75 = 1125$

3. a. Estimated wt in kg: 24.5 kg
   b. Actual wt in kg: 22.27 rounded to 22.3 kg
   c. SDR for this child (IV): 44.6 mcg to 55.8 mcg ($\frac{1}{2}$ of po dose)
   89.2 mcg po dose $\div$ 2 = 44.6 mcg (low safe dose)
   111.5 mcg po dose $\div$ 2 = 55.75 rounded to 55.8 mcg (high safe dose)
   d. Dose ordered: 0.1 mg (100 mcg) IV q am

HAVE	WANT TO HAVE
1 mg : 1000 mcg ::	0.1 mg : x mcg

   $x = 1000 \times 0.1 = 100$ mcg
   e. Evaluation and decision: Hold and clarify promptly (100 mcg is an overdose for IV administration at this child's weight)
   f. Not applicable

4. a. Estimated wt in kg: 40
   b. Actual wt in kg: 36.36 kg rounded to 36.4 kg
   c. SDR for this child: 3.6 to 7.3 mg
   $0.1 \times 36.4 = 3.64$ mg (rounded to 3.6 mg)
   $0.2 \times 36.4 = 7.28$ mg (rounded to 7.3 mg)
   d. Dose ordered: 10 mg
   e. Evaluation and Decision: Hold and clarify (overdose)
   f. Not applicable

5. a. SDR for this child: 40 mg per 0.6 m^2 = 24 mg per day
   b. Dose ordered: 30 mg per day
   c. Evaluation and decision: Hold and clarify promptly (overdose)
   d. Not applicable

6. a. Estimated wt in kg: 11 kg
   b. Actual wt in kg: 10 kg
   c. SDR for this child 500 to 1000 mg per day in 4 divided doses (250 mg each max)
   d. Dose ordered: 0.25 g IV q 6h
   e. Evaluation and decision: Safe to give
   f. Give 1 mL

KNOW	WANT TO KNOW
1000 mg : 1 g ::	x mg : 0.25 g

   $1000 \times 0.25 = 250$ mg

   PROOF
   $1000 \times 0.25 = 250$
   $1 \times 250 = 250$

HAVE	WANT TO HAVE
250 mg : 1 mL ::	250 : x mL

   $250x = 250$
   $x = 1$ mL

   PROOF
   $250 \times 1 = 250$
   $1 \times 250 = 250$

7. **a.** Estimated wt in kg: 3 kg
   b. Actual wt in kg: 2.72 rounded to 2.7 kg
   c. SDR for this child: Up to 8.1 mEq q24h
   $3 \times 2.7 = 8.1$
   d. Dose ordered: 0.9 mEq q8h rounded 2.7 q24h
   e. Evaluation and decision: Safe to give;
   monitor lab potassium values for therapeutic
   range, and assess patient's heart rate, rhythm,
   and muscle tone. May be underdosed.
   f. Add 0.45 mL KCl to compatible IV and mix well.
   HAVE   WANT TO HAVE
   2 mEq : 1 mL :: 0.9 mEq : x mL
   $$\frac{\cancel{2}}{\cancel{2}}x = \frac{0.9}{2} = 0.45 \text{ mL}$$
   PROOF
   $2 \times 0.45 = 0.9$
   $1 \times 0.9 = 0.9$

8. **a.** Estimated wt in kg: 15.5 kg
   b. Actual wt in kg: 14.09 rounded to 14.1
   c. SDR for this child: Up to 1410 mg in
   2 doses or up to 705 mg dose
   $100 \times 14.1 = 1410$
   d. Dose ordered: 600 mg IV q12h or
   1200 mg/day
   e. Evaluation and decision: Safe to give
   f. Use 6 mL after reconstituting
   HAVE   WANT TO HAVE
   100 mg : 1 mL :: 600 mg : x mL
   $$\frac{\cancel{100}}{\cancel{100}}x = \frac{\cancel{600}}{\cancel{100}}$$
   $x = 6$ mL
   PROOF
   $100 \times 6 = 600$
   $1 \times 600 = 600$
   g. Infuse for 30 min at 60 mL/hr
   HAVE   WANT TO HAVE
   30 mL : 30 min :: x mL : 60 min
   $$\frac{\cancel{30}}{\cancel{30}}x = \frac{\cancel{1800}}{\cancel{30}}$$
   $x = 60$ mL/hr
   PROOF
   $30 \times 60 = 1800$
   $60 \times 30 = 1800$

9. **a.** Draw up 0.2 mL in the enclosed dropper.
   b. Use enclosed dropper to administer along the
   inside of the cheek.
   HAVE   WANT TO HAVE
   80 mg : 0.8 mL :: 20 mg : x mL
   $$\frac{\cancel{80}}{\cancel{80}}x = \frac{16}{80}$$
   $x = 0.2$ mL
   PROOF
   $80 \times 0.2 = 16$
   $0.8 \times 20 = 16$

10. **a.** 2 mg per lb of body weight <u>divided</u> into
    2 doses first day 28 mg each
    b. Hold and contact prescriber promptly.
    Overdose (double the recommended
    dose for first day). $\frac{56}{2}$ mg per day $= 28$ mg per
    dose
    c. N/A

WORKSHEET 12I (page 299)

1. **b**
   This is a *two-step* problem.
   Estimated wt in kg: 25 kg
   Step 1:
   2.2 lb : 1 kg :: 50 lb : x kg
   $x = 50 \div 2.2$ or 22.7 kg
   Step 2:
   20 mg : 1 kg :: x mg : 22.7 kg
   $x = 20 \times 22.7$ or 454 mg

   PROOF
   $2.2 \times 22.7 = 49.94$ or 50
   $1 \times 50 = 50$
   PROOF
   $20 \times 22.7 = 45$
   $1 \times 454 = 454$

2. **c**
   30 mg : 1 m² :: x mg : 1.2Ø m²
   $x = 30 \times 1.2Ø$ or 36 mg

   PROOF
   $30 \times 1.2Ø = 36$
   $1 \times 36 = 36$

3. b

5 mL = 1 tsp

5 mL : 1 tsp :: x mL : 1.5 tsp

x = 7.5 mL

Measure 7.5 mL

PROOF

5 × 1.5 = 7.5

1 × 7.5 = 7.5

4. c

This is a *three-step* problem.

Estimated wt in kg: 25 ÷ 2 or 12.5 kg

Step 1:

2.2 lb : 11.4 kg :: 25 lb : x kg

x = 25 ÷ 2.2 or 11.4 kg

PROOF

2.2 × 11.4 = 25

1 × 25 = 25

Step 2:

2 mg : 1 kg :: x mg : 11.4 kg

x = 2 × 11.4 or 22.8 mg *low safe dose*

PROOF

2 × 11.4 = 22.8

1 × 22.8 = 22.8

Step 3:

5 mg : 1 kg :: x mg : 11.4 kg

x = 57 mg *maximum safe dose*

30 mg is within SDR of 22.8 mg to 57 mg.

PROOF

5 × 11.4 = 57

1 × 57 = 57

---

*Note: Concentrated drops are not interchangeable with other liquid medicines.

5. a

Estimated wt: 55/2 or 27.5 kg

Step 1: lb to kg

2.2 lb : 1 kg :: 55 lb : x kg

2.2x = 5.5

x = 25 kg

PROOF

2.2 × 25 = 55

1 × 55 = 55

Step 2: SDR

2 mg : 1 kg :: x mg : 25 kg

x = 2 × 25 or 50 mg *low safe dose*

Compare low SDR with the order. They are equal for the q8h order.

No need to calculate high safe dose. Give the medication.

PROOF

2 × 25 = 50

1 × 50 = 50

6. d

Estimated wt: 5.5/2 or 2.5 kg

Step 1: lb to kg

2.2 lb : 1 kg :: 5.5 lb : x kg

2.2x = 5.5x = 2.2 kg = 2.5 kg actual wt

Step 2: SDR

40 mg : 1 kg :: x mg : 2.5 kg

x = 40 × 2.5   or   100 mg/day

Compare the SDR with the order. The 125 mg order exceeds the 100 mg recommended dose. Clarify with the physician promptly and document promptly.

PROOF

2.2 × 2.5 = 5.5

1 × 5.5 = 5.5

PROOF

40 × 2.5 = 100

1 × 100 = 100

7. b

Estimated wt: 6 ÷ 2 or 3 kg

This is a *three-step* problem

Step 1: lb to kg

2.2 lb : 1 kg :: 55 lb : x kg

$2.2x = 55$

$x = 25$ kg

Step 2: SDR

5 mg : 1 kg :: x mg : 6 kg

$x = 5 \times 6$ or 30 mg

Compare the SDR with the order. 30 mg ÷ 2 = 15 mg bid. The order is 15 mg bid.
The order is safe.

Step 3: Calculate the unit dose.

30 mg : 5 mL :: 15 mg : x mL

$30x = 75 \times 2.5$ mL

Give 2.5 mL using a syringe to measure, if necessary.

PROOF

$2.2 \times 25 = 55$

$1 \times 55 = 55$

PROOF

$5 \times 6 = 30$

$1 \times 30 = 30$

PROOF

$30 \times 2.5 = 75$

$5 \times 15 = 75$

8. d

Metric equivalents

1000 mcg = 1 mg

500 mcg = 0.5 mg

200 mcg = 0.2 mg

Estimate: You want to give *more than double* the 10 mL dose.

HAVE	WANT TO HAVE
200 mcg : 10 mL :: 500 mcg : x mL	

$\dfrac{\cancel{200}}{\cancel{200}}x = \dfrac{50\cancel{00}}{2\cancel{00}}$

$x = 25$ mL

PROOF

$200 \times 2.5 = 500$

$1 \times 500 = 500$

9. d

Estimated wt in kg : 29 kg (58 ÷ 2)

Step 1: lb to kg

2.2 lb : 1 kg :: 58 lb : x kg

$2.2x = 58$

$x = 26.36$ rounded to 26.4 kg

Step 2: Low SDR

Low safe dose range is 0.1 mg per kg or 2.6 mg.
The order is for 5 mg; therefore, continue and
calculate high SDR.

Step 3: High SDR

High safe dose range is 0.2 mg per kg or 5.3 mg.

0.2 mg : 1 kg :: x mg : 26.4 kg

$x = 5.28$ mg rounded to 5.3 mg

The order for 5 mg is within safe range.

(Step 3 Dose Calculation)

You want to give 1/2 of the 10 mg available

HAVE	WANT TO HAVE
10 mg : 1 mL :: 5 mg : x mL	

$\dfrac{\cancel{10}}{\cancel{10}}x = \dfrac{5}{10}$

$x = 0.5$ mL dose

PROOF

$2.2 \times 26.36 = 57.92$ or 58

$1 \times 58 = 58$

PROOF

$0.2 \times 26.4 = 5.28$ rounded to 5.3

$1 \times 5.3 = 5.3$

PROOF

$10 \times 0.5 = 5$

$1 \times 5 = 5$

10. **b**

Estimated wt in kg is 15 kg.

lb to kg

2.2 : 1 kg :: 30 : x kg

$$\frac{2.2}{2.2}x = \frac{30}{2.2}$$

$$x = 13.6 \text{ kg}$$

SDR

25 mg : 1 kg :: x mg : 13.6 kg

$x = 25 \times 13.6$ or 340 mg day in *4 divided*

doses, or 85 mg per dose

50 mg = 2 times the 25 mg dose of 680 mg per day high safe dose per day

Decision: Hold the order. The drug is supposed to be given 4 times a day, not 3 times a day; and the amount ordered, 750 mg per day, exceeds the recommended safe dose of 680 mg per day.

PROOF

$2.2 \times 13.6 = 29.92$

$1 \times 30 = 30$

PROOF

$25 \times 13.6 = 340$

$1 \times 340 = 340$

CHAPTER 12 FINAL: CHILDREN'S DOSAGES (page 303)

1. **a.** Estimated wt in kg: 21 kg
    b. Actual wt in kg: 19.09 rounded to 19.1 kg
    c. SDR for this child: 477.5 to 955 mg per day in 4 divided doses
    d. Dose ordered: 200 mg × 4 or 800 mg/day
    e. Evaluation and decision: Safe to give
    f. Give 8 mL.

2. **a.** Actual wt in kg: 19.09 rounded to 19.1 kg
    b. SDR for this child: 573 to 955 mg/day in 4 divided doses
    c. Dose ordered: 175 mg × 4 or 700 mg/day
    d. Evaluation and decision: Safe to give
    e. Give 4.4 mL.

3. **a.** SDR for this child: 150 mg maximum (6 × 25 mg) in 24 hr in 4-6 divided doses
    b. Dose ordered: 25 mg × 4 or 100 mg per day
    c. Evaluation and decision: Safe to give
    d. Dose to be administered: 2 tsp or 25 mg per dose

4. **a.** SDR for this child: 400 to 800 mg per day
    b. Dose ordered: 2000 mg/day
    c. Evaluation and decision: Overdose. Hold and clarify promptly. Document promptly.
    d. Dose to be administered: Not applicable

5. **a.** Estimated wt in kg: 17.5 kg
    b. Actual wt in kg: 15.9 kg
    c. SDR for this child: 0.3 mg (for 12 to 26 kg child)
    d. Dose ordered: 0.3 mg
    e. Safe to give.
    f. Give 0.75 mL in anterolateral thigh.

6. **a.** Estimated wt in kg: 17.5 kg
    b. Actual wt in kg: 15.9 kg
    c. SDR for this child: 318 to 636 mg/day
    d. Dose ordered: 500 mg × 3 or 1500 mg
    e. Evaluation and decision: Overdose. Hold and clarify promptly. Document promptly.
    f. Dose to be administered: Not applicable

7. **a.** SDR: 159 mg to 318 mg per day divided in 2 to 3 doses.
    b. Dose of 100 mg tid is within safe limits. It is safe to give.
    c. Give one tablet (0.1g = 100 mg) tid.

8. **a.** Actual wt in kg: 15.9 kg
    b. SDR for this child: 0.795 or 0.8 to 1.6 mg q4h
    c. Dose ordered: 5 mg q4h
    d. Evaluation and decision: Hold and clarify promptly (overdose) Document.
    e. Not applicable

9. **a.** BSA in m²: 1.10 m²
    b. SDR for this child: Up to 44 mg per day
    1.10 × 10 × 4 = 44
    c. Dose ordered: 40 mg per day
    d. Evaluation and decision: Safe to give
    e. Give 2 tab.

10. **a.** 1980 mcg (90 mcg × 22 kg)

  b. 1.98 mg rounded to 2 mg

   KNOW   WANT TO KNOW

   $\dfrac{\cancel{1000}}{\cancel{1000}} x = \dfrac{198\cancel{0}}{100\cancel{0}}$

     $x = 1.98$ mg rounded to 2 mg

  c. 2.2 mL

   1 mg : 1.1 mL :: 2 mg : x mL

   $x = 2.2$ mL

  d. 2 vials

  e. 11 calibrations

  f. 0.7 mL per minute

   2.2 mL : 3 minutes :: x mL : 1 minute

   2.2x = 3

     $x = 0.73$ mL per minute or approximately 0.7 mL per minute

  g.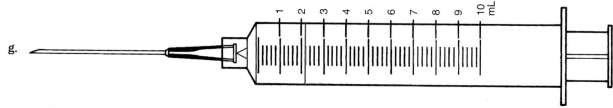

  h. a. 1.5 mL; b. 0.8 ml; c. 0

Multiple-Choice Final

1. c	**2.** c	**3.** a	**4.** c	(page 309)
5. d	**6.** c	**7.** b	**8.** c	
9. d	**10.** a	**11.** c	**12.** b	
13. a	**14.** c; d	**15.** a	**16.** a	
17. b	**18.** c	**19.** d; c	**20.** c; d	
21. a; d	**22.** a	**23.** b	**24.** b; d	
25. d; d	**26.** b	**27.** c	**28.** d	
29. a	**30.** a			

Comprehensive Final

1. 2 tabs   **(page 321)**

2. 1 tab

3. 2 tabs

4. 2 tabs

5. 1 tab

6. 1 tab

7. 7.5 mL

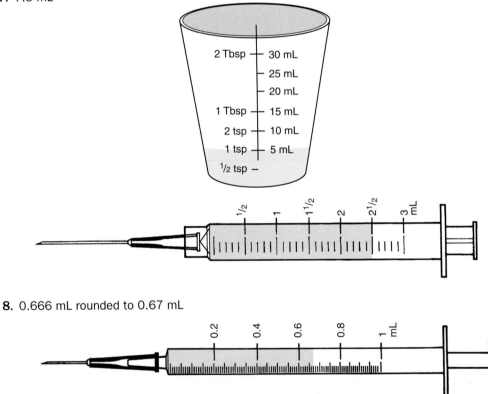

8. 0.666 mL rounded to 0.67 mL

9. *Error:* 0845 Dose given 45 minutes after prior dose. Order stated q4h intervals prn.
    Current Actions: Prescribe complete bed rest for patient, assess mental status and vital signs, notify supervising nurse/charge nurse and physician immediately, and obtain orders for medication to reverse.

Establish a patent IV line according to hospital policy in case emergency care may be needed.

Have crash cart close at hand. Document the error and to whom reported, patient evaluations, and all interventions, and continue to make the above assessments and evaluate. Fill out incident report. Continue to assess and evaluate patient every 5 to 15 minutes until patient is stabilized, then gradually extend assessment time.

Prevention: prn and stat medications must be charted as soon as possible after administration. Nurse A needed to report to Nurse B orally when her patients were due for their next prn medications. Nurse B needed to state she was too busy to care for additional patients beyond her own caseload. Nurse B needed to check record carefully to see when last medication for pain was given. Nurse B needed to ask patient when last medication for pain was received. (This is a recommended double-check but is not always reliable. The accuracy of response depends on the patient's mental status.) Refer to Hand-off Communication Report, Appendix A.

10. 1.16 mL rounded to 1.2 mL

11. 1.5 mL

12. **a.** 250,000 units/mL
    b. Give 1.6 mL.

    c. 500,000 units/mL
    d. Give 0.8 mL.

13. **a.** Add 2 mL of diluent
    b. 4 vials per 24 hr
    c. Give 2.4 mL/dose.

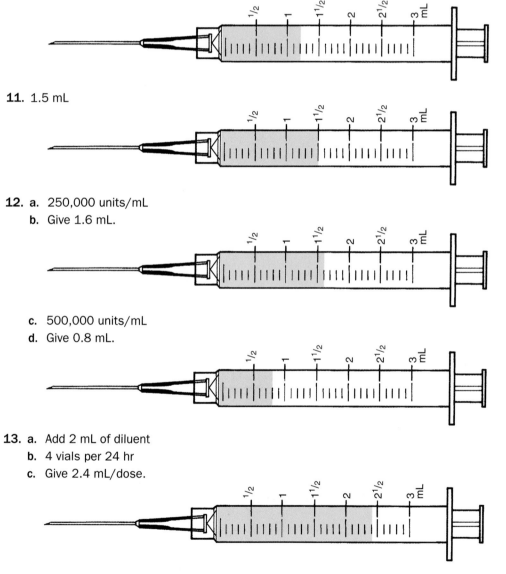

14. **a.** 2.5 mL sterile water for injection

b. Store in refrigerator. Can be at room temperature for only 24 hr.
Last dose will be given in 32 hours.

c. Give 0.8 mL.

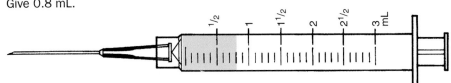

15. **a.** 21 gtt/min

b. 83 mL/hr on infusion device

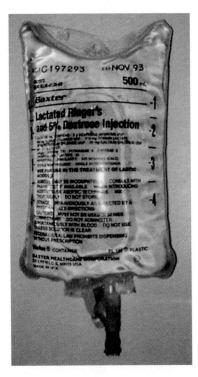

16. **a.** 75 mL/hr

b. 75 gtt/min

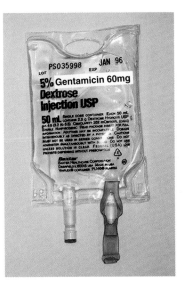

17. **a.** 104 mL/hr
   b. 17 gtt/min

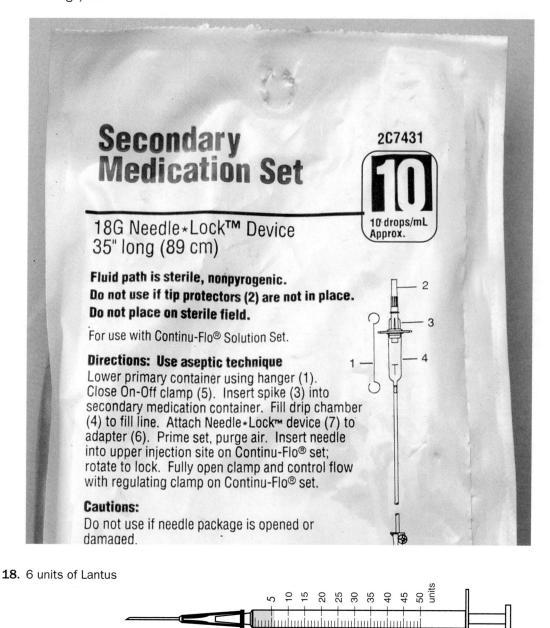

18. 6 units of Lantus

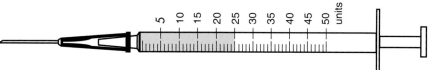

19. 70 mL per hr

20. 25 units of R insulin

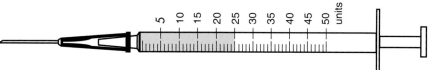

21. **a.** Set infusion rate at 19 mL/hr
   b. IV will be completed at 2139 hours.

22. 0.8 mL Fragmin

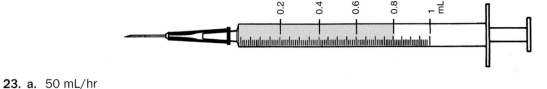

23. a. 50 mL/hr
   b. 20 hr to infuse

24. a. Give 5961 units of heparin for the bolus dose.
   b. 1309 units per hr will infuse
   c. 15 hr 12 min
   d. 33 mL per hr

25. a. 19 g per bag amino acids
   b. 29 g per bag carbohydrates
   c. 14 g per bag lipids

26. a. 76 protein kilocalories
   b. 116 carbohydrate kilocalories
   c. 126 fat kilocalories
   d. Total kilocalories = 318

27. a. 2 mEq per mL
   b. 149 mg per mL
   c. 15 mL

28. a. 2 mL
   b. 120 seconds
   c. 1 mL per min for 2 min
   d. 12 seconds per calibration

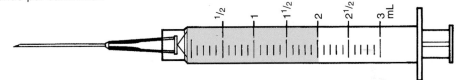

29. 10 mg; 2 tab (based on approximate DSA of 1.1)

30. a. 24,000 mcg per hr (5 mcg × 80 kg × 60 min)
   b. 24 mg per hr
   c. 0.8 mg per mL (200 mg ÷ 250 mL)
   d. Flow rate is correct

Note: Based on national agencies including TJC and ISMP recommendations to reduce medication errors with KCL administration, the pharmacy now supplies KCL premixed solutions. The nurse still needs to check the pharmacy label with the order to be sure the correct amount has been added.
Note: Many EID devices can deliver tenths of a mL per hr.

Index

A

abbreviations
  common IV solutions, 158-161f
  dc use, 45t
  Do Not Use list, 43, 44t
  drug forms, 47
  drug measurements, 46
  errors and, 45-46t
  hs use, 45t
  metric system, 72
  physician's orders, 58f
  qid/qd/qod use, 45t
  time and route, 43
addition
  of decimals, 16-17
  fractions and mixed numbers, 7-8
additives, TPN, 210
ADD-VANTAGE piggyback system, 171, 172f
administration of medications. *see* medication administration
adults
  elderly, 91, 265f, 281, 285
  maximum single injection, 131
allergies
  heparin, 265
  penicillin/cephalosporins, 177, 303, 304f
anaphylactic shock, 135
animal insulin, 225
anticoagulants
  half-life of, 258-259
  injectable, 257-271
  low-molecular-weight, 259-260
  oral, 271-272
  subcutaneous heparin injections, 260-266
antidotes
  to oral anticoagulants, 269
  to warfarin, 271
aqueous suspensions, 49
Arixtra (fondaparinux sodium), 259-260

B

blood sugar levels, 245-247
body surface area (BSA) calculations, 277-279, 281-283
bolus IV administration, 193-196

C

CADD-Prizm infusion pumps, 173
calculating doses. *see* dosage calculations

capsules, 48
carbohydrate intake and insulin dosage, 243-248
catheters (intermittent flushing ranges), 151t
central lines, 150, 151f
central parenteral nutrition (CPN), 206, 211, 212f, 216
cephalosporin allergies, 177, 303, 304f
charting by exception, 57. *see also* documentation
children. *see* pediatric medication administrations
clinical alerts. *see also* error prevention
  abbreviation confusions, 45-46t
  allergies to heparin, 265
  anticoagulants, 259, 260
  body surface area (BSA) calculations, 282, 283
  bolus IV administration, 194
  confusion of similar names, 62
  confusion of units of medication with milligrams, 133
  diabetes mellitus vision loss, 227
  documentation of medication administration, 42, 191
  Do Not Use list, 43, 44t
  drug concentration, 55
  drug sensitivity, 135
  elderly patients, 91, 265
  electronic infusion devices, 175
  elixirs *versus* concentrated drops, 286
  gravity piggyback infusions, 170
  hematomas, 261
  heparin, 259, 265, 266
  high-alert medications, 183
  household measurements, 92
  hyperglycemia, 210, 302
  hypoglycemia, 225
  infants' *versus* childrens' doses, 81, 82
  insulin, 229, 230, 231, 232, 238
  insulin syringes, 231-232
  intramuscular injections, 106, 128, 131
  IV ports, 170
  IV rate, 154, 294
  Lantus insulin use, 231
  liquid medication preparation, 82
  massaging injection sites, 261
  maximum single injections, 131
  measurement utensils, 50
  medication reconciliation, 64
  metric system equivalents, 71
  multiple-dose vials, 121
  needle safety, 106

clinical alerts *(Continued)*
  overdose risk, 13, 82
  patient identification, 64
  pediatric IV medications, 293, 294
  pediatric oral medications, 285, 286
  peripheral lines, 151
  pill cutting, 81
  reconstitution, 126
  resuscitation equipment, 135
  rounding, 76
  safe dose ranges, 63, 284
  second independent nurse checks, 63
  similar names of antibiotics, 293
  single dose vials, 52
  smart pumps, 184
  substitution of forms/utensils, 50
  syringes, 261
  tablets, 50
  titrated infusions, 182, 185
  total dose *versus* unit dose errors, 52
  total parenteral nutrition administration, 205
  TPN administration, 211
  TPN label, 209
  TPN rate, 210
  unit dose, 54
  units of measurement, 74
  verbal and telephone orders, 56
  written ratio and proportion calculations, 77
combined medications, 237
common denominators, 5-6
critical care IV practice, 190-191
crystals, dilution of, 127-129

D

dalteparin (Fragmin), 259, 260
dc abbreviation, use of, 45t
decimal fractions
  addition of, 16-17
  changing fractions to, 20-21
  changing percentages to, 21-23
  comparison of, 12, 16
  division of, 18-20
  multiplication of, 17-18
  rounding, 13-14, 15
  subtraction of, 17
  value of, 12, 14-15
deep vein thrombosis (DVT), 257, 260
delivery sets, IV, 169-175
denominators, 5-6
diabetes mellitus (DM), 223-224. *see also* insulin
diluents, 126

Page numbers followed by *f* refer to figures, *t* refer to tables, *b* refer to boxes

dilution
  pediatric IV medications, 291-294
  piggyback, 170-171
  of powders or crystals, 127-129
division
  of decimals, 18-20
  of fractions and mixed numbers, 10-11
divisors, 10, 18
DM (diabetes mellitus), 223-224. *see also*
    insulin
documentation
  charting by exception, 57
  of IVs, 191
  medical administration records (MARs)
    (*see also* physician's orders)
    examples of, 58-60f
    heparin injection, 258f
    IV therapy, 168f
    overview of, 57-61
    reconstitution, 129
    total parenteral nutrition, 208f, 212-213f,
      212f
  of medication administration (in general), 42
  physicians' orders (*see also* documentation;
    medical administration records (MARs))
    abbreviations used in, 58f
    comparing ordered and available unit dose
      amounts, 79-80
    identifying units and milliequivalents in, 78
    incomplete, 62-63
    insulin, 232
    interpreting, 56
    for total parenteral nutrition, 212f, 215f
    validation of TPN label with, 209
Do Not Use list (abbreviations), 43, 44t
dosage calculations
  comparing ordered and available unit dose
    amounts, 79-80
  elderly patients, 91
  error prevention for, 45-46t
  estimating weight in kg before, 278-279
  heparin, 270-271
  hourly drug and flow rate for titrated infu-
    sions, 184-185
  insulin, 243-248
  intravenous (IV) administration, 151-152
    advanced, 181, 186-187, 189-190
    critical care IV practice, 190-191
    drop factor, 152-153
    drops per minute, 154
    flow meter tape, 154, 155f
    hourly drug and flow rate formula for ti-
      trated infusions, 184-185
    IV drug/flow rates, 184-185, 187-188
    IV push medications, 195-198
    IV solute, 163-168
    medication doses infusing in existing so-
      lutions, 188-189
    for obstetrics, 192
    problems, 156-158
  IV medications, 151-158

dosage calculations *(Continued)*
  maximum single injections, 131
  multidose preparations, 52
  multiple-strength decisions, 130-138
  overdose risks, 13, 79, 82
  pediatric administrations, 295-299
    elixirs *versus* concentrated drops, 286
    infants' *versus* childrens' doses, 81, 82
    injection sites, 288-289
    mg/kg method, 278-279
  ratio and proportion calculation method
    one-step metric, 76-78
    practice, 35-36, 35-37
    setting up, 32-33, 34-35
    two-step, 83-91
  reconstitution, 121-138
  rounding, 74-76
    drops, 75-76
    using metric system, 74-75
  rounding doses
    using metric system, 74-76
  safe practices for, 63
  subcutaneous heparin, 260-266
  unit dose calculations, 54
    for adults *versus* children, 63, 291
    confusion of units of medication with
      milligrams, 133
    definition of, 79
    for elderly patients, 91
    identifying units in, 78
    milliunits, 78
    multiples of unit doses, 75
    total dose *versus* unit dose errors, 52
    use of "unit," 78
double-lumen catheters, 151f
drop factor calculations, 152-154
droppers, 50
drops (gtts)
  concentrated, 286
  drop factor calculations, 152-153
  drops per minute calculations, 154
  elixirs *versus* concentrated, 286
  measurement, 75-76
drug forms abbreviations, 47
drug measurement abbreviations, 46

E
elderly patients
  adverse effects of medications in, 91
  dosage calculations, 265f, 281, 285
electronic infusion devices, 171-173
elixirs, 49, 286
emulsions, 49
Enoxaparin (Lovenox), 259
equivalent fractions
  changing fractions to, 6
  placement of known, 76
  using correct equivalents, 83
equivalent measurements
  metric/apothecary/household, 91-92
  volume and weight, 102

error prevention. *see also* clinical alerts
  caused by abbreviations, 45-46t
  in equivalency calculations, 83
  second independent nurse check and, 63
  total dose *versus* unit dose errors, 52
  web sites related to, 43
extended-release capsules, 49
extracts, 49

F
fat embolus risk, 206
flo meter tape, 154, 155f
flow rates
  compatibility charts and, 182
  estimating hourly, 190
  formula, 187-188
  gravity flow, 153, 170, 175
  hourly drug and flow rate formula, 187-188
  pediatric IV, 294
  titrated infusions, 185
fluid extracts, 49
flushing IV lines, 151
fractions
  adding/subtracting, 5-6
  addition of mixed numbers and, 7-8
  decimal
    addition of, 16-17
    changing fractions to, 20-21
    changing percentages to, 21-23
    comparison of, 12, 16
    division of, 18-20
    multiplication of, 17-18
    rounding, 13-14, 15
    subtraction of, 17
    value of, 12, 14-15
  definition of, 3
  division of mixed numbers and, 10-11
  equivalent, 6
  expressing ratios as, 31
  higher terms, 7
  improper, 4-5
  multiplication of mixed numbers and, 10
  reducing, 6-7
  subtraction of mixed numbers and, 8-9
  value of, 11
Fragmin (dalteparin), 259, 260

G
generic names of drugs, 42, 51
glucagon emergency kit, 224f
glucose levels, 245-247
granules, 49
gravity flow, 153, 170, 175
gtts. *see* drops (gtts)

H
hand-off report, 333-334
hematomas, 257, 261
heparin, 257-259. *see also* anticoagulants
  dosage calculations, 270-271
  IV administration, 266-271

heparin *(Continued)*
  medical administration records (MARs), 258f
  resistance, 265
  saline/heparin locks, 149
  subcutaneous injections, 260-266
HEP-LOCK, 149
high-alert medications, 183t, 335
higher terms (fractions), 7
hospital protocols/policies. *see* protocols/
  policies
hourly drug and flow rate formula, 184-185
household measurements compared with metric measurements, 91-92
hs abbreviation, use of, 45t
human insulin, 225
hyperglycemia, 206, 210-211, 223, 225, 302
hypoglycemia, 225

I

incident reports, 60f
infants. *see* pediatric medication administrations
infusion devices, 149-150. *see also* intravenous
  (IV) administration
  electronic, 171-173
  insulin, 242-243
  pediatric medication administration, 291
  piggyback, 170-171
  smart pumps, 184-185
  and solute calculations, 175-176
injectable anticoagulants, 257-266
injectable liquid forms, 50, 104f
injection sites. *see also* intramuscular (IM) administration; intravenous (IV) administration; subcutaneous (subcut) injections
  heparin, 257, 258f
  insulin, 224
  intradermal, 103, 105f
  intramuscular, 103, 105f
  massaging, 261
  pediatric, 288-289
  subcutaneous, 103, 105f
injuries, needlestick, 106, 107f
INR (international normalized ratio), 271
insertion points for IV lines, 150
insulin
  animal, 225
  diabetes mellitus and, 223-224
  dosage based on carbohydrate intake, 243-
    247
  human, 225
  infusion devices, 242-243
  injection sites, 224
  intermediate-acting, 230
  intermediate- and rapid-acting mixtures,
    230-231
  intravenous, 249-251
  long-acting, 230-231
  mixing, 237-241
  oral diabetes medications (ODMs), 251
  orders, 232

insulin *(Continued)*
  prefilled pens, 226f, 228t, 259f
  rapid-acting, 229-230
  recombinant DNA, 225
  sliding-scale calculations, 241
  syringes, 231-232, 233-236
  types of, 225-231
  U-100, 229-231
  vials, 227
intermediate-acting insulin, 230
intermittent peripheral infusion devices
  (IPIDs), 150
international normalized ratio (INR), 271
international time, 55
interpreting medication labels, 51-55
interpreting orders, 56
intradermal (ID) injections, 103, 105f
intramuscular (IM) administration, 103, 105f,
  128, 131
  aspiration before injecting, 134
  pediatric medications, 288-290
intravenous (IV) administration. *see also* infusion devices; medication administration
  abbreviations related to, 158-161f
  bolus, 193-196
  calculations, 151-152
    advanced, 181, 186-187, 189-190
    critical care IV practice, 190-191
    drop factor, 152-153
    drops per minute, 154
    flow meter tape, 154, 155f
    heparin, 267-269
    hourly drug and flow rate formula for ti-
      trated infusions, 184-185
    insulin, 250-251
    IV drug/flow rates, 184-185, 187-188
    IV push medications, 195-198
    IV solute, 163-168
    medication doses infusing in existing so-
      lutions, 188-189
    for obstetrics, 192
    problems, 156-158
  combining drugs for, 237
  delivery sets, 169-175
  drug sensitivities and, 135
  flushing IV lines, 151
  heparin, 266-271
  insulin, 249-251
  liquid injectables, 50, 104f
  parenteral mixes, 109-112
    reconstitution, 130-133
  pediatric, 291-294
  percentage of solute in IV bags, 161-168
  piggyback, 170-171, 174-175
  reconstituting medications for, 126
  sites, 103
  titrated infusions, 182-183, 184-185
  types of IV lines, 150-151
intravenous (IV) flushes, 151
intravenous piggyback (IVPB), 170-171, 174-
  175

IPIDs (intermittent peripheral infusion de-
  vices), 150
IV nutrition. *see* total parenteral nutrition
  (TPN)
IVPB (intravenous piggyback), 170-171, 174-175

J

Joint Commission on Accreditation of Healthcare Organizations (JCACO)
  Do Not Use list (abbreviations), 43, 44t
  patient identification, 63

K

ketoacidosis, 242
kilocalories (kcal), 210

L

labels
  insulin vials, 227
  interpreting, 51-55
  reconstitution, 121-126
  sample PCN, 217f
  TPN bag, 209
  validation of label with physician's order, 209
Lantus insulin, 231
lipids, 206-210
liquid medication forms, 49-50
  injectable, 50, 104f
  measuring, 50, 119, 120f
  reconstitution, 121-126
long-acting insulin, 230-231
lovenox (enoxaparin), 259
lowest common denominators, 5-6
lowest terms (fractions), 6-7
low-molecular-weight anticoagulants, 259-260

M

manufacturers' drip rates, 154
markers, 195
MARS. *see* medical administration records
  (MARs)
measurement systems
  abbreviations related to, 46
  equivalent measures
    metric/apothecary/household, 91-92
    volume and weight, 102
  household, 91-92
  for liquid medications, 50, 119, 120f
  measurement conversion problems, 83-91
  metric system, 46t
  for oral pediatric medications, 285-289
  syringe amounts, 99-102
measurement utensils, 50
medical administration records (MARs). *see*
  also documentation; physician's orders
  examples of, 58-60f
  heparin injection, 258f
  IV therapy, 168f
  overview of, 57-61
  reconstitution, 129
  total parenteral nutrition, 208f, 212-213f

medication administration. *see also* intravenous (IV) administration; pediatric medication administrations
  abbreviations related to
    Do Not Use list, 43, 44t
    drug forms, 47
    drug measurements, 46
    errors and, 45-46t
    refused/withheld medications, 42
    time and route, 43
  combining drugs for, 237
  delivery and, 48-50
  direct IV bolus, 193-196
  documentation of, 42
  heparin, 257-259
  high-alert medications, 183t, 335
  hourly drug and flow rate formula, 184-185
  incident reports, 60f
  infusions, 149-150
  liquid forms, 49-50
  MAR forms, 57-61
  medication carts, 48
  medication labels, 51-55
  oral
    anticoagulants, 271-272
    calculations, 80-91, 84-91
    for children/infants, 285-289
    oral diabetes medications, 251
    problems, 80-83
    syringes, 120f
  physicians' orders, 56, 62
  polypharmacy and, 266
  prn orders, 59f
  safe practices summary, 62-64
  solid forms, 48-49
  stat, 42, 57
  subcutaneous, 103, 105f, 260-266, 288-290
  time of, 42, 55-56
  total parenteral nutrition (TPN), 205-210
  24-hour clock, 55-56
medication carts, 48
medication labels
  insulin vials, 227
  interpreting, 51-55
  reconstitution, 121-126
  sample PCN, 217f
  TPN bag, 209
meniscus, 50, 119, 120f
mental status, 42
mEq, 78
mEq/L, 78
mEq/mL, 78
metric equivalents, 71-74, 77-78
metric system
  comparing household measurements with, 91-92
  equivalents, 71-74
  location of abbreviations in, 72
  parenteral mixes, 109-112
    one-step and two-step problems, 107-108
  prefixes and values, 72t

metric system *(Continued)*
  ratio and proportion calculations, 34-35, 76-78, 83-91
  rounding medication doses, 74-76
  use of measurements, 46t
mg/kg calculations, 278-279
military time, 55
milliequivalents, 78
milliliters, 75
milliunits, 78
mixed numbers
  addition of fractions and, 7-8
  changing improper fractions to, 4
  changing to improper fractions, 4-5
  division of fractions and, 10-11
  multiplication of fractions and, 10
  subtraction of fractions and, 8-9
mixing insulin, 237-241
mix-o-vial directions, 128f
multiple-dose vials, 121
multiple-strength decisions, 130-138
multiplication
  of decimals, 17-18
  of fractions and mixed numbers, 10

N
needle sizes, 106
needless IV systems, 169
needlestick injuries, 106, 107f
nonogram for body surface area calculations, 281-283
numerators, 5-6
nurse-activated piggyback systems, 171

O
obstetrics, IV calculations for, 192
one-step metric ratio and proportion calculations, 76-78
oral administration
  anticoagulants, 271-272
  calculations, 80-91
  for children/infants, 285-289
  oral diabetes medications, 251
  syringes, 120f
oral diabetes medications (ODMs), 251
oral syringes, 120f
overdose risks, 13, 82

P
pain management systems, 174f
parenteral administration. *see also* central parenteral nutrition (CPN); intravenous (IV) administration; peripheral parenteral nutrition (PPN); total parenteral nutrition (TPN)
partial thromboplastin time (PTT), 258
patient-controlled analgesia (PCA), 174
patient identification, 63
patient medication safety. *see also* clinical alerts
  dosage calculations, 63
  high-alert medications and, 183t, 335

patient medication safety *(Continued)*
  incomplete medication orders and, 62-64
  medication administration, 62-64
  needlestick injuries and, 106, 107f
  patient identification and, 63
  Patient Rights and, 41-43
  resuscitation equipment and, 135
  safety systems for IV ports, 169-170
  summary of safe medication administration practices, 62-64
  verbal communication hand-off report and, 333-334
Patient Rights, 41-43
pediatric medication administrations. *see also* medication administration
  dosages based on body weight and surface area, 277-279
  injection sites, 288-289
  IV medications, 291-294
  oral, 82
  oral medications, 285-289
  safe dose ranges (SDRs), 280-281, 283-284
  subcutaneous and intramuscular medications, 288-290
penicillin, 177, 303, 304f
percentages
  of additives (for TPN), 210
  changing
    to decimals, 21-23
    decimals to, 21-23
    to fractions, 21-23
  finding/converting, 23-24
  of solute in IV bags, 161-168
peripheral inserted central catheters (PICCs), 150, 151f
peripheral lines, 150
peripheral parenteral nutrition (PPN), 205, 214, 215f, 217
physician's orders. *see also* documentation; medical administration records (MARs)
  abbreviations used in, 58f
  comparing ordered and available unit dose amounts, 79-80
  identifying units and milliequivalents in, 78
  incomplete, 62-63
  insulin, 232
  interpreting, 56
  telephone, 56
  for total parenteral nutrition, 212f, 215f
  validation of TPN label with, 209
  verbal, 56, 177
PICC lines, 150, 151f
piggyback (PB) medication infusions, 170-171, 174-175
policies. *see* joint Commission on Accreditation of Healthcare Organizations (JCACO); protocols/policies
polypharmacy, 266
ports, IV. *see* intravenous (IV) administration
powders, 127-129

premixed IV solutions
    pediatric, 291-294
    piggyback, 170-171
    types of diluents, 126
preparation of liquid medications. *see* liquid medication forms
preparation of medication orders, 56
pressure-flow infusion devices, 174
prn caps, 150
prn orders, 59f
proportions, 32-34. *see also* ratio and proportion calculation method; ratios
proprietary (trade) name of drugs, 42, 51
protamine sulfate, 258, 266, 269-270
protocols/policies
    flushing intermittent access locks, 151
    patient identification, 63
    safe medication administration, 43
    syringe sizes for flushes, 194
    verbal/telephone orders, 56, 177
PTT (partial thromboplastin time), 258
push administration (IV bolus), 193-196

Q
qid/qd/qod use, 45t

R
rapid-acting insulin, 229-230
ratio and proportion calculation method
    one-step metric, 76-78
    setting up, 34-35
    two-step, 83-91
ratios
    definition of, 31
    expressing as fractions, 31
reading amounts in syringes, 99-102
recombinant DNA insulins, 225
reconstituted medications, 121-126. *see also* liquid medication forms
    parenteral dosages with multiple-strength decisions, 130-133
    for parenteral use, 126
    pediatric IV medications, 291-294
refused/withheld medications, 42
resistance to heparin, 265
resuscitation equipment, 135
risk factors
    elderly patients, 91
    fat embolus, 206
    hematomas, 257, 261
    overdoses, 13, 82
rounding decimals, 13-14, 15. *see also* dosage calculations
rounding doses, 74-76
routes of medication administration. *see* medication administration

S
safe dose ranges (SDRs), 280-281, 283-284
safe practices
    dosage calculations, 63
    medication administration, 62-64
    safety systems for IV ports, 169-170
SafetyGlide™ needle, 107f, 169
safety systems for IV ports, 169-170
saline/heparin locks, 149
schedule of markers for IV pushes, 194-195
scored tablets, 74, 81
SDRs (safe dose ranges), 280-281, 283-284
sensitivity, drug, 135
SI (Système International d'Unités), 71
single-dose liquid medications, 52
sliding-scale calculations, insulin, 241
smart pumps, 184-185
solid drug forms, 48-49
solute in IV bags, 161-168
S-R (slow-release) capsules, 49
stat medication administration, 42, 57
subcutaneous (subcut) injections, 103, 105f
    heparin, 260-266
    pediatric, 288-290
subtraction
    of decimals, 17
    of mixed numbers and fractions, 8-9
syringes
    BD-Hypak, 108f, 129f
    bolus IV administration with, 193-196
    calibrations on, 76, 231
    for flushing IV lines, 151
    heparin, 260-266
    insulin, 231-232, 233-236
    oral, 120f
    reading/measuring amounts in, 99-102
Système International d'Unités (SI), 71

T
three-in-one solution (for TPN), 206, 216f
time and route, abbreviations related to, 43
time of medication administration, 42, 55-56
timing IV push medications, 195-196
titrated infusions, 182-183, 184-185
total drug/total volume ratio, 182
total parenteral nutrition (TPN)
    administration of, 205-206, 207f, 208f
    device, 174
    kilocalories per bag, 210
    mL/hr to set the pump, 210
    nursing considerations for, 211
    percentage of additives, 210
    percentage of concentration per bag, 210
    three-in-one solution for, 206, 216f
    total grams per bag, 209-210
    validation of label with physician's order, 209

trade (proprietary) name of drugs, 42, 51
traditional time conversions, 55-56
24-hour clock, 55-56
two-step metric ratio and proportion calculations, 83-91
type 1 and 2 diabetes, 223-224. *see also* insulin

U
U-100 insulins, 229-231
unit dose calculations. *see also* dosage calculations
    for adults *versus* children, 63, 291
    confusion of units of medication with milligrams, 133
    definition of, 79
    for elderly patients, 91
    identifying units in physicians' orders, 78
    milliunits, 78
    multiples of unit doses, 75
    total dose *versus* unit dose errors, 52
    use of "unit," 78
unscored tablets, 74, 81

V
values
    decimals, 12, 14-15
    fractions, 11
verbal communication hand-off report, 333-334
verbal physicians' orders, 56, 177
vials
    dilution of powders or crystals in, 127-129
    insulin, 227
vitamin K, 271
volume (milliliters per hour) calculations, 151
volume measurements, 102
volumetric infusion pumps, 182

W
Warfarin (coumadin), 271-272
weight
    insulin dosage based on, 248
    measurements, 162, 280-281
west nomogram (body surface area), 281-283
whole numbers
    changing improper fractions to, 4
    decimals and, 18
withheld/refused medications, 42

X
X factor, 259

Metric Equivalents

Weight	Length
1000 mcg (microgram) = 1 mg (milligram)	10 mm (millimeter) = 1 cm (centimeter)
1000 mg = 1 g (gram)	100 cm = 1 m (meter)
1000 g = 1 kg (kilogram)	1000 mm = 1 m (meter)
	1000 m = 1 km (kilometer)
Pound to Kilogram Conversion	**Volume**
2.2 lb = 1 kg (kilogram)	1000 mL (milliliter) = 1 L (liter)
Household to Metric Length Equivalent	
1 inch = 2.54 cm (centimeter)	
39.37 inches = 1 m (meter)	

Approximate Equivalents of Metric, Household, and Apothecary Measures*

Metric	Household	Apothecary
5 mL	1 teaspoon (tsp)	
15 mL	1 tablespoon (tbs)	½ ounce
30 mL	2 tablespoons (tbs)	1 ounce
240 mL	1 measuring cup	8 ounces
500 mL	1 pint	1 pint or 16 ounces
1000 mL (1 liter)	1 quart	1 quart or 32 ounces
4 liters	1 gallon (gal) or 4 quarts	1 gallon (gal) or 4 quarts

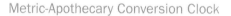

Metric-Apothecary Conversion Clock

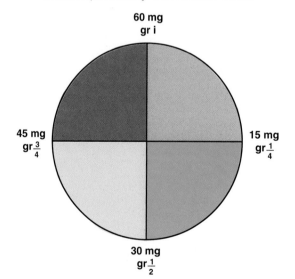

*Household equipment and apothecary measurements are not a substitute for metric measurements. The volume capacity of household equipment varies greatly. The apothecary measurements are imprecise and not equal to the metric measurements. **Use Metric**. Clarify unfamiliar abbreviations with the prescriber.